Endocrinology Research and Clinical Developments Series

ESTROGENS: PRODUCTION, FUNCTIONS AND APPLICATIONS

ENDOCRINOLOGY RESEARCH AND CLINICAL DEVELOPMENTS SERIES

Estrogens: Production, Functions and Applications
James R. Bartos (Editor)
2009. ISBN: 978-1-60741-086-7

Errata for *Estrogens: Production, Functions and Applications*

Editor: James R. Bartos

ISBN: 978-1-60741-086-7

p.183 The second author's affiliation should be:

Department of Anatomy, Faculty of Pindamonhangaba (FAPI), Pindamonhangaba, São Paulo, Brazil

p.203, 5th paragraph should read:

According Lill et al. [156] clinical experience is inconsistent regarding a possible delay of healing in osteoporosis. To our knowledge, until recently, research concerning the influence of estrogen deficiency in the wound healing of alveolar bone and periapical lesions was not performed in humans.

p.203, 7th paragraph should read:

Yamazaki et al. [164] investigated the reaction of bone tissue after implant insertion in the tibiae of osteopenic rats. The results suggested that a decrease in bone mass causes a decrease in the contact area between implant and bone and may also result in a reduction in the supporting capability of the implant, because of thinning of the surrounding bone trabeculae. Motohashi et al. [165] observed that ovariectomy did not seriously affect bone healing after the placement of implants in cortical bone areas, but did reduce the bone contact ratio and the bone in the cancellous bone area.

p.206, reference 27 should read:

Olea N, Pulgar R, Pérez P, Olea-Serrano F, Rivas A, Novillo-Fertrell A, et al. Estrogenicity of resin-based composites and sealants used in dentistry. *Environ. Health Perspect.* 1996 Mar;104(3):298-305.

p.208, reference 58 should read:

Lindhe J, Attsfröm R. Gingival exudation during the menstrual cycle. *J. Periodontal. Res.* 1967;2(3):194-8.

p.208, reference 59 should read:

Holm-Pedersen P, Löe H. Flow of gingival exudate as related to menstruation and pregnancy. *J. Periodontal Res.* 1967;2(1):13-20.

Endocrinology Research and Clinical Developments Series

ESTROGENS: PRODUCTION, FUNCTIONS AND APPLICATIONS

JAMES R. BARTOS
EDITOR

Nova Biomedical Books
New York

For permission to use material from this book please contact us:
Telephone 631-231-7269; Fax 631-231-8175
Web Site: http://www.novapublishers.com

Library of Congress Cataloging-in-Publication Data

Estrogens : production, functions and applications / [edited by] James R. Bartos.
p. ; cm. -- (Endocrinology research and clinical developments)
Includes bibliographical references and index.
ISBN 978-1-60741-086-7 (hardcover)
1. Estrogen--Therapeutic use. I. Bartos, James R. II. Series: Endocrinology research and clinical developments.
[DNLM: 1. Estrogens--therapeutic use. 2. Estrogens--pharmacology. 3. Estrogens--physiology. WP 522 E824 2009]
RM295.E884 2009
615'.36--dc22

2009010504

Published by Nova Science Publishers, Inc. ✝ New York

Contents

Preface

Estrogens are a group of steroid compounds, named for their importance in the estrous cycle, and functioning as the primary female sex hormone. Estrogens are used as part of some oral contraceptives, in estrogen replacement therapy of postmenopausal women, and in hormone replacement therapy for transwomen.

Like all steroid hormones, estrogens readily diffuse across the cell membrane; inside the cell, they interact with estrogen receptors. Additionally, estrogens have been shown to activate a G protein-coupled receptor. This new book gathers leading research from around the world.

Chapter I - Phytoestrogens are naturally occurring, plant-derived, non-steroidal phytochemicals. The major structural classes of phytoestrogens are the isoflavones and lignans found at high levels in various plants such as soybeans, clover or flax. Since their chemical structures are similar to endogenous estrogens, they are able to bind to human estrogen receptors (ERα and ERβ) and act as selective estrogen receptor modulators (SERMs).

Epidemiological data support the idea that consumption of phytoestrogens could be associated with beneficial effects regarding the prevention or inhibition of carcinogenesis of hormone-dependent malignancies. Furthermore, clinical studies have demonstrated that phytoestrogens are potentially beneficial in treating osteoporosis and arthrosis, as well as mammalian and endometrial carcinoma (primary and secondary prevention). Due to an apparent increase in the incidence of breast cancer in the Western World compared to most countries in Asia the interest in phytoestrogens has increased tremendously. However, up to now the modes of action of the different phytoestrogens at the molecular and cellular level are not well understood.

To enlighten the mechanisms underlying phytoestrogen function, we investigated the effects of synthetic isoflavones and lignans, and of phytoestrogen extracts from various plants in comparison to synthetic estrogens and antiestrogens in human mammalian, endometrial and trophoblast tumor cells as well as primary cells (cell vitality, cell proliferation, cytotoxicity and gene expression). The extracts from flax roots of *Linum usitatissimum* and from the bark of *Ulmus laevis* inhibited the cell vitality and cell proliferation in a concentration-dependent manner without showing strong cytotoxicity. Concentrations >100 μg/ml induced oncocidal effects in our tumor cells.

To analyze the substance classes of the flax root and elm bark extracts Pyrolysis Field Ionization Mass Spectrometry (Py-FIMS) was performed. Flax root extracts are composed mainly of phenols and lignans, while elm bark extracts contained primarily sterols, phenols, lignans and flavonoids. Furthermore, HPLC-MS analysis demonstrated that the flax root extracts are comprised of more representatives of lignans compared to isoflavones. Considering also that the metabolism of phytoestrogens in the human organism is little-known, further research in clinical studies needs to be conducted to develop strategies in the prevention and treatment of cancer.

Chapter II - *Introduction.* Cardiovascular disease (CVD) is the leading killer of women (aged over 18 years) in United States, with an annual mortality rate of over 450,000, and a majority of deaths attributable to heart disease. One in 30 female deaths is due to breast cancer in contrast to one in six deaths from heart disease. Declining ovarian estrogen levels during perimenopause and menopause have been implicated in the development of CVD. The Women's Ischemic Syndrome Evaluation (WISE) is a National Heart, Lung and Blood Institute (NHLBI)-sponsored, multi-center study designed to optimize the symptom evaluation, and diagnostic testing for ischemic heart disease. A specific aim within WISE is to study the influence of reproductive hormones on pathophysiology, symptoms and diagnostic test response of myocardial ischemia. In this chapter we discuss new data on the role of estrogen in CVD obtained from the WISE study.

A synopsis and discussion of new reproductive hormone data from ten WISE publications are organized into four categories: A) Pre- and perimenopause; B) Postmenopause; C) Hormone Therapy; D) Phytoestrogens as Selective Estrogen-Receptor Modulators (SERMs). The chapter begins with a description of the WISE method of determining menopausal status. New data is presented on the topics of hypothalamic hypoestrogenemia (HHE) and coronary artery discase (CAD), including women with diabetes mellitus (DM), polycystic ovary syndrome (PCOS) and CAD, estrogen levels and statin lipid lowering medication, estrogen levels and obesity patterns, past oral contraceptive (OC) use and CAD, estrogen hormone therapy on psychological factors among women of different ethnic backgrounds, and dietary phytoestrogen-rich products relations to blood lipoproteins and coronary microvascular function.

Conclusions. New research from the WISE study suggests that estrogen plays a role in CVD in women. Specific findings include: 1) the use of a simple WISE hormone algorithm can improve the accuracy of menopausal status classification for research purposes; 2) disruption of ovulatory cycling characterized by HHE appears to be associated with angiographic CAD; 3) the presence of DM and HHE predicts a greater burden for angiographic CAD; 4) in postmenopausal women with past OC use is associated with less angiographic CAD; 5) clinical features of PCOS are associated with more angiographic evidence of CAD and worsening CVD event-free survival; 6) blood estrogen levels vary according to central vs. general obesity; 7) there are ethnic differences observed between HT use and psychological health; 8) higher blood levels of the phytoestrogen, daidzein, are associated with beneficial lipoprotein levels in women with low blood estrogen; 9) higher blood level of the phytoestrogen, genistein, are associated with impaired non-endothelial–dependent and endothelial-dependent coronary microvascular function; 10) use of statins, and resultant lower cholesterol levels, are not associated with lower levels of reproductive hormones. New data from WISE study suggests that estrogen play a role in CVD in women. Ongoing research is directed at further understanding.

Chapter III - Chronic infections with hepatitis C virus (HCV) and hepatitis B virus (HBV) appear to progress more rapidly in males than in females. Nonalcoholic fatty liver disease (NAFLD), cirrhosis and hepatocellular carcinoma (HCC) are predominately diseases of men and postmenopausal women. Female sex hormone, estrogen is a potent endogenous antioxidant. Estrogen suppresses hepatic fibrosis, or the collagen deposition, in animal models, and attenuates induction of redox sensitive transcription factors, and hepatocyte apoptosis by inhibiting the generation of reactive oxygen species in primary cultures. Hepatic steatosis is observed in aromatase-deficient mice, and it is shown to decrease in animals after estrogen treatment. In addition, estrogen has salutary effects on various hepatic stresses including ischemia/reperfusion, hemorrhagic shock-resuscitation, and hepatectomy. Variant estrogen receptors are expressed to a greater extent in male patients with chronic liver disease than in females. Better knowledge of the basic mechanisms underlying the sex-associated differences during the progression of liver disease may open up new avenues for the prevention and treatment of chronic liver disease.

Chapter IV - Postpartum period represents one of the most critical phases of a woman's life. A percentage ranging between 10% and 20% of mothers may develop psychiatric disorders after parturition. Postpartum disorders with psychiatric symptoms are represented by three main syndromes: postpartum blues, postpartum depression, and postpartum psychosis.

One of the most exhaustive theories about the etiology of postpartum psychiatric disorders speculates that their onset may be due to the physiological changes in maternal estrogen levels during pregnancy and the first weeks after parturition.

However, in assessing available literature information about the role of estrogen-therapy in preventing and treating puerperal psychiatric diseases, all reviewed studies were found to suffer from severe methodological limitations. For this reason, further, well-designed, and strictly focused multi-center trials are warranted in order to firmly establish the effectiveness of estrogen-therapy in puerperal psychiatric disorders.

Chapter V - There is a wealth of historical and circumstantial evidence to suggest that women patients with schizophrenia may suffer from a deficit in estrogenic function. The prolactin inducing properties of the majority of antipsychotic drugs, and subsequent negative feedback on estrogen levels, is in keeping with this. The functions of estrogen, its complex receptor organization and its numerous actions are the focus of ongoing research activity. Of particular interest are its neuroprotective properties, particularly with regard to cognitive impairment, and its involvement with neurotransmitter systems which are the substrate for psychotropic drugs. Estrogen has now been used as an adjunct to standard antipsychotic medication in quite a few studies of women schizophrenia patients. Most of these are, however, not double blind randomized controlled trials. Only three relatively small double blind RCTs returned positive results: one long term study which selected for hypoestrogenism reported negative findings. Furthermore, recent evidence of the risks of long term hormone replacement therapy is of concern. The advent of specific estrogen receptor modulators, which may avoid excess risks of cancer and cardiovascular events, will have little to add to schizophrenia treatment if estrogen is, essentially, devoid of any specific antipsychotic or adjuvant mechanism of action relevant to the pathophysiology of this disorder.

Chapter VI - Estrogen treatment is rarely indicated during childhood. A limited number of patients requires either topical or systemic estrogens in selected cases. Labial adhesions in which the labia minora fused over the vestibule is the most common indication for topical estrogen treatment in children. Although the most accepted theory of labial adhesions is low estrogen levels, the use of topical estrogen treatment is still controversial.

The systemic application of estrogen is used in girls with hypogonadism. Either in hypo or hypergonadotropic hypogonadism, low doses of estrogen treatment is initiated at pubertal age as a replacement treatment, to mimic normal puberty. In Turner syndrome, which is an example of hypergonadotropic hypogonadism, estrogen treatment should be also initiated at pubertal age in addition to growth hormone replacement. Although in girls, 'constitutional growth and pubertal delay' is not observed as frequently as in boys, very low doses of estrogen therapy for a short duration can be considered to induce normal puberty. Another indication of systemic estrogen treatment is for tall stature in carefully selected cases to fuse epiphysis.

Though topical estrogen treatment in labial adhesions is preferred and used by many practitioners, systemic use of this hormonal therapy is only constituted by pediatric endocrinologists. In this chapter, our aim is to discuss the estrogen treatment in children with special emphasis on indications, treatment doses and results.

Chapter VII - The connection between estrogens and oral health has been a concern and the subject of much research in several areas of dentistry, such as periodontology, implantodontology, endodontology, prosthodontics, orthodontics, maxillofacial surgery, and oral pathology. However, this link still remains controversial. Therefore, the purpose of this chapter is to review and summarize the available literature regarding the role of estrogen in stomatognathic tissues and the consequences of estrogenic variations to this system. Estrogen depletion results in bone loss and may lead to a reduced bone repair capacity, which has been implicated in several clinical complications experienced by postmenopausal women. Among them, a residual alveolar ridge reduction increases the difficulty of dental prosthesis adaptation. Delayed bone repair may modify the wound healing process after intraosseous neoplasm removal or alter the course of endodontic treatment of periradicular lesions, as well as for implant osseointegration. Estrogen deficiency could be an aggravating factor in periodontal diseases and may cause significant rapid orthodontic tooth movement. Estrogenic action has been suggested to be responsible for the high prevalence of autoimmune diseases in women, such as Sjogren's syndrome; the occurrence of burning and dry mouth seems to be generally associated with climacteric symptoms, which are related to estrogen deficiency. Temporomandibular disorders, common clinical conditions involving pain, are more prevalent in women of reproductive-age than in men. Furthermore, women may present different patterns of periodontal disease during pregnancy, the menstrual cycle, or when using contraceptives or hormone replacement therapy. In conclusion, estrogens significantly affect the oral cavity, but further studies are needed to elucidate the extension and molecular mechanisms of those interactions.

Chapter IX - The pharmacology of the human Estrogen Receptor α (ERα) depends on a large number of parameters such as post-traductional modifications, nature of ligands and associated ERα conformational changes, intracellular localization of ERα as well as estrogenic pathways that are activated for specific co-regulators recruitment. In this context, a number of amino-acids that constitute the ERα Ligand Binding Domain (LBD) have been shown to play crucial functions. Unfortunately, most data covering these topics are reported in a huge amount of literature not easily accessible to all investigators. We, therefore, attempt to extract essential informations from this literature to constitute a useful database describing the functions ascribed to key residues.

Chapter X - The action of estrogens is mediated through the estrogen receptor alpha (ERα) and the more recently discovered estrogen receptor beta (ERβ). These estrogen receptor (ER) subtypes have distinct functions and differential tissue distribution patterns. Tissue- or cell-specific estrogenic activity of receptor ligands have become targets of drug research due to the potential to affect and control physiological and disease states such as breast and endometrial carcinoma, osteoporosis, and menopause. Receptor-ligand activity can be achieved in different ways such as by selective binding or selective modulation. These, in turn, are governed by the intermolecular interactions between estrogen receptors and their ligands.

The estrogen receptor ligand binding pocket has a degree of flexibility enabling binding of endogenous and synthetically-derived steroids, as well as non-steroidal molecules. Ligand fit is dependent upon aspects of size, polarity, and specific subsitution on ring and sidechain structures. Selectivity of a ligand for the estrogen receptor subtypes can be explained on the basis of differences in ligand-binding affinity, ligand potency, or ligand efficacy. In addition, molecular characteristics can lead to selective antagonism by ligands as well as antiestrogen character. Determinants of selectivity and antagonism have been elucidated using x-ray crystallography revealing various intermolecular and steric features of importance.

The present review will examine aspects of estrogenic binding including non-selective binding, and ERα/ERβ selectivity. Various chemical classes are critically examined including endogenous compounds, phytoestrogens, and other classes of interest to drug discovery and pharmaceutical product development.

Chapter XI - The estrogen receptor is an important receptor in human beings. It relates to the physiological function of estrogen as well as to some specific pathological disorders. In this article, the author will briefly review and discuss the estrogen receptor. The structure of the estrogen receptor will be focused upon in depth. Important analyses of the structural component of an estrogen receptor will be demonstrated and presented. In addition, details on the clinical importance of an estrogen receptor laboratory test and examples of experience in cases of breast cancer will be reported in this article.

Chapter XII - Estrogen is classified as a feminine hormone although it can be found in both sexes. Excessive estrogen in men can be problematic. However, in some situations, intended administration of estrogen in men can be seen. The best scenario is the use of estrogen in gays, with the aim of achieving a feminine appearance. In this article, the author will focus on this extraordinary application and other transsexual procedures for gays.

In: Estrogens: Production, Functions and Applications
Editor: James R. Bartos, pp. 1-53
ISBN: 978-1-60741-086-7

Chapter I

Molecular and Cell Biological Investigations of the Mode of Action of Established and Potential Phytoestrogens for the Development of Strategies in the Prevention and Treatment of Cancer

Volker Briese[1]*, Sibylle Abarzua*[2]*, Dagmar-Ulrike Richter*[1]*, Birgit Piechulla*[2]*, and J. Barbara Nebe*[3]

[1]University of Rostock, Dept. of Obstetrics and Gynecology, Südring 81, D-18059 Rostock, Germany
[2]University of Rostock, Institute of Biological Sciences, Albert-Einstein-Str. 3, D-18059 Rostock, Germany
[3]University of Rostock, Center for Medical Research, Dept. of Cell Biology, Schillingallee 69, D-18057 Rostock, Germany

Abstract

Phytoestrogens are naturally occurring, plant-derived, non-steroidal phytochemicals. The major structural classes of phytoestrogens are the isoflavones and lignans found at high levels in various plants such as soybeans, clover or flax. Since their chemical structures are similar to endogenous estrogens, they are able to bind to human estrogen receptors (ERα and ERβ) and act as selective estrogen receptor modulators (SERMs).

Epidemiological data support the idea that consumption of phytoestrogens could be associated with beneficial effects regarding the prevention or inhibition of carcinogenesis of hormone-dependent malignancies. Furthermore, clinical studies have demonstrated that phytoestrogens are potentially beneficial in treating osteoporosis and arthrosis, as well as mammalian and endometrial carcinoma (primary and secondary prevention). Due to an apparent increase in the incidence of breast cancer in the Western World compared to most countries in Asia the interest in phytoestrogens has increased tremendously. However, up to now the modes of action of the different phytoestrogens at the molecular and cellular level are not well understood.

To enlighten the mechanisms underlying phytoestrogen function, we investigated the effects of synthetic isoflavones and lignans, and of phytoestrogen extracts from various plants in comparison to synthetic estrogens and antiestrogens in human mammalian, endometrial and trophoblast tumor cells as well as primary cells (cell vitality, cell proliferation, cytotoxicity and gene expression). The extracts from flax roots of *Linum usitatissimum* and from the bark of *Ulmus laevis* inhibited the cell vitality and cell proliferation in a concentration-dependent manner without showing strong cytotoxicity. Concentrations >100 μg/ml induced oncocidal effects in our tumor cells.

To analyze the substance classes of the flax root and elm bark extracts Pyrolysis Field Ionization Mass Spectrometry (Py-FIMS) was performed. Flax root extracts are composed mainly of phenols and lignans, while elm bark extracts contained primarily sterols, phenols, lignans and flavonoids. Furthermore, HPLC-MS analysis demonstrated that the flax root extracts are comprised of more representatives of lignans compared to isoflavones. Considering also that the metabolism of phytoestrogens in the human organism is little-known, further research in clinical studies needs to be conducted to develop strategies in the prevention and treatment of cancer.

1. Introduction

1.1. Medical Background and Therapeutic Goals

Of all malignant tumors in women, those of the breast (mammary carcinoma) have the highest annual incidence rate, around 25 new cases per 100,000 females. Mammary carcinomas have thus become a key theme in the fields of gynecology and oncology. In 1990, 38,000 cases were registered in Germany whereas by 2002 the number had risen to 55,100, making it clear that preventive research must be given priority. Despite the introduction of new adjuvant and palliative chemotherapeutic treatments and the establishment of primary tumor surgery, a favorable prognosis can hardly be expected in the near future [Page 1996, Kuo et al. 2006]. Up to now, there have been no consolidated findings on the prevention (chemoprevention) of mammary carcinomas, even though environmental and nutritional factors play an important role. Epidemiological studies have revealed that Asian women, compared to European or North American women have a significantly lower incidence of mammary carcinomas and lower mortality rates for hormone-dependent tumors. They also suffer less from climacteric symptoms and have high phytoestrogen levels in their urine. These effects are attributed to the high dietary intake of soy-based products, which are rich in isoflavones [Steinmetz et al. 1991]. Japanese women who migrated to Hawaii had a three-fold higher breast cancer risk. Foods and supplements containing phytoestrogens could thus constitute the basis for a chemoprevention (prophylaxis) of mammary carcinoma in the future.

It has been discussed for several years whether fruits, vegetables, or whole-grain foods have a high potential for cancer prevention and whether the increase in diet-dependent tumors is caused by a lack of protective constituents in the diet, e.g., vitamins, minerals, trace elements, fiber, secondary plant metabolites. Secondary plant metabolites can thus be considered for their role in cancer prevention as well as in modulation of tumor growth [Mothes 1980, Nahrstedt 1990, Knight and Eden 1996]. Approximately 30,000 secondary plant metabolites are known to date, of which 5,000–10,000 are found in the diet [Ames et al. 1990].

Within the past ten years, interest in the physiological role of bioactive compounds in plants has increased sharply, especially with regard to the group of substances known as phytoestrogens in relation to human health. The phytoestrogens are compounds from several diverse classes of non-steroidal secondary plant metabolites, including isoflavones, lignans, and coumestans, exhibiting clinical efficacies similar to those of estrogens [Adlercreutz et al. 1991, 1992, 1995, Adlercreutz 1995] because of structural similarities (Figure 1). They bind to estrogen receptors (ERα, ERβ) and, in addition, exert an estrogenic and/or antiestrogenic effect on various target organs by influencing the biosynthesis and metabolism of endogenous hormones. Previous findings have shown that phytoestrogens exhibit only 0.1% the efficacy of human estrogens, but it is interesting to note that the concentration of phytoestrogens in human urine is 10 to 10^3 times that of endogenous human estrogens [Setchell und Adlercreutz 1988]. However, with an appropriate diet, it is possible to reach phytoestrogen plasma levels of 50-800 ng/ml, which is 10^3 to 10^4 times that of estradiol plasma levels. Compounds that fail to exert all of the effects of estradiol but exhibit a more or less selective activity profile in a given organ are called “Selective Estrogen Receptor Modulators” (SERMs). This term, when applied to phytoestrogens, has lead to the classification of some phytoestrogens as phytoSERMs.

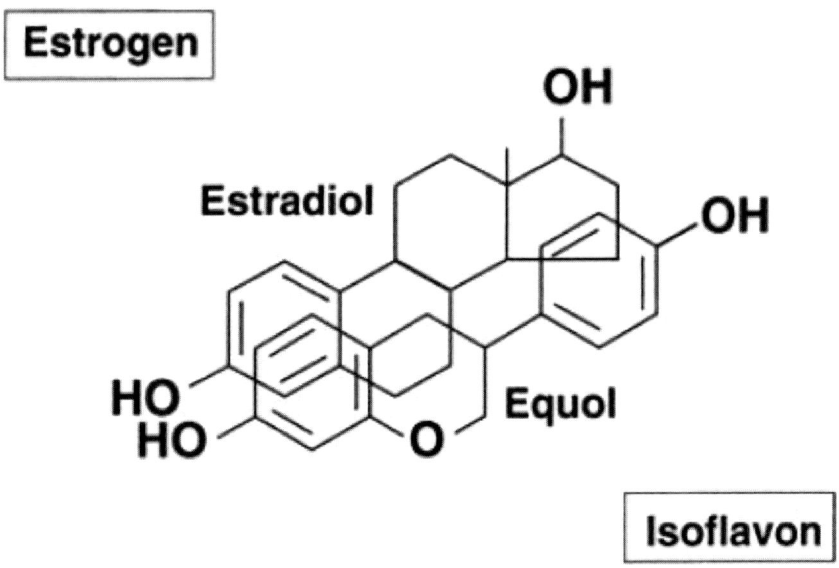

Figure 1. Structural similarities of estrogens and phytoestrogens (e.g. isoflavones).

1.2. Impacts of Phytoestrogen-Rich Diets

"Let food be thy medicine and medicine be thy food"— this advice given 2500 years ago by Hippocrates has never been more relevant than it is today [Kleine-Gunk 2008].

There are promising epidemiological studies that associate a phytoestrogen-rich diet with fewer deaths due to chronic diseases, such as breast and prostate cancer, cardiovascular disease, and osteoporosis [Messina 1999, Clarkson 2002, Setchell et al. 2003]. Studies involving immigrants have shown that a diet containing soy products reduces the breast cancer risk, especially when soy intake took place before puberty or during adolescence [Adlercreutz 2003, Stephens 1997]. According to our present state of knowledge, the premenopausal risk of mammary carcinoma can be reduced by isoflavones (incidence lowered by 50%). Opposing results were obtained in a comprehensive retrospective study on isoflavone intake by 16,165 Dutch women, which found no evidence for a protective effect of phytoestrogens with regard to cardiovascular disease [van der Schouw and Grobbee 2005]. Phytoestrogens may also play a role in brain development and in the prevention of neurodegenerative disease [Branca and Lorenzetti 2005, Kreijkamp-Kaspers et al. 2005, Patisaul 2005, Schreihofer 2005]. Setchell et al. [1997] reported on soy-based infant formula diets. Children on a soy-rich diet had levels of serum isoflavone between 10^6 and 10^7 pg/ml, whereas in adults it was between 10^4 und 10^6 pg/ml, so it is possible to achieve high isoflavone serum concentrations. In a 14-day case-control study, 35 women were given a daily dietary supplement of 60 g soy protein (45 mg isoflavone). After 2 weeks, significantly higher serum concentrations of both genistein and daidzein could be detected [Harding et al. 1997]. The biological effects of genistein have been studied most extensively. Investigations have shown that genistein, which can be detected in human urine after soybean intake [Adlercreutz et al. 2004b], suppresses the growth of new blood vessels *in vitro*. Tumor growth and metastasis thus could be blocked [Fotsis et al. 1993]. Since 1991, five case-control studies on the problem of soy-based diet and mammary carcinomas are known [Messina et al. 1997]. Three of these studies, in which soy was part of the regular diet, showed that the risk for premenopausal mammary carcinomas was substantially lowered, whereas only one of the studies confirmed this effect for postmenopausal mammary carcinomas. Mammary carcinomas in younger women (< 35 years of age) differ biologically from those of older women: the proliferation rate is higher and the differentiation stage is lower. The surface marker p53 is more often expressed [Henderson und Patek 1997]. It could be shown that a soy-rich diet increased the menstrual cycle length in proband women. Other clinical investigations, if only involving a small number of cases, showed that within the menstrual cycle progesterone, estrogen, and androgen levels can be lowered by a daily isoflavone intake of 100 mg daidzein and 100 mg genistein [Lu et al. 1996]. In the premenopausal phase, the serum concentrations of FSH and LH were lowered significantly. Ingram et al. [1997] published a case-control study on the relation between isoflavone intake and mammary carcinoma risk. This study has a definite advantage over the sole use of diet anamneses because objective criteria, i.e., measurement of isoflavone metabolites in the urine, were used for the evaluation. The measurement of isoflavones in the urine provides information on the dietary intake of these plant metabolites as well as on their metabolism by intestinal bacteria (flora) and their bioavailability. Between 1992 and 1994, 149 patients (from the Perth area, Western Australia) who had been diagnosed with mammary carcinomas were admitted. Urine collected over a 72-hour period and a venous blood sample were used to determine FSH and estradiol levels in the laboratory. Control patients exhibited a higher median excretion of all isoflavones, and the median excretion of the mammalian lignan enterolactone was even 50% higher in the control group. High urinary equol and enterolactone excretions could thus be associated with reduced breast cancer risk. When evaluating the results, it should be taken into consideration that the study participants were subjected to exceptional stress (a mentally stressful situation in this case) and it is presently unknown if this has an effect on phytoestrogen excretion. In addition to the beneficial effects of isoflavones on health, i.e., cancer, osteoporosis, and possibly cardiovascular diseases, they also relieve premenstrual and climacteric symptoms during the premenstrual or climacteric phase. This is of clinical relevance because more than half of the women suffer from premenstrual symptoms, e.g., depressed mood, irritability, aggressiviness, breast tenderness, headaches, having to deal with weight gain as well. Besides, 30% of the women in Germany are in the postmenopausal phase of life. Due to large-scale studies in the past few years, hormone replacement therapy (HRT) is no longer generally recommended; besides, fewer than 5% of the women use HRT for more than 5 years. Prospective controlled, randomized studies have demonstrated the favorable effect of functional food (soy bread) and a dietary supplement on subjective discomfort in the climacterium. In addition, the serum levels of bone-specific alkaline phosphatase increased (osteoblast activity) and pyridinoline/deoxypyridinoline (osteoclast activity) decreased. None of the „soy-diet experiments“ had a detectable influence on thyroid gland, prolactin, FSH, LH, testosterone, insulin, or progesterone parameters. In single cases, an increase in serum DHEA-S and serum estradial concentrations was observed.

In animal experiments on the influence of the glucosinolate metabolite indole-3-carbinol in the diet, the formation of estrogens (e.g., catechol estrogen) increased to a level only slightly beneficial to tumor growth. In a clinical study, the daily administration of an estimated 500 mg indole-3-carbinol (equivalent to 400 g white cabbage) led to a 50% increase of catechol estrogen synthesis after 7 days and to its urinary excretion [Michnovicz and Bradlow 1990].

Phytoestrogens possess antiangiogenic and estrogenic as well as antiestrogenic properties due to competitive binding on estrogen receptors and activation of metabolizing enzymes such as aromatase and the estrogen-specific 17ß-hydroxysteroid oxidoreductase [Santti et al. 1998]. Phytoestrogens reduce by way of an aromatase inhibition the conversion of androstendion, so the concentration of circulating estrogens is lowered. *In vitro* studies have shown that phytoestrogens inhibit the binding of xenestrogens (DDT) to target cells [Zava et al. 1997, Zava and Duwe 1997]. Xenestrogens on the other hand could be important for carcinogenesis. Furthermore, phytoestrogens induce in humans the synthesis of the "Sex - Hormone - Binding - Globulin (SHBG)“ in the liver, so more of the circulating estrogens are bound to this transport protein, rendering them biologically inactive [Watzl et al. 1994, Watzl and Leitzmann 1995]. In women of various age groups, the plasma SHBG concentration correlated positively with the excretion of phytoestrogens in urine [Adlercreutz et al. 1987, Chie et al. 2002], whereby vegetarian women showed a higher excretion rate than non-vegetarian women.

However, within this spectrum of investigations, the results are sometimes opposing and at present difficult to interpret [Adlercreutz et al. 2004a, Sacks 2005]. Current retrospective analyses of diets with regard to fruit, vegetables, and fiber also are controversial. In a recent review summarizing prevention studies published to date, clear-cut relations have not yet been proven [Gikas et al. 2005]. This could be explained especially by the diversity of the phytoestrogens consumed and by their individual absorption behaviors [Hanf and Gonder 2005]. In a similar sense, this is also true for extracts containing phytoestrogens. Therefore, further extensive research is required.

1.3. Phytoestrogens – Isoflavones and Lignans Isolated from Plants

An important area of biomedical research is the search for new active ingredients (especially natural substances). The *in vitro* testing of supposedly active ingredients from plants is carried out if possible in stages, progressing from a multiconstituent mixture with many constituents to one with one or a few constituents (single constituent). Depending on the manufacturing process used, different active ingredients could be obtained from the same starting material and these may differ in their pharmaceutical, pharmacotoxological, and clinical properties. The various constituents of a plant extract may exhibit differing biopharmaceutical properties and pharmacological activities, which as a whole account for the therapeutic efficacy. The isoflavones and lignans are two groups of chemical compounds that are of special importance acting as phytoestrogens.

The soybean is the main source of isoflavones, a group of phenolic compounds found in nature that belong to the flavonoids [Coward et al. 1993]. Around 100 natural isoflavones and structurally related compounds, such as isoflavones, isoflavanes, and complex isoflavanes, have been isolated from higher plants, especially leguminoses (pulses/legumes). The isoflavones mainly differ structurally on the 3rd ring at the position of the hydroxyl and methoxy groups. The complex isoflavones also contain one to several isoprenoid substituents. Carbohydrate components are in particular glucose and rhamnose. Well-known isoflavones include the widely occurring genistein from various broom species. At present, the soybean is the most important source of these nutritionally essential compounds, together with the glycosides of genistein, daidzein and glycitein, which in part are bound to proteins. There are dietary supplements on the market made from red clover, which is rich in phytoestrogens, particularly glycosides of the isoflavones formononetin und biochanin A. These compounds are converted to daidzein und glycitein by intestinal bacteria. Genistein has also been found in curry, among other sources, so apparently phytoestrogen intake is more complex than previously assumed [Clarke et al. 2004].

The biotransformation of isoflavone glycosides from soybeans is carried out by intestinal microflora. Absorption in the small intestine is followed by transport to the liver (enterohepatic circulation) [Setchell und Adlercreutz 1988, Wang 2002]. Glucosidases from intestinal bacteria split off carbohydrate, leading to the formation of the biologically active isoflavones daidzein and genistein as well as enterolactone und enterodiol (phase II des enterolactone and enterodiol metabolism). In phase I, the formation of enterolactone sulfate, enterolactone glucuronide, and enterodiol glucuronide takes place in the colon epithelium [Jansen et al. 2005]. In adults, these compounds are converted to the metabolites equol, ortho-desmethylangolensin (o-DMA), and p-ethylphenol, whereby the conversion to equol (30–50%) and o-DMA (80–90%) is partial [Atkinson et al. 2005]. Additional compounds in urine samples could be identified by mass spectroscopy, for example, 3‘-methoxy-3‘-hydroxy-equol, 6‘-methoxy-equol, α-methyl-deoxy-benzenoid, angiolensin, und 6‘hydroxy-o-DMA [Heinonen 2004]. In contrast to other mammals, only 30–50% of humans are capable of converting isoflavones to other metabolites [Frankenfeld et al. 2004, Wiseman et al. 2004].

Lignans are present in a number of plants in the diglucosidic form and play an important role in cell-wall structure [Peeters et al. 2003]. The best-known representatives of the lignans are secoisolariciresinol (SECO) and matairesinol (MATA), whereas a number of additional lignan structures should exist, some of which have been described and some whose structure has not yet been clarified [Ho et al. 1998]. The intestinal microflora convert by demethylization SECO, MATA, and the isoflavones to the body's own, so-called "mammalian lignans" [Adlercreutz 1995, Nesbitt et al. 1999, Bowey et al. 2003]. These compounds, as do their chemical precursors, have inhibitory effects on tumor growth. The quantitative analysis of these compounds in urine or serum is used to predict the metabolizing capability of the organism [Yamamoto et al. 2001, Kilkkinen et al. 2001]. At present, the lignans known are found in grain kernels and fruit, whereby linseeds (flax) are the best source of lignans [van Kranen 2003]. Linseeds contain approximately 53 μg lignan per 100 g linseed flour, based on the phytoestrogen content [Stark et al. 2002]. Lignans inhibit the growth of tumor cells in mammary-carcinoma cell lines [Chen et al. 2004] and trophoblast Jeg3 cell lines [Abarzua et al. 2007]. Concentrations between 1 μmol/ml and 100 μmol/ml exhibited a concentration-dependent activity [Adlercreutz et al. 1993]. By combining the use of linseed metabolites and the antiestrogenic tamoxifen, metastasis processes (cell adhesion, invasion, and migration) were arrested [Chen et al. 2003]. It thus becomes clear that phytoestrogens can develop completely different efficacies, depending on the receptor status and the individual hormone constellation. When administered together, however, both active substances inhibited tumor-cell proliferation. This indicates that both active substances are agonists in competition for estrogen receptor occupancy.

1.4. Phytoestrogens Tested in Cell Cultures

Many investigations and studies with humans have shown in some cases a correlative relation between a diet containing phytoestrogens and beneficial effects on health. Causal relations however can be better demonstrated by using *in vitro* tests. For this reason, experiments with cancer cell lines are the method of choice. By using different cell lines, the efficacies of phytoestrogens could be tested and, above all, detailed cellular and molecular effects analyzed.

An extract from *Epimedium brevicornum*, a medicinal plant in traditional Chinese medicine, proved to be effective on the proliferation of mammary carcinoma cells [Yap et al. 2005]. Low doses (1,3 μg/ml) caused a stimulation of the estrogen-receptor activity and, on the other hand, higher dosages inhibited growth. Following fractionation, a new prenylflavone, breviflavon B, as active substance was found. High breviflavone dosages led to elimination of the α-ER protein, an occurence that should be viewed in connection with increased proteasome degradation. Similar dose-dependent results were obtained with MCF-7 cell lines and biochanin A [Hau et al. 1999]. At biochanin A concentrations less than 10 μg/ml, cell proliferation and the de novo DNA synthesis were enhanced. On the other hand, concentrations between 30 und 40 μg/ml resulted in an inhibition of cell growth and DNA synthesis. It was also demonstrated on MCF-7 cells that a low concentration of genistein stimulated the cell proliferation but a higher concentration inhibited proliferation. It is not yet known, which effect varying concentrations of phytoestrogens have on normal breast tissue and on triggering of precancers, especially of importance for long-term use [Dimitrakakis et al. 2004]. A potential anticancerogenic effect on mammary carcinoma cell lines (for example, MCF-7) turned out with the antiproliferative effect of genistein und daidzein (concentration 1 μmol/ml) [Hawrylewicz et al. 1995]. Inhibition of the tyrosine-specific protein kinase and of angiogenesis by genistein could be demonstrated [Akiyama et al. 1987, Fotsis et al. 1993]. In experiments with mammary carcinoma cell lines treated with phytoestrogens, receptor-dependent as well as receptor-independent mechanisms affected DNA synthesis, and inhibition of cell growth was dependent on the phytoestrogen concentration [Wang and Kurzer 1997]. At low concentrations (0,01 - 10 μmol/ml) of genistein and coumestrol, there was an increase in estradial-induced tyrosine kinase-dependent DNA synthesis in mammary carcinoma cell lines. At high concentrations, there was inhibition [Wang and Kurzer 1998]. Further tests demonstrated that especially the isoflavone genistein in physiologial concentrations is capable of inhibiting cell growth of mammary carcinoma cell lines and is thus a potent estrogen agonist [Zava et al. 1997, Zava and Duwe 1997]. Both genomic and non-genomic mechanisms have been made responsible for the anticarcinogenic properties of the phytoestrogens, including induction of apoptosis, inhibition of tyrosine kinases, and inhibition of DNA topoisomerases [Lechner et al. 2005].

When interpreting *in vitro* assays of active substances of plant origin, it must be kept in mind that the actual *in vivo* concentrations of relevant constituents are unknown because they are affected in their biopharmaceutical properties by other constituents (cofactors) and/or are subject to metabolic processes. The conclusions based on results from *in vitro* systems must therefore take the biopharmaceutical properties and metabolism of the substances being studied into consideration, e.g., the evaluation of the biological functions, in addition to quantitative assertions, should address factors such as food intake, metabolism, and bioavailability with regard to the mechanisms of action of phytoestrogens on mammary carcinomas. Investigations along this line are thus absolutely necessary before any soy products or products of other plants could be recommended for the prevention of mammary carcinoma.

2. Results

2.1. Anticancerogenic Effects of Phytoestrogens at the Cellular Level

2.1.1. Phytoestrogens from Plant Extracts

2.1.1.1. Flax (Linum usitatissimum) Extracts

The major classes of phytoestrogens are the isoflavones and lignans found at high levels in legumes such as soybean, chickpea, clover, flax and in various plant parts, including roots, stems, leaves, flowers, fruits and seeds [Kulling and Watzl 2003, Lee and Xiao 2003, Rickard-Bon and Thompson 2003]. The addition of flaxseed products reduced tumor incidence or cell multiplicity in tumor models of the breast, colon, prostate, liver, oesophagus and lung [Rickard-Bon and Thompson 2003, Westcott and Muir 2003]. Because of these anticancerous effects of the seeds, other organs of the flax plant might also be biologically effective. Therefore we isolated and identified potential phytoestrogens from leaves, stems and roots of the flax plant *Linum usitatissimum* and tested their effect on human trophoblast and mammalian tumor cell lines in *in vitro* cell cultures.

Effects on Human Trophoblast Tumor Cell Lines
Preparation of phytoestrogen extracts from leaves, stems and roots of L. usitatissimum:

The seeds, cultivar Barbara, were obtained from the Agricultural Research Institution Mecklenburg-Vorpommern (LUFA), Rostock, Germany, sown on soil and grown under field conditions. When the plants reached a height of about 1 m, they flowered and the leaves, stems and roots were harvested. These plant organs were frozen in liquid nitrogen and stored at –70°C till extraction. Different extraction methods [Franz and Köhler 1992, Luyengi et al. 1996, Windhövel et al. 2003] were performed to obtain either isoflavones or lignans from the various plant organs of *L. usitatissimum* [Abarzua et al. 2007]. The most effective extraction procedure was the lignan extraction method according to Luyengi et al. [1996].

It is known from other studies that isoflavones and lignans occur in glycosilated forms in planta and are therefore often biologically inactive [Muir and Westcott 2003, Rickard-Bon and Thompson 2003]. To improve the bioavailability *in vitro*, nonspecific HCl hydrolysis and specific β-glucosidase hydrolysis were used to release the aglycons [Abarzua et al. 2007].

Identification of isolated phytoestrogens with HPLC-MS:

The phytoestrogen extracts were dissolved in methanol and used for analysis. Chromatographic separation of the isolated phytoestrogen fractions was performed using reversed-phase HPLC using a gradient elution program: 0.2 ml/min, 20% methanol (A), 80% water with 0.1% formic acid (B), linearly to 80% A: 20% B in 15 min, followed by a hold for 25 min to reach initial conditions for an additional 10 min. A Discovery C18 (15 cm x 2.1 mm) column produced by Supelco (Taufkirchen, Germany) was used.

For MS analysis a LCQ-Advantage (Thermo Finnigan, San Jose, USA) mass spectrometer was used. Identification of the compounds was obtained by ion trap technology;

using the ESI mode and positive ion. The source voltage was 4.5 kV and a mass range of 150 – 2000 amu was used for detection.

Table 1. Classes, representatives and forms of phytoestrogens identified in leaf, stem and root extracts of *Linum usitatissimum* using HPLC-MS analysis. Phytoestrogen extracts were prepared according to Franz and Köhler [1992], Luyengi et al. [1996] and Windhövel et al. [2003] with and without HCl-or β-glucosidase hydrolysis [Abarzua et al. 2007].

Class of phytoestrogen	Representative	Chemical form
Isoflavones	Genistein Daidzein Biochanin A	Aglycone Glycoside Diglycoside Dimer Glycoside dimer Deoxydiglycoside
Lignans	Secoisolariciresinol Matairesinol Pinoresinol Lariciresinol Isolariciresinol Arctigenin 6-Methoxypodophyllotoxin	

The leaf, stem and root extracts from the flax species, *L. usitatissimum*, contain measurable concentrations of isoflavones such as genistein, daidzein and biochanin A, and lignans such as secoisolariciresinol, matairesinol, pinoresinol, lariciresinol, isolariciresinol and arctigenin. All extracts contain more representatives of lignans compared to isoflavones, as has been shown for other *Linum* species [Westcott and Muir 2003]. The compounds were found in the extraction procedure as aglycones or as glycosides, independently of whether additional HCl- or enzyme hydrolysis was used or not. Therefore it can be concluded that isoflavones and lignans were present in the flax extracts prior to hydrolysis as aglycons and glycoside derivates. In the case of the special lignan/toxin extraction [Windhövel et al. 2003] the aryltetralin lignan, 6-methoxypodophyllotoxin, was additionally found in the leaf extracts (Table 1). The lignan podophyllotoxin is of special interest, since its derivatives such as Etopophos are presently used in anticancer therapy [Fuss 2003]. One of the future tasks will be to determine the quantity of 6-methoxypodophyllotoxin and other lignans and isoflavones in plant extracts.

In Vitro Cell Studies:

The *in vitro* cell studies were performed with the human trophoblast tumor cell line Jeg3, obtained from the Department of "Human and Animal Cell Cultures" Braunschweig, Germany. Cells were cultured in Dulbecco's Modified Eagle's medium (DMEM, BioWhittaker) with 10% inactivated fetal calf serum and antibiotics (1% penicillin/streptomycin) and antimycotic (0.5% amphotericin) at 37°C and 5% CO_2.

As a representative cell study test the cell proliferation and viability assay (MTT test), based on the activity of mitochondrial dehydrogenases, was used. Cell viability was analyzed using an MTT-kit according to the instructions of the manufacturer (Roche, Germany) [Abarzua et al. 2007]. The test conditions were optimized in preliminary experiments and the optimal cell number was found to be $1x10^6$ Jeg3 cells/ml.

The phytoestrogen extracts were dissolved in 1% DMSO to get a stock solution of 100 mg/ml. From this stock solution, aliquots were taken and added to 0.1 ml supplemented culture medium producing final concentrations of 0.05 mg/ml, 0.5 mg/ml, 1 mg/ml and 5 mg/ml (0.05% final concentration of DMSO). Jeg3 cells ($1x10^5$/0.1 ml supplemented culture medium) were grown in 96-well tissue culture plates for 48 h in the absence (controls) and presence of different concentrations of phytoestrogen extracts at 37°C and 5% CO_2. Two negative controls were prepared with (i) Jeg3 cells in DMEM and (ii) Jeg3 cells in DMEM and DMSO (0.05% final concentration of DMSO). In general, the negative controls 1 and 2 did not differ in absorbance values, indicating that 0.05% DMSO did not inhibit cell growth (data not shown). After incubation with MTT for 4 h at 37°C and 5% CO_2, solubilization solution was added and the plates were incubated in a humidified atmosphere (37°C, 5% CO_2) overnight. The spectrophotometrical absorbance of the purple formazan crystals was measured at 570 nm using a microplate ELISA reader (BioRad, Hercules, California, USA). The reference wavelength was 670 nm.

All lignan extracts obtained from leaves, stems and roots of *L. usitatissimum* with and without HCl hydrolysis revealed significant inhibition of cell viability. The strongest decrease in cell growth was induced by treatment of Jeg3 cultures with root extracts which had not undergone HCl hydrolysis (Figure 2). Incubation of Jeg3 cells with these extracts at 1 and 0.5 mg/ml reduced cell viability by about 93%. Most lignan extracts exhibit concentration-dependent effects. Since extractions performed with and without HCl hydrolysis result in extracts which are effective to different extents, it can be concluded that several different compounds in the extracts are responsible for the bioactivity.

Statistical analysis was performed using the Student´s *t*-test for comparison of the means. Data were presented as mean ± standard deviation (SD) of mean. A p value of < 0.01 was considered as being statistically significant and denoted by an asterisk.

Effects on Human Mammalian Tumor Cell Lines

The aim of this study was to prepare flax leaf, stem and root extracts from *L. usitatissimum* (Figure 3) and to test their effects in cell studies *in vitro* in ER positive and ER negative human mammalian cancer cell lines to distinguish between ER dependent and independent effect mechanisms of the flax extracts tested. The different role of estrogen receptor dependent and independent effect mechanisms of phytoestrogens has so far only been poorly investigated. We therefore started a systematic investigation to test the influence of the flax extracts on the receptor positive mammalian cell line MCF 7 and the receptor negative mammalian cell line BT 20 (Marlen Szewczyk, Sibylle Abarzua, André Schlichting, Dagmar-Ulrike Richter, Barbara Nebe, Birgit Piechulla, Volker Briese, unpublished results 2009).

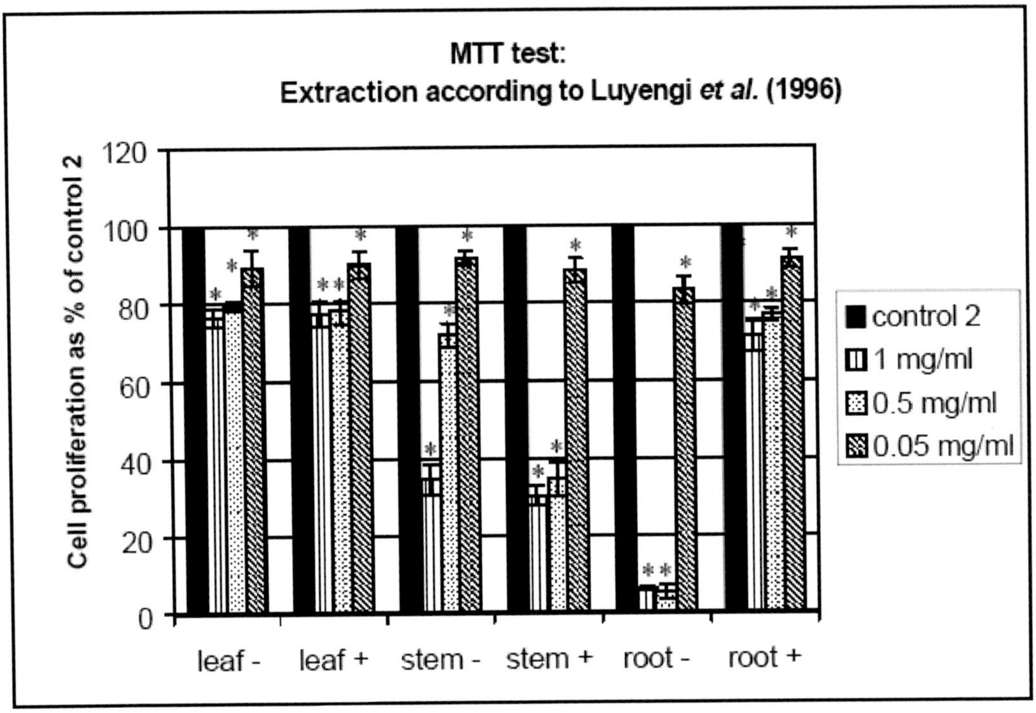

Figure 2. Effect of different concentrations of leaf, stem and root extracts from *Linum usitatissimum* on the cell proliferation and viability of Jeg3 cell lines measured by the MTT test. Extracts were prepared according to Luyengi et al. [1996] with (+) and without (-) hydrolysis with 1 M HCl. Data (mean±SD) represent relative formation of formazan from MTT in % in comparison to negative control 2 (100%) obtained in at least 3 experiments. Asterisks (*) indicate significant differences between treated Jeg3 cell lines and the negative control 2 (p<0.01) [Abarzua et al. 2007].

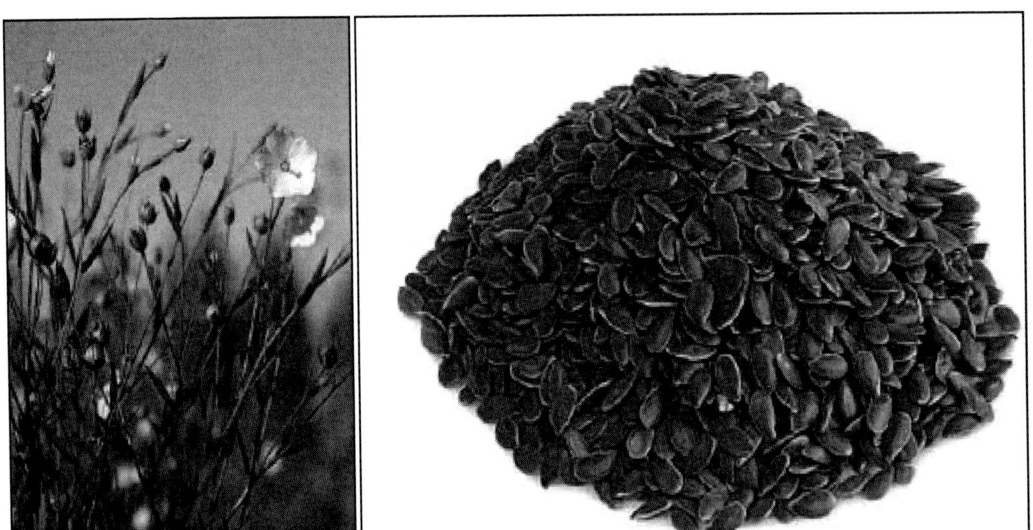

Figure 3. *Linum usitatissimum*.

In Vitro Cell Studies:

The *in vitro* cell studies were performed with the human mammalian cancer cell lines MCF 7 (ER positive) and BT 20 (ER negative), obtained from the Department of "Human and Animal Cell Cultures" Braunschweig, Germany. The cell cultivation procedure was the same as for the human trophoblast cell line Jeg3 (see above).

As representatives for the *in vitro* cell studies the cell vitality (also designated cell proliferation and cell viability test, see before), proliferation and cytotoxicity of the human mammalian cell lines MCF 7 and BT 20 (5×10^5 cells/ml) treated with different concentrations of phytoestrogen extracts from *L. usitatissimum* were analysed. For these studies the MTT, the BrdU Cell Proliferation ELISA kit (colorimetric) and the cytotoxicity detection kit (LDH kit) were used as recommended by the manufacturer (Roche, Germany). The phytoestrogen extracts were dissolved in 100% ethanol to provide a stock solution of 100 mg/ml. Aliquots from this stock solution were added to the supplemented culture medium to give final concentrations of 0.01, 0.1, 1, 10, 50, 100, 500 and 1000 μg/ml (final concentration of ethanol: 1%). Two negative controls were examined in all tests: (i) cells in DMEM (control 1) and (ii) cells in DMEM and ethanol, final concentration of ethanol: 1% (control 2).

Flow Cytometric Measurement of Apoptosis:

MCF 7 cells (5×10^5 cells/ml) were grown to confluence for 24 h in 6-well-plates. After refreshing the medium, root extracts and the negative controls 1 and 2 (see above) were added and incubated for 24 h at 37°C and 5% CO_2. Cells were washed with PBS, trypsinized, centrifuged and washed again. Cells were treated with 1 mg/ml RNase at 37°C for 20 min and incubated with propidium iodide (50 μg/ml) for 3 h on ice. Measurements were performed on BD FACSCalibur, equipped with an argon-ion laser of the wavelength 488 nm (BD Bioscience). For data acquisition, the software CellQuest Pro 4.0.1 (BD Bioscience) was used.

The Influence of Flax Extracts on Cell Viability and Proliferation of MCF 7 and BT 20:

The leaf, stem and root extracts from *L. usitatissimum* at low concentrations nearly did not affect the cell vitality and cell proliferation of MCF 7 and BT 20 cell lines. However, at higher concentrations of the root extract a significant inhibition of the cell activity and cell proliferation was found. BT 20 cells were repressed stronger in comparison to MCF 7 ones.

These differences point out that flax root extracts probably can affect the growth of MCF 7 and BT 20 carcinoma cell lines through ER mediated as well as ER independent mechanisms of action, whereby the ER independent mechanisms of action seem to play a greater role. On the other hand the differences could also indicate a higher sensitivity for flax root extracts in the ER negative BT 20 cell lines than in the ER positive MCF 7 cells.

Our results are in line with an *in vitro* study which showed that the mammalian lignans have stimulatory as well as inhibitory effects on the cell growth of breast cancer cells, depending on the concentrations used. Using DNA synthesis as a marker of cell growth, 1-10 μmol/l of the mammalian lignan enterolactone was found to be stimulatory in the breast cancer cell line MCF 7 [Wang and Kurzer 1997, 1998], but higher levels (>50 μmol/l) were inhibitory [Wang and Kurzer 1997]. In terms of cell proliferation, 0.5 to 10 μmol/l enterolactone was found to stimulate the growth of MCF 7 cells, whereas concentrations above 10 μmol/l were inhibitory [Mousavi and Adlercreutz 1992].

Statistical analysis was performed as described before.

The Effect of Flax Extracts on Cytotoxicity of MCF 7 and BT 20 Cells:

Low concentrations of flax leaf stem and root extracts did not induce cytotoxic effects in MCF 7 and BT 20 cell lines. However, higher concentrations of the stem and leaf extracts caused a significant cytotoxicity. By contrast over the whole range of flax root extract concentrations there were no cytotoxic effects on MCF 7 cells. However, in BT 20 cell lines the addition of high flax root extract concentrations caused significant cytotoxic effects. These results correlate with the strong inhibition of cell vitality of the BT 20 cells after the addition of high flax root extract concentrations.

Induction of Apoptosis:

Flow cytometric analyses were performed for examining induction of apoptosis induced by flax root extracts. Addition of low flax root extract the percentage does not increase apoptotic cells, however high concentrations of flax root extracts resulted in a significant increase of apoptosis.

Several studies described the induction of apoptosis as a respond to phytoestrogens [Jo et al. 2005, Danbara et al. 2005]. We suggest that apoptosis of MCF 7 cells might be induced by the phytoestrogens found in the flax root extract of *L. usitatissimum* (Table 1).

Since flax root extracts of *L. usitatissimum* induce significant inhibition of cell vitality and proliferation without performing strong cytotoxicity in the human mamma carcinoma cell lines MCF 7 the potential phytoestrogens in flax roots could have beneficial effects for the prevention of hormone-dependent tumors. Forthcoming research will be directed at identifying the active molecules, testing the flax root extract effects in hormone-dependent and independent mechanisms of action and finally disclosing the relevant intracellular processes.

2.1.1.2. Elm Bark (Ulmus laevis) Extracts

Traditional Chinese medicine indicates that the bark of *Ulmus sp.* has positive effects against oedema, mastitis, inflammation and cancer [Wang et al. 2004]. Elm bark extracts also provide resources for anticancer drug recovery [Tai and Cheung, 2005, Kulp et al. 2006]. Elm tree components are present in different herbal teas, which are available as medical-tea products. An *in vitro* study found out that FlorEssence (herbal remedy tea) significantly inhibits the proliferation of human breast cancer (MCF7, MDA-MB-468) and leukaemia cells (Jurkat, K562) [Tai and Cheung 2005].

At present, the substances responsible for these effects are unknown. Naturally occurring substances such as terpenes [Wattenberg 1983), glycopeptides [Dong et al. 1997], polyphenols [Gamet-Payrastre et al. 1999, Caltagirone et al. 2000] and phytoestrogens [Adlercreutz 1995, Rickard-Bon and Thompson 2003, Abarzua et al. 2007] have been considered to have anti-cancerogenic effects. The cytostatic agent Taxol A is a diterpene-polyester from the bark of *Taxus brevifolia* and has been successfully applied against mammalian and ovarial carcinoma [Ofir et al. 2002]. Bark of the regional elm (*Ulmus laevis*) may also contain substances with anti-cancerogenic potential against hormone-dependent gynaecological tumors. Therefore, the aim of the present study has been to identify potentially active substances of crude extracts from bark of *Ulmus laevis* (Figure 4) and to analyse their effects on cell vitality, cell proliferation and cytotoxicity in human chorion carcinoma cell lines Jeg3 and BeWo and the human endometrial cell line RL95-2. The placental cell culture model is suitable for the direct comparison of the human tumor cell lines Jeg3 and BeWo with a primary cell culture under *in vitro* conditions [Jeschke et al. 2003].

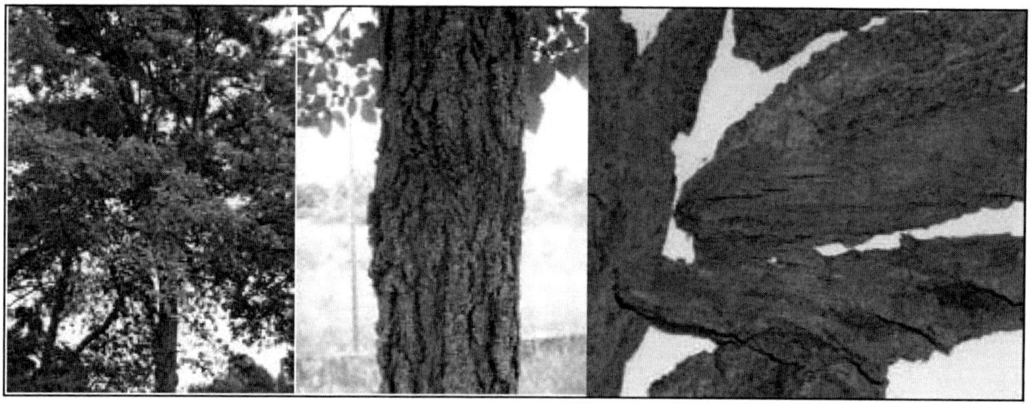

Figure 4. *Ulmus laevis*.

Effects on Human Trophoblast Tumor Cell Lines
Extract Preparation from Elm (Ulmus laevis) Bark:

Bark was collected from *Ulmus laevis* Pallas (identified by Prof. Porembski, Botany, University of Rostock) in a forest near Rostock (Mecklenburg-Western Pomerania, Germany). A voucher specimen of *U. laevis* from individuum studied was deposited at the Herbarium of the Department of Botany, University of Rostock. The extracts were prepared according to Luyengi et al. [1996] as modified by Matscheski et al. [2006]. The extracts were dissolved in 100% ethanol to provide a stock solution of 100 mg/mL. Aliquots of this stock solution were added to the supplemented culture medium to give final concentrations of 0.25, 0.5, 1, 5, 10, 50, 100, 150, 250 and 500 µg/ml (final concentration of ethanol: 1%) (Anna-Maria Hartmann, Sibylle Abarzua, André Schlichting, Marina Chwalisz, Dajana Domik, Kai-Uwe Eckhardt, Dagmar-Ulrike Richter, Peter Leinweber, Volker Briese, unpublished results, submitted for Planta Medica 2009).

Chemical analysis with pyrolysis-field ionization mass spectrometry (Py-FIMS):

For Py-FIMS, about 5 µL of the extract was transferred to a quartz crucible that was placed in the micro-oven of the direct inlet system of a double-focusing Finnigan MAT 900 mass spectrometer (Finnigan, MAT, Bremen, Germany). The analyte was evaporated to dryness in the fore-vacuum (10^{-1} hPa). The micro-oven heated the sample from 110 to 700°C at 20 K-increments in 12 min, and 91 magnetic scans were recorded for the mass range 15 to 900 Dalton (single spectra). These were combined to obtain one thermogram of total ion intensity (TII) and an averaged Py-FI mass spectrum. For each of the single scans, the absolute and relative ion intensities of 14 classes of chemical compounds were calculated by summation of the ion intensities of 8 to 39 indicator signals [Schulten and Leinweber 1999], including the protonated molecule ion mass signals ((M+H)+) if present. All Py-FIMS data were normalised per mg sample. This procedure was carried out for each of five replicate measurements per sample and the results were averaged for statistical analyses. Py-FIMS of the crude bark extract of Ulmus laevis isolated by the Luyengi-procedure [Luyengi et al. 1996] indicated mainly triterpenes and sterols, fatty acids with lower amounts of lignans. These results are in agreement with the findings of Martin-Benito et al. [2005] and Rowe et al. [1972].

In Vitro Cell Studies:

The *in vitro* cell studies were performed with the chorion carcinoma cell lines Jeg3 and BeWo (Figure 5), obtained from the LGC Standards GmbH, Wesel, Germany. Cells were cultured in Dulbecco`s Modified Eagle`s Medium (DMEM, Bio Whittaker) with 10% inactivated fetal calf serum (FCS) and antibiotics (penicillin/streptomycin) and an anti-mycotic (amphotericin) at 37°C and 5% CO_2. The primary trophoblast cell culture was directly isolated from the placenta according to Jeschke et al. [2003]. As representatives of the *in vitro* cell study the MTT test was performed as described before. Additionally two positive controls, dissolved in ethanol were examined: 1 μg/ml 17β-estradiol (estrogen) and 10 μg/ml tamoxifen (anti-estrogen).

Statistical analysis was performed as described before.

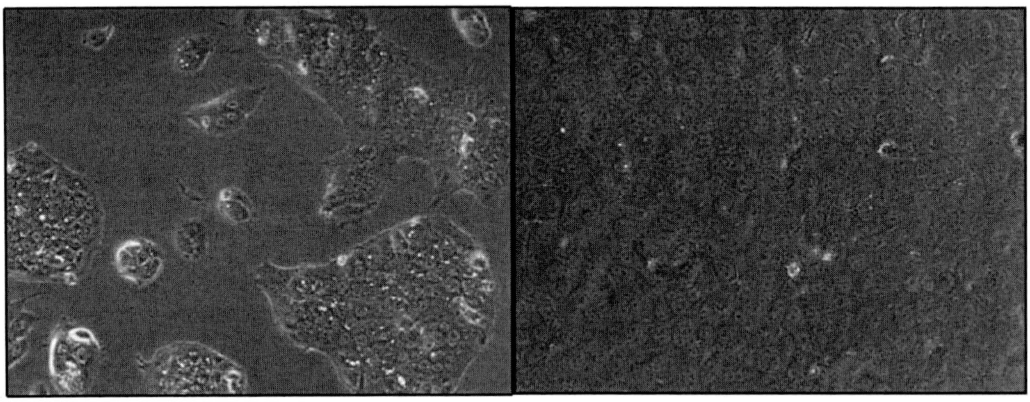

Figure 5. Cell morphology of the chorioncarcinoma cell line BEWO (left) and the endometrial cell line RL 95-2 (right). Light microscopy, magnification 10x.

The Effect of Elm Bark Extracts in Vitro:

It was shown that the vitality of Jeg3 and BeWo cells (MTT test) decreased significantly in a concentration-dependent manner, after application of elm bark extracts, relative to the negative control 2. The strongest inhibition of cell vitality was measured in the Jeg3 culture. The addition of 17β-estradiol did not affect the vitality of Jeg3 and BeWo cells, but the application of tamoxifen significantly inhibited the uptake of MTT by the Jeg3 and BeWo culture. The vitality of the primary trophoblast cells was increased by all concentrations of elm bark extracts and 17β-estradiol. By contrast, tamoxifen significantly reduced their vitality. Cell vitality can be enhanced by estrogens (17β-estradiol) and reduced by anti-estrogens (tamoxifen) *via* the activity of the estrogen–receptor (ER). Primary trophoblast cells and the Jeg3 and BeWo carcinoma cell lines have been found to be positive for ERα and ERβ [Szewczyk 2007, Ho et al. 1998, Jiang et al. 1997]. The positive ER mediation becomes obvious by the significantly contrasting estradiol and tamoxifen effect on the vitality of primary trophoblast cells.

Effects on Human Endometrial Tumor Cells
In Vitro Cell Studies:

The *in vitro* cell experiments were performed with the non-polar human uterine epithelial cell line RL95-2, purchased from the American Type Culture Collection (ATCC; Rockville, MD, USA). This cell line was maintained in a 1:1 mixture of Dulbecco's modified Eagle's medium (Gibco-Life Technology, Eggenstein, Germany) and Ham's F12 medium (Sigma, Taufkirchen, Germany), supplemented with 10% fetal calf serum (FCS) (Gibco), 10 mmol/l HEPES pH 7.4 (Sigma), 5 μg/ml insulin (Sigma), 2.0 g/l $NaHCO_3$ (90%), 1% penicillin/streptomycin (Sigma) and 0.5% amphotericin B (Sigma). The cells were cultured in a humidified atmosphere at 37°C with 5% CO_2. As representatives of the *in vitro* cell studies the MTT-, BrdU- and LDH tests with statistical analysis were performed as described before (Daniel Paschke, Sibylle Abarzua, Andre Schlichting, Dagmar-Ulrike Richter, Peter Leinweber, Volker Briese, unpublished results, submitted for European Journal of Cancer Prevention 2008).

Effects of Elm Bark Extracts on Cell Vitality and Proliferation of RL 95-2 Cells:

Our experiments demonstrated a significant inhibition of cell viability and cell proliferation after application of elm bark extracts in a dose-dependent manner measured by the MTT and BrdU assay. These results suggest that elm bark extracts have tumor growth inhibiting properties as indicated by an inhibition of mitochondrial activity (MTT test) as well as decreased DNA synthesis (BrdU test).

To test the possibility that the inhibition of cell viability and cell proliferation in the presence of elm bark extract is due to cell lethality of the human endometrial carcinoma RL 95-2 cell lines the cytotoxicity of the extracts was measured by the LDH activity. It was shown that elm bark extracts did not induce cytotoxic effects. These results lead to presumption that elm bark extracts did not have lethal properties on endometrial carcinoma cells.

Different phytoestrogens have been found in the elm tree root and bark in the form of lignan xylosides and neolignan glycosides [Lee et al. 2001]. It has been suggested that plant cell walls containing significant amounts of phenolic components may be the most likely to protect against cancer (dietary fiber hypothesis) [Ferguson et al. 2001, Dembitsky and Maoka 2007]. The other analysed substance classes from elm bark could be also potent agents possessing high anticancer activities. Anticancer effects of free fatty acids were estimated using a rabbit liver cancer model [Hayashi et al. 1992]. Palmitic acid and octadecenoic acid as well as oleic acid resulted in apoptosis – inducing activity in colon tumor cells [Waterman and Lockwood 2007, Yoo et al. 2007]. Recently Juan et al. [2008] detected antiproliferative and apoptosis-inducing effects of maslinic and oleanolic acids, two pentacyclic triterpenes from olives on HT-29, on colon cancer cells. In summary, many substance classes we had found in elm bark by Py-FIMS are described as potential anti-cancer products on different tumor cell lines. According to the incidence of the main fractions, we suggest a main responsibility for observed effects by sterols, triterpenes, free fatty acids and phytoestrogens. Single substances as well as a combined action of the analysed substance classes could be responsible for the decreased cell vitality and cell proliferation.

Conclusion

In this study we demonstrated inhibitory effects of flax root and elm bark extracts obtained from *Linum usitatissimum* and *Ulmus laevis* on trophoblast, mammalian and endometrial tumor cell lines. The observations displayed considerable significance from an oncological and botanical standpoint for future investigations into the usefulness of flax root and elm bark extracts for cancer prevention and treatment as well as drug candidates.

2.1.2. Synthetic Phytoestrogens

There is accumulating evidence that phytoestrogens, which are naturally occuring, plant-derived phytochemicals, could inhibit tumorigenesis during the development of breast cancer. Tumor metastasis and the proliferation of cells resulting in tumor cell growth in breast cells is directly connected with cell adhesion receptors, such as integrin and hyaluronan receptor expression. In maintaining tissue architecture, e.g. of the mammary gland, the integrin receptor- and steroid hormone-signaling pathways play an important role. Disruption of the delicate balance of signaling can result in dramatic changes in thc cellular interactions, which might lead to breast cancer [Hansen and Bissell 2000]. The adhesion receptors of the integrin family are transmembrane receptors consisting of an α- and a β-subunit and exert important functions in signal transduction via the actin cytoskeleton [Wiesner et al. 2005, Dedhar and Hannigan 1996, Nebe et al. 1995]. With their extracellular domain, integrins bind to extracellular matrix proteins (ECM) like fibronectin (FN) as a prime target of α5β1 [Hynes 1999]. Integrins transduce extracellular signals via the cytoplasmic domain and facilitate downstream signalling cascades by organizing the cytoskeletal 'scaffold' for intracellular signaling components [Aplin et al. 1999, Nebe et al. 1996]. Thus, integrin-mediated cell adhesion and resulting cytoskeletal dynamics lead to an early cell response like intracellular calcium mobilization [Sjastaad and Nelson 1997, Pommerenke 1996] and to the control of focal adhesion kinase, which activity is sufficient for cell growth [Hansen et al. 1994], and gene expression [Roskelley et al. 1994].

The integrin function can also be influenced by other receptors, like the adhesion receptor CD44 [Wang et al. 2005]. CD44, a transmembrane glycoprotein, binds hyaluronan and plays a major role in cell-cell adhesion and cell-substrate adhesion. CD44 is also expressed in differentiated epithelial cells [Speranza et al. 2005]. This receptor is associated with tumor metastasis as demonstrated in experiments of CD44 cross-linking-induced upregulation of integrins resulting in increased adhesion of breast cancer cells (MDA-MB-435S) [Wang et al. 2005]. The direct linkage between integrins and cell growth has also been clearly indicated in recent experiments on breast cancer cells in which the inhibition of the β3-integrin function by antagonists was correlated with a decrease of proliferative subpopulations [Vellon et al. 2005]. Tumor metastasis and the enhanced motility of mammary carcinoma cells are associated with integrin-mediated adhesion and hyaluronan receptor expression. It is important to get deeper insights into the behavior of cells and their cellular structure-cell function-dependencies under estrogen influence. The reason is that synthetic estrogens are able to modulate *in vitro* the β1-integrins, alter the cell-matrix-interaction, increase the adhesion contact numbers and are responsible for more organized F-actin in the lamellipodia of motile cells [DePasquale et al. 1999, Iype et al. 2001]. Migrating mammary epithelial cells stimulated *in vitro* with estrogens (17β-estradiol) demonstrate more so called footprints of the integrin residues (see scheme Figure 6). Less is known how phytoestrogens act in these cellular adhesion receptor dependent processes. The aim of our studies is to unravel the mode of action of phytoestrogens and the regulation of adhesion receptors like integrins and the hyaluronan receptor.

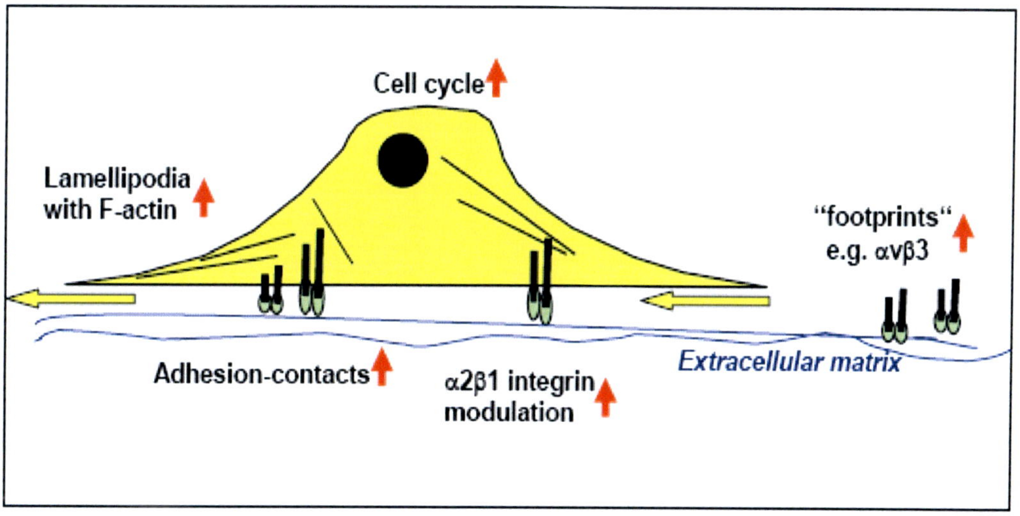

Figure 6. Schematic presentation how synthetic estrogens influence mammary epithelial cells possibly resulting in enhanced motility of the tumor cells: 17β-estradiol modulates the β1-integrins, alters the cell-matrix-interaction, increases the adhesion contact numbers and is responsible for more organized F-actin in the lamellipodia of motile cells.

In Vitro Cell Studies:

First experiments using estrogen-sensitive breast cancer cells MCF-7 (ATCC no. HTB-22) indicated that the integrin adhesion receptors were significantly up-regulated with 17β-estradiol but in contrast, genistein and daidzein did not affect the expression, which was concentration dependent [Nebe et al. 2006]. The MCF-7 cells express the integrin receptors α2, α3, β1 in the same intensity as observed in primary mammary epithelial cells [Nebe et al. 2006]. Therefore, this cell line is well suited for the phytoestrogen studies. The hyaluronan receptor CD44 was significantly increased with 17β-estradiol (1 μM) compared to untreated control cells. In contrast, the synthetic phytoestrogen genistein increased CD44 expression only at lower concentrations, whereas CD44 remained unaffected at 100 μM. The phytoestrogen daidzein did not affect the CD44 expression level at any of the concentrations tested [Nebe et al. 2006].

We also determined the influence of phytoestrogens on cell growth. In all proliferation experiments with a significant stimulation of the primary mammary epithelial cells due to 17β-estradiol, genistein and daidzein did not influence S- and G2/M-phase cells. Additionally, the stimulative effect of 17β-estradiol could be inhibited.

Our contemporary, preliminary investigations using matairesinol (MATA) and secoisolariciresinol (SECO) seem to confirm that estrogens upregulate the adhesion receptor CD44 of mammary epithelial cells, whereas phytoestrogens do not (Figure 7). However, for statistical achievements further experiments are necessary. MCF-7 cells were cultured in DMEM (Invitrogen, Karlsruhe, No. 31966) at 37°C and in a 5% CO_2 atmosphere. The cells were cultured in serum free DMEM for 24 h before incubation with the phytoestrogens Mata and Seco (further 48 h) to avoid unspecific stimulation. Integrin preparation was according Nebe et al. [2006]. Briefly, MCF-7 cells were trypsinized, washed and sedimented cells were incubated with the monoclonal anti-CD44 (Immunotech), or for control with mouse IgG_1 (BD Biosciences). For fluorescence labelling a FITC-conjugated anti-mouse IgG (Fab_2 fragment, Sigma) was used and cells were measured by flow cytometry.

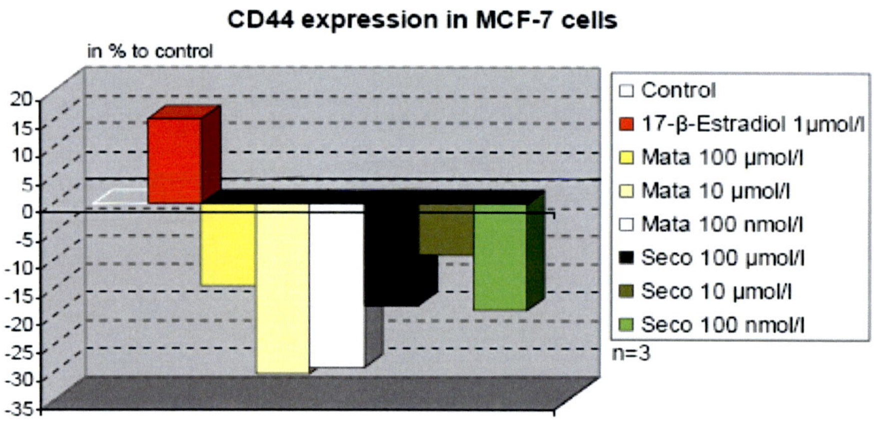

Figure 7. The CD44 hyaluronan receptor is upregulated after 17β-estradiol application and downregulated due to the influence of the phytoestrogens matairesinol and secoisolariciresinol.

It is possible that the action of estradiol is due to the expression of the estrogen receptor α and β (ER) in these cells (Figure 8). Immunocytochemical characterization of estrogen receptors were proven with cytospins [Nebe et al. 2006]. Briefly, 300 μl of suspended cells ($3x10^5$) per slide were centrifuged for 1 min at 1000 rpm. The slides were air dried, fixed with 3.7% formalin and permeabilized with cold methanol, followed by incubation with 0.1 % hydrogen peroxide (H_2O_2). After rinsing with PBS the slides were incubated with normal serum from the Vectastain ABC-Kit (Vector Laboratories, Dako, Hamburg) followed by incubation with the primary antibodies mouse anti-human estrogen receptor α (1:10, Dako) and anti-human estrogen receptor β (1:10, Serotec).

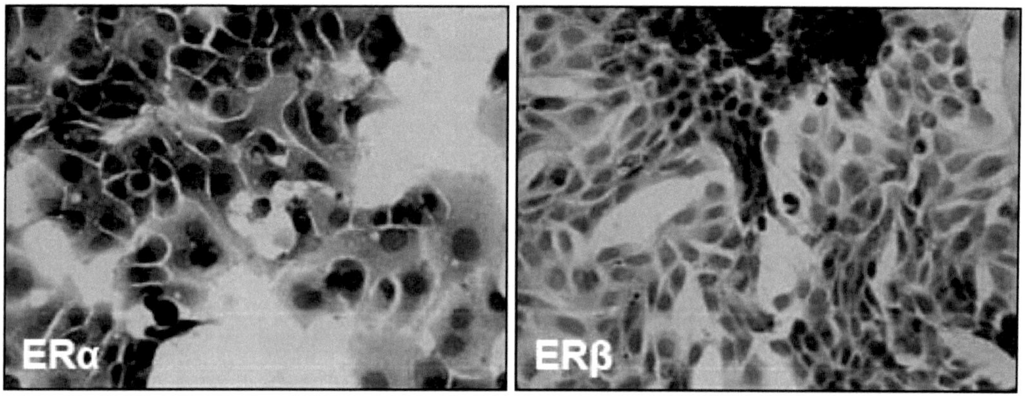

Figure 8. Estrogen receptor (ER) expression in mammary epithelial cells MCF-7. The ERα and the ERβ both are expressed (brownish color).

2.2. Anticancerogenic Effects of Phytoestrogens at the Molecular Level

Lignans are primarily found in flax, whole rye flour, pumpkin seeds, cereals and fruits. These are products that, in contrast to soy, are part of a healthy diet in Western countries. Lignans also mainly act through the estrogen receptor β (ERβ). The gene for the ERβ is located on the human chromosome 14, and is expressed in the testicles, the ovaries, the lung, the kidney, the prostate and the thymus. Five isoforms of ERβ have been found. Only isoform 1 (ERβ1) is able to produce homodimers and thus has an own function. Isoforms 2, 4 and 5, however, are able to produce heterodimers with isoform 1 and thus increase the ligand-dependant activation of transcription. Only homodimers can attach to the corresponding ERE promoter sequence. The ERα/ERβ ratio is additionally important for cellular proliferation or inhibition. Furthermore, gene activation through estrogen receptors has also been observed with genes without ERE responsive elements. It can be concluded that other ways of activation exist, e.g. the binding of complexes to AP-1 (activator protein) binding sites or of other transcription factors (e.g. NFκB, SP1).

For the present work, we investigated the activation of estrogen-sensitive genes through lignan-containing extracts of flax root and pumpkin seeds in *in vitro* settings. Previous studies have shown that extracts of these raw extracts significantly inhibit the proliferation of tumor cells (MCF7, Jeg3) in a cytotoxicity test (MTT). The trefoil factor 1 (TFF1), the estrogen receptors α and β, the progesterone receptor (PR) and the insulin receptor were selected as estrogen-sensitive genes. Increased expressions of TFF1, ER and PR would constitute favorable prognosis factors. Trefoil factor 1 is a small secretory protein consisting of 60 amino acids. It belongs to the trefoil family of which three proteins are known (TFF1, TFF2, and TFF3) and is expressed mainly in healthy tissue in the gastrointestinal tract. TFF1 is known to stimulate intestinal repair. If the expression of TFF1 in the mamma carcinoma is increased, a favorable effect on the further course of the disease and a response to the hormone therapy can be expected.

Material and Methods

Extracts from the root material of flax, *Linum usitatissimum*, variety: Barbara, and shelled pumpkin seeds of the variety Gele Centenaar were produced. The cell cultures used included the chorioncarcinoma cell line Jeg3 and the human mamma carcinoma cell line MCF7. 100 ml serum and 2 g activated carbon are incubated for 24 h at 4°C with mild rotation in order to filter the majority of the steroid hormones out of commercial fetal calf serum (FCS). For the examination of gene expression, the cells are prepared in a concentration of 300,000 cells per well.

Estradiol is used in the concentration of 1 µg/ml, secoisolariciresinol in the concentration of 10 µg/ml. The flax root extract is used in two different concentrations - 500 µg/ml and 100 µg/ml-; the pumpkin seed extract is used in the concentration of 5000 µg/ml.

Further steps comprise RNA extraction and cDNA synthesis. An oligo-d(T)$_{12}$ primer is used to this effect. A survey of the primers for real-time PCR, in part derived using the Primer3 program (http://frodo.wi.mit.edu/cgi-bin/primer3/primer3.cgi) or taken from other publications, is shown in the table 2.

Table 2. *Primers.* Number of base pairs, annealing temperature and sequence, HPRT: Hypoxanthine - phosphoribosyltransferase, TFF1: trefoil factor 1; INSR: insulin receptor, PGR: progesterone receptor, ESR1: estrogen receptor α, ESR2: estrogen receptor β

Gene	Primer designation	Length (bp)	Annealing temp.	Sequence
HPRT	HPRTup	21	61°C	TGTAATGACCAGTCAACAGGG
	HPRTdw	21		TGGCTTATATCCAACACTTCG
TFF1	TFF1up	22	65°C	GTGAGCCGAGGCACAGCTGCAG
	TFF1dw	22		TGACTCGGGGTCGCCTTTGGAG
INSR	INSRup	18	61°C	TCGTCCCCAGAAAAACCT
	INSRdw	19		GATAGCCCGTGAAGTGTCG
PGR	PRGup	24	61°C	CACAAAACCTGACACCTCCAGTTC
	PRGdw	22		GCAAAATACAGCATCTGCCCAC
ESR1	ESR1up	20	61°C	AGCCCGCTCATGATCAAACG
	ESR1dw	23		GGATCATACTCGGAATAGAGAAT
ESR2	ESR2up	20	61°C	AACCTCCTGATGCTCCTGTC
	ESR2dw	21		GCCCTCTTTGCTTTTACTGTC

For relative quantification, the concentrations of the unknown samples to be measured are analyzed in comparison to a reference gene (housekeeping gene). The ΔΔCT method is used to this effect.

We used the absolute quantification for evaluating the data collected here since the standard gene did not show any stable expression. The concentrations were related to the ethanol control which is set to one. The significances were determined using the Tukey-Kramer test (statistics program: SAS).

Results

In the hormone receptor-positive mamma carcinoma cell line MCF7, a dose-related increase in the expression of the trefoil factor 1, the insulin receptor, the progesterone receptor and the estrogen receptor α was observed after addition of the flax root extract. The gene expression was less pronounced in the hormone receptor-positive Jeg3 cell line than in the MCF7 cell line. The flax root extract resulted in an increased gene expression. At present it cannot be distinguished which compounds of the extract are responsible for the results achieved. But it can be assumed that in particular the flax root extract as a multicomponent mixture is able to support an expression of therapeutically important receptors and thus can be considered in concomitant therapies.

2.3 Clinical Studies

2.3.1. The Treatment of Climacteric Symptoms by Isoflavones Using a Prospective, Randomized, Placebo-Controlled Double-Blind Study

We performed a prospective, randomized double-blind study on a product made of soybean extract, vitamins and other nutrients.

66 peri- and postmenopausal women were randomized into the study. The treatment group included 29 participants, the placebo group 37 participants.

The treatment group received the micronutrient combination with 50 mg soy isoflavones daily for 6 months; the control group received a corresponding placebo. The patients were called in at the beginning of the study, after 6 and after 12 weeks as well as after 6 months.

The climacteric symptoms were objectivized using Hauser's Menopause Rating Scale / MRS II. The bone metabolism was examined through cross-links and ostase. Pyridinoline and deoxypyridinoline, markers for the absorption of bone, i.e. for osteoclast activity, were analyzed in urine samples. Ostase, a marker of bone formation, i.e. for osteoblast activity, was determined in serum samples.

The intensity of the following complaints was determined using the menopause rating scale as clinical standard of valuation: hot flushes, breaking out into a sweat, cardiac complaints, sleep disorders, depressive moods, irritability, timidness, physical and mental exhaustion, sexual problems, urinary tract problems, dryness of the vagina as well as joint and muscular complaints.

Results

The entirety of these subjective complaints showed a significant reduction in both groups after 6 months compared with the baseline value with statistically relevant benefit for the treatment group compared with the placebo group ($p < 0.001$).

The laboratory chemical analyses showed an improvement of the bone metabolism in the treatment group. Ostase showed a significant increase in the treatment group ($p = 0.003$), deoxypyridinoline showed a significant drop in the treatment group ($P = 0.007$).

Conclusion

The study results show that the intake of the used product containing soybean extract, vitamins and other nutrients relieves the entirety of the subjective climacteric complaints. Furthermore, the study demonstrated that the product has a positive influence on the bone metabolism. Thus, soy isoflavones constitute a useful dietetic therapy option for menopausal complaints [Anderson et al. 1999, Barnes 2003].

2.3.2. Quantitative Detection of the Phytoestrogens Daidzein and Genistein in the Urine in a Placebo-Controlled Double-Blind Study on Osteoporosis Prevention

Phytoestrogens, in particular the isoflavones daidzein and genistein present in soy, are currently in the centre of interest of scientists doing research on plant agents for the prevention and therapy of the climacteric syndrome. Up to now, isoflavone ingestion has been assessed mainly on account of diet protocols, intestinal absorption and metabolism not being taken into consideration [Yan et al. 2007]. Phenotypical differences are not identified [Pineda et al. 2001, van der Heide et al. 2003].

In the context of the present work, we have developed a method for the determination of free daidzein and genistein in the urine by means of HPLC (high performance liquid chromatography with UV detection) as well as of conjugated daidzein and genistein after splitting of the conjugates by means of acid hydrolysis. 492 urine samples of 80 participants in the "randomized placebo-controlled double-blind study on the realization of osteoporosis prophylaxis and relief of climacteric complaints using nutrient-enriched food" of the Department of Obstetrics and Gynecology of the University Rostock were examined for their content of isoflavones.

In all, 89 women were included in the study, including 23 women who have already been receiving an HRT and continued it during the study. Six women discontinued the study prematurely. The study participants were aged between 43 and 66 years (∅ 53.1 years), the women were postmenopausal and had at least one climacteric symptom. The body mass index (BMI) was between 18 and 40 (∅ 26.3).

In the randomized, placebo-controlled double-blind study, a bread enriched with 750 mg calcium, 2,5μg vitamin D, 80 mg isoflavones, 200 mg lignans, 250 mg magnesium and 1 mg fluoride for the corresponding daily quantity (250 g) was regularly sent to the women over a period of six months. The symptoms were recorded monthly by means of a standardized questionnaire and serum and urine samples were collected.

We used specific bone markers for recording the dynamics of bone metabolism: pyridinoline as well as deoxypyridinoline (cross-links) for bone resorption and ostase for bone formation [Poulsen and Kruger 2008]. In addition, triglyceride, HDL, LDL and cholesterol were determined in the serum for lipid metabolism and FSH, LH and estradiol for hormonal balance.

Urine measurements of the isoflavones daidzein and genistein:

The used HPLC (high performance liquid chromatography) method is briefly described:

- Separation procedure according to substance-specific retention times and measurement of UV detection.
- Qualitative and quantitative analysis using peak height and retention time compared with standardized chromatograms.
- 2 ml safe-lock reaction vessels + 1000 µl urine + 20 µl 4-hydroxybenzophenone (0.2 µmol/ml) + 400 µl sulfuric acid, shaking for 1 min in the gyrator.
- Extraction at room temperature by adding 500 µl diethyl ether.
- Processing of the upper organic phase after centrifugation 14,000 rpm, injection volume 10 µl.
- An isocratic ammonium formate / formic acid buffer in acetonitrile that is pumped through the column system at a pressure of 170 bars and a flow rate of 0.7 ml/min is used as mobile phase, wave length at the UV detector 260 nm.
- Collection of urine samples according to clinical study: pre-phase, six-month study phase, three-month post-phase.
- Collection of 24 h-urine in the pre-phase as "blank sample" (U1), during the study phase, one urine sample per month (U2 – U7). After another 3 months, "control sample" U8.

Results of the Clinical Study

Regarding the subjective symptoms, we found that the climacteric symptoms decreased in all three groups. Nevertheless, a significant reduction of several symptoms was detected in the treatment group compared to the placebo group. For example, the complaints of hot flushes ($p = 0.02$), heart hurry ($p = 0.03$) and attacks of vertigo ($p = 0.04$) clearly decreased both regarding number and frequency. Sleep disorders ($p = 0.01$) and irritability ($p = 0.02$) improved in the treatment group as well. Complaints in the genital area such as pruritus ($p < 0.01$) and dry vagina ($p = 0.01$) occurred less commonly, which certainly also explains the higher desire for sexuality ($p \leq 0.01$) in the treatment group.

Table 3. Determination of genistein and daidzein in urine samples - frequencies of sample evaluation

Isoflavones measured	Treatment group	Control group
Positive	240	30
Questionably positive	22	8
Negative	47	145
Total	309	183

Figure 9 shows the time course of daidzein concentrations. Clear differences compared with the placebo group are identified. Please note that the group of patients with hormone related therapy (HRT) received both the classical hormone and the phytoestrogens.

The laboratory chemical analyses showed a clear improvement of the bone metabolism in the treatment group. The bone resorption markers decreased significantly more strongly in this group than in the placebo group (PYD $p = 0.02$; DPD $p = 0.04$). The ostase level did not show any significant change. Regarding the lipid metabolism, it becomes clear that a drop in the triglyceride and cholesterol levels occurs in the treatment group. This, however, does not become significant on account of the high variance and the small number of cases. No changes were found in the hormone analyses for the two groups.

The women under HRT have to be considered as a separate group. Laboratory parameters change only marginally under the additional therapy. However, a clear improvement of the complaints takes place in this group as well.

Results of the determination of daidzein and genistein concentrations in the urine samples of the nutrition study revealed isoflavone concentration (daidzein, genistein) in the treatment group (Table 3).

Summary of the Clinical Study on a Soy Supplementation:

Up to present, mainly diet protocols have been used in clinical studies on the effect of isoflavones on climacteric complaints for assessing the exposure to isoflavones. No general standard for the determination of isoflavones has been found yet. As a reasonable objective alternative, we determined the concentration of free daidzein, total daidzein, free genistein and total genistein in the urine without and with acid hydrolysis by means of high performance liquid chromatography (HPLC). Regular soy consumption was identified for 45 test persons of the treatment group. Significant quantities of isoflavones were detected irregularly in the urine of 3 test persons. It is unclear whether these results are explained by irregular soy consumption or special features of the metabolism of the test persons. For 25 of the 28 test persons in the control group, isoflavones were detected rarely or never in the urine samples during the study phase. This also means that we have to assume a small current intake of isoflavones in the population. Isoflavones were detected irregularly for 3 test persons so that food intake has to be assumed in these cases. This emphasizes that special phenotypic characteristics have to be taken into account with regard to the phytoestrogen metabolism. An administration of a certain quantity of isoflavones alone does not mean that this quantity is of biological relevance.

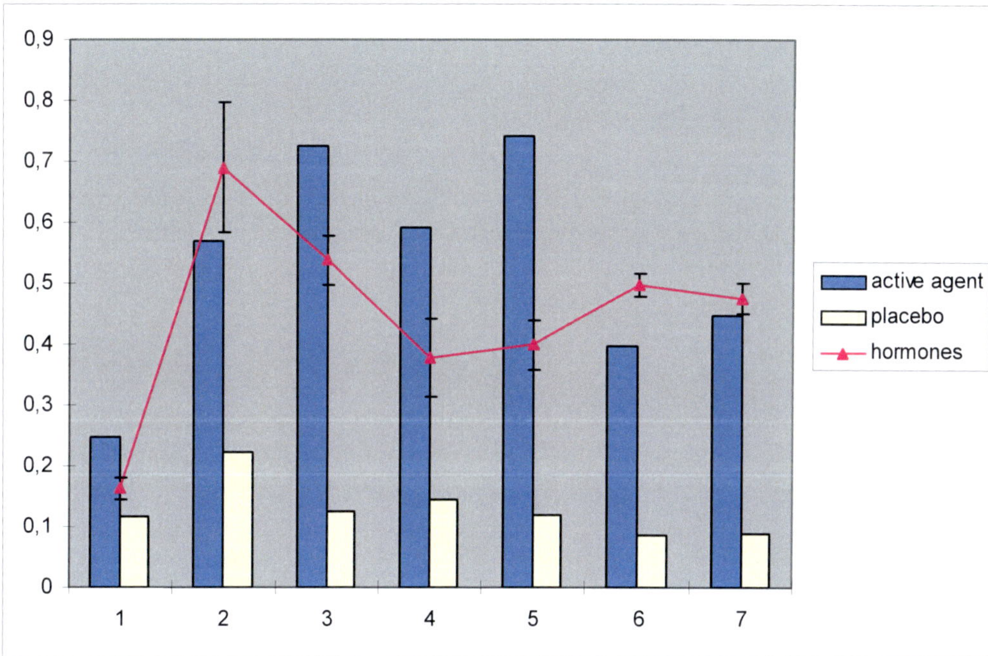

Figure 9. Presentation of daidzein concentrations (nmol/ml) in the course of the study.

Figure 10 shows the time courses of genistein concentrations. The differences between treatment and placebo group are smaller. Please note again that the hormone group additionally received the phytoestrogens.

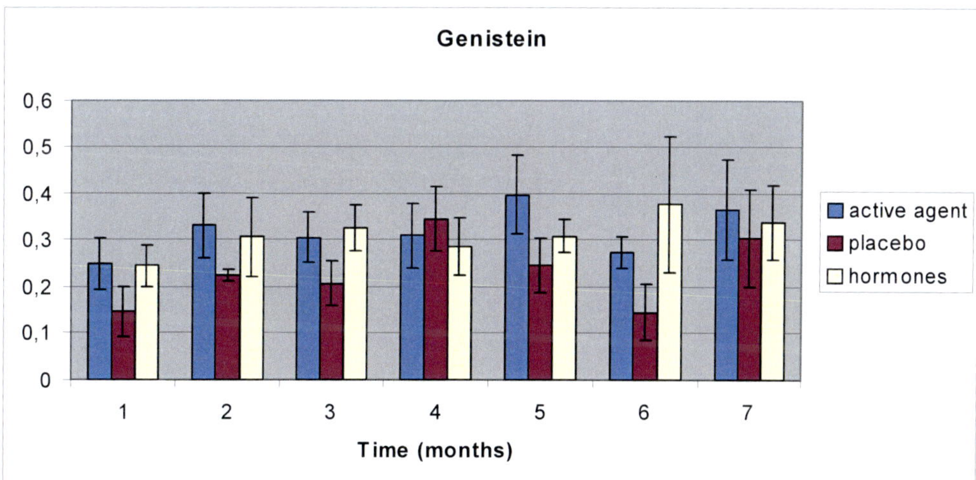

Figure 10. Presentation of genistein concentrations (nmol/ml) in the course of the study.

The evaluation of our results makes clear that the determination of isoflavones in the urine without and with acid hydrolysis by means of HPLC is well suitable for studies including a large number of samples since the presence of significant quantities of free unconjugated daidzein and genistein in the urine can be quantified relatively simply and quickly. This is how the exposure to isoflavones can be assessed in an objective way. These results constitute decisive preparations for further studies.

A significant reduction of the climacteric complaints compared to the placebo groups was proven in the present treatment groups. For example, the complaints of hot flushes, heart hurry and attacks of vertigo clearly decreased both regarding number and frequency. Sleep disorders and irritability improved in the treatment group as well. The laboratory chemical analyses showed a clear improvement of the bone metabolism in the treatment group. There was a trend towards an increase in ostase in the serum and towards a decrease in pyridinoline (cross-links). In particular the concentration of triglycerides, but also of total cholesterol, was reduced, whereas no changes were found in the placebo group.

Thus, we can establish that prevention and therapy of the climacteric syndrome are possible both using food supplements and functional food enriched with phytoestrogens.

2.3.3. Remifemin – Prospective Cohort Study

Medicinal products that contain extracts of black cohosh (*Cimicifuga racemosa*) enjoy more and more popularity for the therapy of climacteric complaints. The two established products Remifemin® and Remifemin® plus are the subject matter of a worldwide clinical research program.

Remifemin® contains the isopropanolic extract of back cohosh. Remifemin® additionally contains an ethanolic extract of St. John's wort (*Hypericum perforatum*). Randomized, placebo-controlled clinical trials have proven the efficacy of both products.

Our study is a prospective, controlled post-authorization study [Briese et al. 2007]. More than 1,000 gynecological surgeries throughout Germany have participated in this study. Considering this great participation and the study period of two years, the random test has to be considered to be representative.

Patients with climacteric complaints who have not been treated with the study drugs during the last 6 months or with hormones during the last 4 weeks were included in the study.

The findings were established at the beginning of the study, after 3 and after 6 months. The climacteric symptoms were measured using the Menopause Rating Scale I (MRS I).

As expected, the two treatment groups showed minor differences regarding the individual demographic and anamnestic data. On average, Remifemin® patients were a bit younger slightly more frequently premenopausal. Nevertheless: Both drugs are used both for pre- and postmenopausal women.

The intensity of the dominant symptoms of hot flushes and sleeping disorders was approximately identical in both groups. On the contrary, Remifemin® plus was used more frequently in patients suffering from more intense depressive moods or nervousness / irritability than the drug containing only a single active agent.

The comparison of the therapy groups is in the center of interest. In this comparison, Remifemin® plus proves to be highly significantly superior to Remifemin® regarding the influence on the MRS subscore of psychological symptoms.

2.4. Prevention and Therapy with Phytoestrogens (Basic Research and Clinical Aspects)

Orthodox medicine as well is increasingly discovering the potential for health offered by plant hormones. Long-term hormone replacement therapy (HRT) has come under criticism [Kleine-Gunk 2008, Rohr 2004]. Therefore, a more careful and differentiated assessment of the necessity of such a therapy is required in future. Alternatives to classical hormone replacement therapy (HRT) are called for. At present, phytoestrogens constitute the most promising option [Branca and Lorenzetti 2005, Gebhardt 2008]. Phytoestrogens have many of the positive effects – albeit in a weaker form – that classical hormone preparations show as well; but without their undesired risks and side effects. Orthomolecular medicine has discovered in which way vitamins and trace elements can have a selective influence on our immune system. At present we are not sure if phytoestrogens are generally safe food additives or dangerous drugs [Wuttke 2007]. In this context, dose-effect relationships, period of administration and interindividual differences of the metabolic characteristics have to be taken into account. Phytoestrogens reveal new possibilities: plants have an influence on our hormone system. They produce hormones similar to human hormones - hormone-related substances - and, as a result, have hormone-like effects in the human body [Adlercreutz 1997, 2000, 2002]. According to human estrogens, we have to assume genomic and non-genomic mechanisms of action mainly through ERß, but also through ERα [Cabanes et al. 2004]. It has not been discovered yet to which extent the hypothalamo-hypophyseal-ovarial axis is influenced.

From the clinical point of view the phytoestrogens are weak estrogens. They act by estrogen receptors predominantly. We don't know which the crucial conditions are for their estrogenic or antiestrogenic activity, respectively. However, there are conflicting results related to differences in study design, estrogen status of the body, metabolism of isoflavones among individuals, and other dietary factors. Thus must be understandably for the clinically active physician that basic research results are needed before standards for prevention could be recommended.

The positive influence of phytoestrogens on the cardiovascular system is caused mainly by the action via the endothelial membrane sex steroid receptors. This receptor is likely to the estrogen receptor α (ERα). The activated palmityolated membrane sex steroid receptor induces the endothelial nitric oxide synthesis (eNOS) via an intracellular signal cascade [Nakaya et al. 2007].

Experiments in adult female animals have shown that estrogen induces endothelium-dependent vascular relaxation via the nitric oxide (NO), prostacyclin, and hyperpolarization pathways. Also, surface membrane estrogen receptors (ERs) decrease intracellular free Ca^{2+} concentration and perhaps protein kinase C-dependent vascular smooth muscle contraction [Oia et al. 2008]. On the other side a phytoestrogen antagonism on homocysteine-induced endothelin-1 gene expression and on reactive oxygen species accumulation could be responsible for vasodilatation. Anti-inflammatory effects of phytoestrogens are also of interest. Phytoestrogens are hypothesized to act through inflammation pathways [Pan et al. 2008]. It could be demonstrated that a consumption for 6 week of a 500 mg/d of secoisolariciresinol diglucoside may reduce CRP (c-reactive protein) serum concentrations but had no effect on plasma lipid concentrations, serum lipoprotein oxidation resistance, or plasma antioxidant capacity [Hallund et al. 2006, Hallund et al. 2008]. No significant effects of phytoestrogens on other plasma inflammatory markers were observed [Hall et al. 2005].

Present is to be assumed that phytoestrogens are acting at the molecular level regarding to the protection of degenerative and cancer diseases. Recently, Park et al. [2008] determined the effect of genistein on adipogenesis and estrogen receptor (ER) alpha and beta expression during differentiation in primary human preadipocytes. Their study adds to the elucidation of the molecular pathways involved in the inhibition of adipogenesis by phytoestrogens. The inhibition of lipid accumulation was associated with inhibition of glycerol-3-phosphate dehydrogenase activity and down-regulation of expression of adipocyte-specific genes, including peroxisome proliferator-activated receptor gamma, glycerol-3-phosphate dehydrogenase, adipocyte fatty acid binding protein, fatty acid synthase, sterol regulatory element-binding protein 1, perilipin, leptin, lipoprotein lipase and hormone-sensitive lipase. These effects of genistein during the differentiation period were associated with down-regulation of ERα and ERβ expression.

Review of the existing literature suggests that consumption of soy foods or an exposure to a soy isoflavone genistein during childhood and adolescence in women, and before puberty onset in animals, reduces later mammary cancer risk. A meta-analysis of human studies indicates a modest reduction in pre- and postmenopausal risk when dietary intakes are assessed during adult life. These findings concur with emerging evidence indicating that timing may be vitally important in determining the effects of various dietary exposures on the susceptibility to develop breast cancer. The biochemical pathway for cancer prevention are based the ability of phytoestrogens to bind preferentially to estrogen receptor ß (ERß), inhibit enzymes that convert circulating steroid precursors into estradiol and inhibit cell signalling pathways of growth factors [Rica and Whitehead 2008]. Chen et al. [2007] indicated that genistein is involved in mechanisms in activation of insulin-like growth factor 1 receptor expression in human breast cancer cells. The studies have shown that genistein can enhance the insulin-like growth factor (IGF)-1 receptor signalling pathway via an estrogen receptor (ER) in human breast cancer MCF-7 cells. The results indicated that the induction of IGF-1 receptor promoter activity by genistein required the action of ER while the stimulatory actions of genistein on IGF-1 receptor expression required the activity of the IGF-1 receptor and de novo protein synthesis (cross-talk between IGF-1 receptor and the ER-dependent pathways). The new focus is on changes in gene expression, such as those involving BRCA1 and PTEN. Warri et al [2008] debated whether mammary stem cells are the targets of genistein-induced alterations and also whether the alterations are epigenetic. We propose that the effects on mammary gland morphology and signalling pathways induced by pubertal exposure to genistein mimic those induced by the oestrogenic environment of early first pregnancy.

Metabolism of dietary soy isoflavones to equol by human intestinal microflora [Yan et al. 2007]:

In vivo studies have shown variations in health benefits of isoflavones among individuals, which have been attributed to dissimilarities in the population of colonic bacteria responsible for isoflavone conversion [Rafii et al. 2003, Setchell et al. 2002].

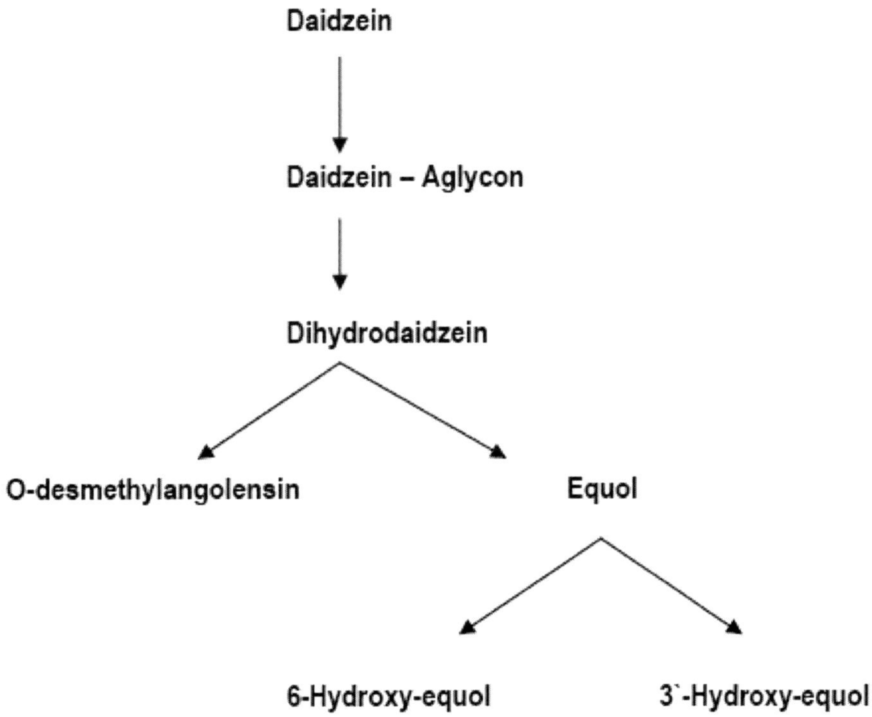

Figure 11. Bioavailability – daidzein is converted to O-desmethylangolensin and equol via the action of intestinal ß-glycosidase from bacteria.

Isoflavones (genistein, daidzein) can be metabolized by intestinal microflora and converted to dihydrodaidzein, O-desmethylangolensin, equol or 4-hydroxyequol, significantly altering its biological properties [Hedlund et al. 2003]. The bioavailability of soy isoflavones strongly depends on the activity of intestinal bacteria. The intestinal microflora plays a crucial role in the metabolism of isoflavones. The underlying interactions remain poorly understood [Clavel et al. 2005]. Equol suggests a major role as a biomarker for the effectiveness of soy isoflavones. Despite this known biological and clinical importance of equol, there have been limited studies of equol effects in vivo because of the high cost of equol and its limited availability [Selvaraj et al. 2004]. The bioavailability of isoflavone glycosides requires the conversion of glycosides to aglycones via the action of intestinal ß-glycosidase from bacteria that colonize the small intestine for uptake into the peripheral circulation. Genistein is converted to p-ethyl phenol and 4-hydroxyphenyl-2-propionic acid, while daidzein is reduced to O-desmethylangolensin and equol (Figure 11) [L`homme et al. 2002, Bowey et al. 2003].

The distinction between equol producers and equol nonproducers can be derived from urine. An equol producer is defined as someone excreting > 1000 nmol/L [Setchell 2002]. The physiologic differences between equol producers and nonproducers have not been fully elucidated [Blair et al. 2003]. However, it is clear that nutritional diets influence the metabolism of isoflavones. The role of prebiotics comes also into the question.

Phytoestrogens as Anti-Menopausal Agents

Female ovaries are designed as "temporary organs". The endocrine function significantly reduces approximately in the late forties, at the latest however in the mid-fifties, individual very indifferently. The feed back mechanisms of the hypothalamo-hyophyseal-ovarial axis are detoriated irreversibly. This concerns autocrine, paracrine cerebral and endocrine central and peripher mechanisms. This results in the great variety of climacteric symptoms, e.g. due to the impairment of cerebral centers such as the centre for temperature, the limbic system, autonomic nervous system. About 30% of all women experience a significant impairment of their quality of life due to daily and undulant hot flushes. Only one third of women can live without any treatment. Recently symptoms of depression move into the foreground [Briese et al. 2007]. In addition to hot flushes, other psycho-autonomic complaints include sleep disorders, heart hurry or latent and obvious depressions. From numerous experiences and reports we can conclude that by means of phytoestrogens easy symptoms can be covered well.

The cancer preventive effect of phytoestrogens allows women suffering from a mamma carcinoma to take this substance for menopausal complaints. In contrast to hormone replacement therapy performed up to now, phytoestrogens constitute a therapy option during the critical stage at the beginning of the menopause as well since they do not cause hormone substitution, but hormone modulation (SERMS = selective estrogen receptor modulators). Phytoestrogens have a weak estrogen effect. Their hormone receptors are identical to the body's own hormones. They unfold their estrogen effect in case of endogenous hormone deficiency [Anderson et al. 1999, Jungbauer and Pfitscher 2005, Kleine-Gunk 2008]. On the contrary, in case of excessively high estrogen levels, phytoestrogens act as antiestrogens so that the essentially stronger endogenous hormones cannot unfold their proliferative effect. Thus, their use for the premenstrual syndrome seems to be possible as well [Kleine-Gunk 2008]. However new studies are to be considered, which warn of uncontrolled application of phytoestrogens. In our region (Germany) we dedicate ourselves at present excellently lignans.

What to Do for Women Suffering from Persistent Climacteric Complaints that Cannot Be Managed Through Phytodrugs?

We recommend first a phytoestrogen application over 6 - 12 weeks. We vary the dose of isoflavons pray if 50 and 100 mg and change then on another preparation, for example black cohosh. In some cases, the classical hormone replacement therapy (HRT) should be applied - at least for some time. The application of HRT for treating acute complaints is very effective. Then, a switchover of therapy to phytoestrogens should be tried by slowly reducing the dose, e.g. reduction from 2 mg estradiol to 1 mg estradiol with simultaneous administration of phytoestrogen [Kleine-Gunk 2008]. Under in vitro conditions genistein and daidzein could decrease proliferation rates of mammary epithelial cells stimulated by estradiol [Nebe et al. 2006].

Protection Against Osteoporosis

According to epidemiologic studies from the Asian region, we can conclude that a long-term diet rich in soy can prevent osteoporosis [Barnes 2003, Branca and Lorenzetti 2005]. In Asia the osteoporosis occurs very rarely. Just like the actual estrogens, phytoestrogens inhibit osteoclast activity. In addition, osteoblast activity is stimulated so that real new bone formation can be promoted. In the meantime, the positive effects of phytoestrogens on the bones have been proven in animal experiments. Laboratory rats in which estrogen deficiency was established developed osteoporosis. The now started administration of genistein, the most important soy phytoestrogen, prevented the development of an osteoporosis. Human studies showed that biomarkers such as pyridinoline and osteocalcin can verify this effect of phytoestrogens after approx. 6 weeks. Women who keep to a diet rich in phytoestrogens had less products of bone absorption (pyridinoline) in their urine and more bone-stimulating substances (osteocalcin) in their blood. In accordance with our in vitro cell culture investigations we assume, which also the arthritis are favorably affected through phytoestrogens (genistein, daidzein) [Claassen et al. 2008]. Proteoglycans consisting of low and high sulfated glycosaminoglycans are the main components of articular cartilage matrix, and their synthesis is increased by insulin in growth plate cartilage. We have investigated whether glycosaminoglycan synthesis and sodium [(35)S]sulfate incorporation in female bovine articular in chondrocytes are affected by daidzein, genistein, and/or insulin. However, the stimulating effect of insulin on sulfate incorporation was enhanced significantly after preincubation of cells with 10(-11) M-10(-5) M daidzein or 10(-9) M-10(-5) M genistein but not by 17β-estradiol was estimated. In view of the risks of long-term estrogen replacement therapy, further experiments should clarify the potential benefit of phytoestrogens in articular cartilage metabolism.

In the meantime, a synthetic phytoestrogen, ipriflavone, has become available and has already been used for osteoporosis treatment in 20 countries [Kleine-Gunk 2008]. A daily dose of 600 mg ipriflavone for a period of 2 years is recommended. In addition to phytoestrogens, soy protein is associated with a positive effect on the preservation of the bone structure. The absorption of soy protein needs 30% less calcium than the absorption of animal proteins. However, we have to add that a sufficient resorption of soy proteins and phytoestrogens is attached to a well functioning intestinal flora.

Lipid Metabolism and Cardiovascular Protection

Animal experimental and human studies indicate that a reduction of high cholesterol levels and the improvement of the LDL-HDL-ratio are widely demonstrated effects of phytoestrogens. Phytoestrogens are highly effective radical scavengers (antioxidants) and can reduce the oxidation of LDL cholesterol. Oxidation of LDL cholesterol mainly is a result of aggressive molecules, the so-called free radicals. Like heparins, phytoestrogens contribute to the improvement of the thinning of the blood. They have a mild anticoagulant effect. This is why phytoestrogen, unlike the classical estrogens, are not associated with an increase in the risk of thrombosis, but with a reduction of the risk of thrombosis. With regard to the protection of the cardiovascular system, soy protein contains less homocysteine than animal protein. Soy protein is rich in B vitamins and folic acid. It is generally known that folic acid strongly reduces high homocysteine levels. The positive influence of phytoestrogens on the cardiovascular system can be explained by means of the membrane estrogen receptor. In its parmitoylated form, the membrane estrogen receptor is associated with the cell membrane and activates the endothelial nitrogen oxide synthetase (eNOS). On account of the similarity with the estrogen receptor, phytoestrogens also act through the membrane estrogen receptor or through non nuclear pathways and can thus effect a dilatation of the vessels and also contribute to a reduction in blood pressure [Ho and Liao 2002, Klinge et al. 2003].

Anticancerogenic Properties of Phytoestrogens

Cancer initiation and cancer promotion constitute the two most important steps in carcinogenesis. So-called carcinogenic as well as cancerogenic substances in the form of pollutants and so-called free radicals play a role in cancer initiation. This results in an initial damage to the hereditary material of a cell so that growth-promoting substances (promoters) can advance the further cancerogenic degeneration. As radical scavengers, phytoestrogens can prevent the malignant degeneration in both stages - both during cancer initiation and cancer promotion - in particular of hormone-dependent tumors. Furthermore, phytoestrogens act as aromatase and angiogenesis inhibitors [Chen et al. 2003]. The antiangiogenic properties of phytoestrogens have been proven by means of experiments [Fotsis et al. 1995].

Breast cancer prevention through phytoestrogens should already start before puberty [Controneo et al. 2002]. This statement is corroborated by the known Asian migration studies [Luo et al. 2004]. Asian women usually eat food rich in phytoestrogens. After migration to Western countries, the "protection against carcinoma" was preserved [Pineda et al. 2001]. Their daughters (next generations) who have grown up with food adapted to Western culture and thus poor in phytoestrogen had lost this protection.

Maskarinec and Noh [2004] compared cancer incidence trends among Japanese in Japan, and Japanese and Caucasians in Hawaii, between 1960 and 1997, and estimated the impact of migration on the incidence of different cancers. Among the 5 more common cancers, the migrant effect was strongest for colon and stomach cancers, prostate and breast cancers were affected to a lesser degree, and lung cancer risk differed little between Japanese in Japan and Hawaii. Migration led to lower risk of stomach, esophageal, pancreatic, liver, and cervical cancers, but to higher rates for all other cancers. Although the migration effect can be partially explained by known etiologic factors, a large proportion of the changing risk remains unexplained. Recently, cancer rates for Korean-American immigrants have increased for prostate, breast, colon, and rectal cancers [Lee et al. 2007].

Experiments with prepubertal rats showed that a complete differentiation of the mammary glands takes place in case of exposure to isoflavones. This "complete" differentiation is considered to be an important factor for the prevention of breast cancer. Phytoestrogens contribute to the upregulation of the expression of the mRNA for the marker protein BRCA1.

According to the Asian studies more than 15 (20) mg isoflavones per day are considered to be the ideal quantity for the prevention of mamma carcinoma. A daily intake of isoflavones of under 1 mg is assumed in the industrial nations of the US, Canada and Australia. It is essential that the intake of isoflavones is started in childhood and continued throughout life [Wu et al. 2008].

Catechins are said to have anticancerogenic properties as well. Catechins belong to the secondary plant substances and, according to their structure, to the polyphenols. An ointment for local application, the polyphenon ointment, has been available since 2007. The polyphenon ointment has indications in gynecology and dermatology for HPV viral infections (genital warts, *Condylomata acuminata*). Only few experiences are available at present. Studies indicate that catechins have a primary and/or secondary preventive effect for cardiac diseases and tumor diseases. Studies of cell cultures showed that the proliferation of tumor cells is inhibited [Cooper et al. 2005]. On the other hand, apoptosis is induced. Especially green tea has demonstrated promise in the prevention of several cancers. Green tea contains several components including catechins, a category of polyphenols that have chemopreventive properties [Lee et al. 2006]. Besides, in vitro studies indicate that tumor suppressor genes are expressed to an increased extent. The gene expression of EGF – and of the tumor necrosis factor α (TNFα) is reduced significantly [Adachi et al. 2007]. With regard to mamma carcinoma, we currently have to assume that the prognosis can be improved by secondary preventive application of catechins in particular in stages 1 and 2. Furthermore, it is assumed for catechins that anti-inflammatory and anti-stress properties might be responsible for the prevention of degenerative diseases.

Protection of the Skin Through Phytoestrogens

The experience with hormone replacement therapy (HRT) has shown that estrogens can have a large number of positive cosmetic effects. Exactly the critical studies have shown that estrogens cannot be applied without hesitation, they remain a medicinal measure. Local creams and ointments, but also phytoestrogens offer an alternative to this systemic hormone replacement therapy. The first cosmetic containing phytoestrogen – a skin care cream produced by Vichy Company – is available on the marked under the name of Novadiol®. Further experiences in dermatology remain to be seen.

What Clinicians Need to Know According to the Newest Literature? What's the Meaning of Protective Features of Phytoestrogens against Prostate Cancer?

Accumulating epidemiological data suggest that Asian men have lower incidences of prostate cancer and benign prostate hyperplasia compared with American and European populations and may have benefited from their higher intake of phytoestrogens in their diet. However, how these phytochemicals affect prostatic diseases is still unclear [Gaynor 2003]. To determine the clinical effects of soy isoflavones on prostate cancer Hussain et al. [2003] conducted a pilot study in patients with prostate cancer who had rising serum prostate-specific antigen (PSA) levels. Patients with prostate cancer were enrolled in the study if they had either newly diagnosed and untreated disease under watchful waiting with rising PSA (group I) or had increasing serum PSA following local therapy (group II) or while receiving hormone therapy (group III). The study intervention consisted of 100 mg of soy isoflavone (Novasoy) taken orally twice daily for a minimum of 3 or maximum of 6 months. Serum genistein and daidzein levels increased during supplementation from 0.11 to 0.65 μM. The follow up of the PSA levels suggests that soy isoflavones may benefit some patients with prostate cancer. There was a decrease in the rate of the rise of serum PSA in the whole group with rates of rise decreasing from 14 to 6% in group II and from 31 to 9% in group III following the soy isoflavone intervention. It can be postulated, dietary intervention with isoflavone supplementation may have biologic activity in men with biochemical active prostate cancer as shown by a decline in the slope of PSA in pilot studies.

Pendleton et al. [2008] evaluated the efficacy of isoflavones in patients with PSA recurrent prostate cancer after prior therapy. They postulated that isoflavone therapy would slow the rate of rise of serum PSA. Twenty patients with rising PSA after prior local therapy were enrolled in this open-labeled, Phase II, nonrandomized trial. Patients were treated with soy milk containing 47 mg of isoflavonoid three times per day for 12 months. Nearly two thirds of the patients were noted to have significant levels of free equol in their serum while on therapy. The slope of PSA after study entry was significantly lower than that before study entry in 6 patients and the slope of PSA after study entry was significantly higher than before study entry in 2 patients. For the remaining 12 patients, the change in slope was statistically insignificant.

Kumar et al. [2007] evaluated the safety of 80 mg of purified isoflavones regarding to men with early stage prostate cancer. A total of 53 men with clinically localized prostate cancer, Gleason score of 6 or below, were supplemented with 80 mg purified isoflavones or placebo for 12 wk administered in 2 divided doses of 40 mg. Changes in plasma isoflavones, and clinical toxicity were analyzed at baseline, 4, and 12 wk. A continuous, divided-dose administration of 80 mg/day of purified isoflavones at amounts that exceeded normal American dietary intakes significantly increased ($P < 0.001$) plasma isoflavones in the isoflavone-treated group compared to placebo and produced no clinical toxicity.

Which Actual Statements about Phytoestrogens and Breast Cancer Prevention Are Meaningful at Present?

Scientific achievements in the last two decades have revolutionized the treatment and prevention of breast cancer. This is mainly because of targeted therapies and a better understanding of the relationship between estrogen, its receptor, and breast cancer. One of these discoveries is the use of synthetic selective estrogen modulators (SERMs) such as tamoxifen or raloxifen in the treatment strategy for estrogen receptor (ER)-positive breast cancer. The potential effects of phytoestrogens may alter the risk of breast cancer, but only a limited range of phytoestrogens has been examined in prospective cohort studies. Serum and urine samples from 237 incident breast cancer cases and 952 control individuals (aged 45 to 75 years) in the European Prospective into Cancer-Norfolk cohort were analysed for seven phytoestrogens (daidzein, enterodiol, enterolactone, genistein, glycitein, o-desmethylangolensin, and equol) using liquid chromatography/mass spectrometry [Ward et al. 2008]. In summary, urinary or serum phytoestrogens were not associated with protection from breast cancer. Breast cancer risk was marginally increased with higher levels of total urinary isoflavones (odds ratio = 1.08 (95% confidence interval = 1.00 to 1.16), $P = 0.055$); among those with estrogen receptor-positive tumors, the risk of breast cancer was increased with higher levels of urinary equol (odds ratio = 1.07 (95% confidence interval = 1.01 to 1.12), $P = 0.013$). There was limited evidence of an association between phytoestrogen biomarkers and breast cancer .risk in the present study.

The observation that some phytoestrogen biomarkers may be associated with slightly greater risk of breast cancer warrants further studies. At present, it remains uncertain whether the different phytoestrogens are chemo protective or whether they may produce adverse outcomes related to breast carcinogenesis.

Recently Helferich et al. [2008] reported results of animal breast cancer model focused on the effects of dietary genistein on the growth of estrogen dependent mammary tumors both in vitro and in vivo. Genistein enhances the proliferation of estrogen dependent human breast cancer tumor growth. In a similar manner, dietary genistein stimulates tumor growth in the chemically-induced mammary cancer rodent model. Genistein, the glycoside of genistein, simulates growth similar to that of genistein and withdrawal of either genistein or genistein results in tumor regression. The extent of soy processing modulates the effects of dietary genistein *in vivo* as soy protein isolate, a highly purified and widely used source of protein that is processed to contain low, medium, and high amounts of isoflavones, stimulate the growth of the estrogen dependent mammary tumors in a dose dependent manner. In contrast to the more purified diets, studies with soy flour of equivalent genistein levels did not stimulate the growth of estrogen dependent breast cancer tumors in vivo.

There is conflicting evidence from epidemiological, intervention and experimental animal studies regarding the chemo preventing effects of soy isoflavones in breast cancer. Isoflavones are weak estrogens and their effect depends upon the dose, time of exposure and species involved. It would, therefore, not be safe to indisputably accept soy or red-clover as a source of isoflavone resource to prevent breast cancer [Tomar and Shian 2008].

Should We Recommend Adult Women in Western Countries Take a Daily Phytoestrogen Application for Breast Cancer Prevention?

Studies conducted in Asian populations have suggested that high consumption of soy-based foods, at the beginning of childhood, that are rich in isoflavone phytoestrogens is associated with a reduced risk of breast cancer. At present it must be pointed out that no context exists regarding an association between phytoestrogen rich diets and successful breast cancer prevention in Western countries. Because one of the biological effects of phytoestrogens is probably estrogenic, it is possible that the preventive effect on breast cancer differs by estrogen receptor (ER) or progesterone receptor (PR) status of the tumor. High dietary intakes of plant lignans and high exposure to enterolignans were associated with reduced risks of ER- and PR-positive postmenopausal breast cancer in a Western population that does not consume a diet rich in soy. Touillaud et al. [2007] prospectively examined associations between the risk of postmenopausal invasive breast cancer and dietary intakes of four plant lignans (pinoresinol, lariciresinol, secoisolariciresinol, and matairesinol) and estimated exposure to two enterolignans (enterodiol and enterolactone), as measured with a self-administered diet history questionnaire, among 58,049 postmenopausal French women who were not taking soy isoflavone supplements. During 383,425 person-years of follow-up (median follow-up, 7.7 years), 1469 cases of breast cancer were diagnosed. Compared with women in the lowest intake quartiles, those in the highest quartile of total lignan intake (>1395 μg/day) had a reduced risk of breast cancer (RR = 0.83, 95% CI = 0.71 to 0.95, p (trend) = 0.02, 376 versus 411 cases per 100,000 person-years), as did those in the highest quartile of lariciresinol intake (RR = 0.82, 95% CI = 0.71 to 0.95, P(trend) = 0.01). The inverse associations between phytoestrogen intakes and postmenopausal breast cancer risk were limited to ER- and PR-positive disease.

Hedelin et al. [2008] evaluated the associations between dietary phytoestrogen (isoflavonoids, lignans, and coumestrol) intake and risk of breast cancer and whether the ER/PR statuses of the tumor influence this relationship. In 1991-1992 a prospective population-based cohort study among Swedish pre- and postmenopausal women was performed, making questionnaire data available for 45,448 women. A total of 1014 invasive breast cancers were diagnosed until December 2004. However, intake of coumestrol was associated with decreased risk of receptor negative tumors (ER-PR-) but not positive tumors. The risk of ER-PR- tumors was significantly lower (50%) in women with intermediate coumestrol intake compared with those who did not consume any. In addition, the authors found no association between intake of isoflavonoids or lignans and breast cancer risk.

Are Synthetic SERMS (Tamoxifen) and Phytoestrogens Applicable in Combined Form in the Secondary Prevention of Breast Cancer?

Not enough clinical trials exist. Label use applications are present, but no data base of follow-up observations. Dietary genistein can negate the inhibitory effects of tamoxifen on estradiol stimulated growth of MCF-7 cell tumors implanted into ovariectomized athymic mice [Helferich 2008]. An increasing number of breast cancer patients seek to take supplements together with their standard treatment in the hope that these will either prevent recurrence or treat their menopausal symptoms. Observational studies suggest a protective effect of isoflavones on breast cancer risk and the case may be similar for increasing lignan consumption although evidence so far is inconsistent. In contrast, short-term intervention studies suggest a possible stimulatory effect on breast tissue raising concerns of possible adverse effects in breast cancer patients. However, owing to the dearth of human studies investigating effects on breast cancer recurrence and survival the role of phytoestrogens remains unclear. So far, not enough clear evidence exists on which to base guidelines for clinical use, although raising patient awareness of the uncertain effect of phytoestrogens is recommended [Valentzis 2008]. Hormonal replacement therapy (HRT) is contra indicated in breast cancer survivors [Holmberg et al. 2008].

Should We Recommend Adult Women in Western Countries Take a Daily Phytoestrogen Application Regarding the Prevention of Osteoporosis?

In vitro, phytoestrogens promote osteoblastogenesis and inhibit osteoclastogenesis [Poulsen and Kruger 2008]. Human studies support a long-term substitution with phytoestrogens against osteoporotic progression [Rohr 2004]. The recommended daily dosages of isoflavone applications amounted to 40–100 mg in most studies. On the other side a relatively large number of intervention studies have been undertaken in animals and humans, the efficacy of phytoestrogens as bone-protective agents *in vivo* remains unclear. Differences in the bioactivities of individual phytoestrogens, differences in phytoestrogen metabolism and bioavailability within different study populations, and imprecise reporting of the dose of phytoestrogens administered in intervention studies may have contributed to the disparity in study findings.

What Is the Usefulness of Phytoestrogens in Reduction of Blood Pressure?

To determine whether treatment with phytoestrogens or soy proteins succeeds in lowering blood pressure, Rosero et al. [2008] evaluated all the observation studies and clinical trials in a systematic review. No significant variations in blood pressure were found, whether systolic (-1.20 mm Hg; 95% CI, -2.80 to 0.41 mm Hg) or diastolic (-1.31 mm Hg; 95% CI, -2.73 to 0.11). If there were any variations, they are clinical of little importance. There are no statistically significant or clinically important differences in blood pressure between patients treated with phytoestrogens and those not treated.

Are Isoflavones Able to Decrease Serum Total and LDL Cholesterol Concentrations in Humans?

Clinical trials have reported the cholesterol-lowering effects of soy protein intake, but the components responsible are not known. Taku et al. [2007] performed a meta-analysis to evaluate the precise effects of soy isoflavones and soy proteins on lipid profiles. Eleven studies were selected for the meta-analysis. Soy isoflavones significantly decreased serum total cholesterol by 0.10 mmol/L (3.9 mg/dL or 1.77%; $P = 0.02$) and LDL cholesterol by 0.13 mmol/L (5.0 mg/dL or 3.58%; $p < 0.0001$); no significant changes in HDL cholesterol and triacylglycerol were found. Isoflavone-depleted soy protein significantly decreased LDL cholesterol by 0.10 mmol/L (3.9 mg/dL or 2.77%; $p = 0.03$). Soy protein that contained enriched isoflavones significantly decreased LDL cholesterol by 0.18 mmol/L (7.0 mg/dL or 4.98%; $p < 0.0001$) and significantly increased HDL cholesterol by 0.04 mmol/L (1.6 mg/dL or 3.00%; $p = 0.05$). The reductions in LDL cholesterol were larger in the hypercholesterolemic subcategory than in the normocholesterolemic subcategory.

Weggemans and Trautwein [2003] identified literature to the relation between soy associated isoflavones and LDL and HDL cholesterol concentrations in humans. A total of ten studies were adapted in a meta-analysis. Studies were included if they had a control group or treatment, experimental diets only differed in the amounts of soy protein and isoflavones and were each fed for at least 14 days. Studies comprised 959 subjects (336 men and 623 women), average age ranged from 41 to 67 years and baseline cholesterol concentration from 5.42 to 6.60 mmol/l. The intake of soy-associated isoflavones increased by 1–95 mg/day and the intake of soy protein increased by 19–60 g/day. Feeding daily 36 g soy protein with 52 mg soy-associated isoflavones on average decreased low-density lipoprotein (LDL) cholesterol by -0.17+/-0.04 mmol/l and increased high-density lipoprotein (HDL) cholesterol by 0.03+/-0.01 mmol/l. There was no dose-response relation between soy-associated isoflavones and changes in LDL cholesterol or HDL cholesterol. Consumption of soy-associated isoflavones is not related significantly to changes in LDL or HDL cholesterol.

Thorp et al. [2008] examined the contributions of soy protein, isoflavones and equol to the hypocholesterolemic effects of soy foods in a prospective study. Nonsoy consumers (33 men, 58 women) with a plasma total cholesterol concentration > 5.5 mmol/L participated in a double-blind, placebo-controlled, crossover intervention trial. The subjects consumed 3 diets for 6 wk each in random order, which consisted of foods providing a daily dose of 1) 24 g soy protein and 70-80 mg isoflavones (diet S); 2) 12 g soy protein, 12 g dairy protein , and 70-80 mg isoflavones (diet SD); and 3) 24 g dairy protein without isoflavones (diet D). Total cholesterol was 3% lower with the S diet (-0.17 +/- 0.06 mmol/L; $p < 0.05$) than with the D diet, and triglycerides were 4% lower with both the S (-0.14 +/- 0.05 mmol/L; $p < 0.05$) and SD (-0.12 +/- 0.05 mmol/L; $p < 0.05$) diets. There were no significant effects on LDL cholesterol, HDL cholesterol, or the total cholesterol:HDL cholesterol ratio. On the basis of urinary isoflavones, 30 subjects were equol producers. Lipids were not affected significantly by equol production. Equol, a gut bacterial metabolite of isoflavone daidzein, may improve health through changes in vascular function and in estrogen metabolism. The individual function is unclear. The authors concluded that regular consumption of foods providing soy protein and isoflavones had no significant effect on plasma LDL cholesterol in mildly hypercholesterolemic subjects, regardless of equol-producing status.

Are Phytoestrogen Supplements Standardized and Comparable Among Themselves Respectively?

For guarantee of quality of isoflavone-rich supplements, raw material standards are needed. The main isoflavones must be identified and marked.

For example, the investigations of Thompson et al. [2007] clearly demonstrated that supplements regarding their phytoestrogen content are incomparable. Twenty one nonvitamin, nonmineral dietary supplements commonly consumed by women in Canada were analyzed for isoflavones (formononetin, daidzein, genistein, glycitein), lignans (pinoresinol, lariciresinol, secoisolariciresinol, matairesinol), and coumestrol. Supplements containing soy or red clover had the highest concentrations of total isoflavones (728.2-35,417.0 μg/g) and total phytoestrogens (1030.1-35,517.7 μg/g) followed by licorice and licorice-containing supplements (41.3-363.3 μg/g isoflavones; 56.5-370.0 μg/g total phytoestrogens). Other supplements had considerably less isoflavones (</= 19.0 μg/g) and total phytoestrogens (</= 44.2 μg/g). Lignans were present in all (</= 298.9 μg/g), whereas coumestrol was either not present or present in only small amounts (</= 3.0 μg/g). Supplements differed in phytoestrogen profiles.

Another problem is “functional foods”. In the United States, about 25% of infant formula sold is based on soy protein, which is an important source of estrogenic isoflavones in the human food supply [Cao et al. 2008]. Urinary concentrations of genistein and daidzein were about 500 times higher in the soy formula-fed infants than in the cow milk formula-fed infants.

It Is Possible to Guarantee a Significant Lignan Substitution by Rye Bread?

Lignins are basic substances of plant scaffolds derived from lignans. They are part of high-fibre substances. Main sources of lignans are rye and flaxseed. In processed flours lignans are hardly available.

Is the Knowledge Regarding the Content of Lignans in Foods of Western Countries Extensive Enough?

Accurate information about dietary phytoestrogens is important, but there are very limited data concerning food content. Lignans were the main type of phytoestrogens detected for instance in different regions in Germany, but exact information is often absent. Tea and coffee contained up to 20 μg/100 g phytoestrogens and beer (except bitter) contained up to 71 μg/100 g, mainly lignans [Kuhnle et al. 2008].

3. Conclusion

In clinical endocrinology, phytoestrogens (isoflavones, lignans) — estrogen-like substances — are considered to be a “gentle alternative” to classical estrogen therapies. Areas of indication include: protection against hormone-dependent tumors, protection against osteoporosis and cardiovascular protection, relief of climacteric complaints, protection of the skin. Phytoestrogens prove to be an interesting group of substances in particular in oncology since they can act as anti-estrogens, aromatase inhibitors and angiogenesis inhibitors. At present, it still has to be taken into account that the study data from experimental and human biological trials in part is inconsistent. Dose-effect relationships are particularly considered to be not clear.

According to the data available up to now, the absorption of phytoestrogen before puberty is not associated with damage to the reproductive system. A diet rich in phytoestrogen is recommended for prepubertal girls. The situation for prepubertal boys still is not clear. The question of what consequences would result from an exposure to phytoestrogen in this case cannot be answered definitely yet. The exposure to isoflavones during pregnancy and lactation in rats showed a demasculinization of the reproduction system of the offspring. Other groups did not show any influence.

Final Statements on Flax and Elm Bark Extracts as Anticancerogenic Substances

Flax root and elm bark are potential candidates for anticancerogenic active agents for hormone-dependent gynecological tumors. Two strategies could be pursued based on the *in vitro* studies realized by us together with the corresponding results:

1) Check food chemistry and food technology for processing flax root and elm bark (tea etc.).
2) Identification of subfractions of extracts and single substances and elucidation of action mechanisms.

Although we have to assume that phytoestrogens display a favorable anticancerogenic effect in combination with other active agents, no sufficient statements on the dose dependency in human biology are possible at present.

Acknowledgements

We thank the University of Rostock, FORUN-programs no. 989008 and no. 989039, for supporting these investigations. The authors are very thankful to Ute Kringel, Ulf Kringel, Gunther Bruer, Wolfgang Ruth, André Schlichting, Susann Gailus, Marlen Szewczyk, Anna-Maria Hartmann, Daniel Paschke, Christel Bauer, Erika Greschkowitz, Petra Müller, Friederike Behler, and Annelie Peters.

4. References

Abarzua S, Szewczyk M, Gailus S, Richter D-U, Ruth W, Briese V. Effects of phytoestrogen extracts from *Linum usitatissimum* on the Jeg3 human trophoblast tumor cell line. *Anticancer Res.* 2007;27:2053-8.

Adachi S, Nagao T, Ingolfsson HI, Maxfield FR, Andersen OS, Kopelovich L, Weinstein IB. The inhibitory effect of epigallocatechin gallate on activation of the epidermal growth factor receptor is associated with altered lipid order in HT29 colon cancer cells. *Cancer Res.* 2007; 67: 6493-501.

Adlercreutz, H. Phytoestrogens: epidemiology and a possible role in cancer protection. *Environ. Health Perspect.* 1995;103:103-12.

Adlercreutz H. Phyto-oestrogens and cancer. *Lancet Oncol.* 2002;3:364-73.

Adlercreutz H. Phytoestrogens and breast cancer. *J. Steroid Biochem. Mol. Biol.* 2003;83:113-8.

Adlercreutz H, Bannwart C, Wähälä K, Mäkelä T, Brunow G, Hase T. Inhibition of human aromatase by mammalian lignans and isoflavonoid phytoestrogens. *J. Steroid Biochem. Molec. Biol.* 1993;44:147-53.

Adlercreutz H, Goldin BR, Gorbach SL, Hockerstedt KA, Watanabe S, Hamalainen EK. Soybean phytoestrogen intake and cancer risk. *J. Nutr. 1*995;125:757-70.

Adlercreutz H, Heinonen SM, Penalvo-Garcia J. Phytoestrogens, cancer and coronary heart disease. *Biofactors.* 2004b;22:229-36.

Adlercreutz H, Hockerstedt K, Bannwart C. Effect of dietary components, including lignans and phytoöstrogens on enterohepatic circulation on liver metabolism of estrogens and on sex hormon binding globulin (SHBG). *J. Steroid. Biochem.* 1987;27:1135-44.

Adlercreutz H, Honjo H, Higashi A, Fotsis T, Hämäläinen E, Hasegawa T. Urinary excretion of lignans and isoflavonoid phytoestrogens in Japanese men and women consuming a traditional Japanese diet. *Am. J. Clin. Nutr.* 1991;54:1093-100.

Adlercreutz H, Kiuru P, Rasku S, Wahala K, Fotsis T. An isotope dilution gas chromatographic-mass spectrometric method for the simultaneous assay of estrogens and phytoestrogens in urine. *J. Steroid Biochem. Mol. Biol.* 2004a;92:399-411.

Adlercreutz H, Mazur W. Phyto-oestrogens and Western diseases. Ann Med. 1997;2:95-120.

Adlercreutz H, Mazur W, Stumpf K. Food containing phytoestrogens, and breast cancer. *Biofactors.* 2000;12:89-93.

Adlercreutz H, Mousavi Y, Clark J, Hockerstedt K, Hamalainen E, Wahala K. Dietary phytoestrogens and cancer: in vitro and in vivo studies. *J. Steroid Biochem. Mol. Biol.* 1992;41:331-7.

Akiyama T, Ishida J, Nakagawa S. Genistein, a specific inhibitor of tyrosin-specific protein kinase. *J. Biol. Chem.* 1987;262:5592-5.

Ames BN, Profet M, Gold LS. Dietary pesticides (99,99% all natural). *Proc. Natl. Acad. Sci. USA.* 1990;87:7777-81.

Anderson JJ, Anthony MS, Cline JM, Washburn SA, Garner SC. Health potential of soy isoflavones for menopausal women. *Public Health Nutr.* 1999;2489-504.

Aplin AE, Howe AK, Juliano RL. Cell adhesion molecules, signal transduction and cell growth. *Curr. Opin. Cell Biol. 1*999;11:737-44.

Atkinson C, Frankenfeld CL, Lampe JW. Gut bacterial metabolism of the soy isoflavone daidzein: exploring the relevance to human health. *Exp. Biol. Med.* 2005;230:155-70.

Barnes S. Phyto-oestrogens and osteoporosis: what is a safe dose? Br J Nutr. 2003;89: 101-8.

Blair RM, Appt SE, Franke AA, Clarkson TB. Treatment with antibiotics reduces plasma equol concentration in cynomolgus monkeys (Macaca fascicularis). *J. Nutr.* 2003;133:2262-67.

Bowey E, Adlercreutz H, Rowland I. Metabolism of isoflavones and lignans by the gut microflora: A study in germfree and human flora associated rats. *Food Chem. Toxicol.* 2003;41:631-36.

Branca F, Lorenzetti S. Health effects of phytoestrogens. *Forum Nutr.* 2005; 57: 100-11.

Briese V, Stammwitz U, Friede M, Hennecke-von Zeppelin HH. Black cohosh with or without St. John`s wort for symptom-specific climacteric treatment-results of a large-scale, controlled, observational study. *Maturitas* 2007;405-14.

Cabanes A, Wang M, Olivo S. Prepubertal estradiol and genistein exposures up-regulate BRCA1 mRNA and reduce mammary tumorigenesis. *Carcinogenesis.* 2004;25:741-8.

Caltagirone S, Rossi C, Poggi A, Raneletti FO, Natali PG, Brunetti M. Flavonoide apigenin and quercitin inhibit melanoma growth and metastatic potential. *Int. J. Cancer.* 2000;87:595-600.

Cao YA, Calafat AM, Doerge DR, Umbach DM, Bernbaum JC, Twaddle NC. Isoflavones in urine, saliva, and blood of infants: data from a pilot study on the estrogenic activity of soy formula. *J. Expo Sci. Environ. Epidemiol.* 2008;30.

Chen J, Hui E, Ip T, Thompson LU. Dietary flaxseed enhances the inhibitory effect of tamoxifen on the growth of estrogen-dependent human breast cancer (mcf-7) in nude mice. *Clin. Cancer Res.* 2004;10:7703-11.

Chen J, Thompson LU. Lignans and tamoxifen, alone or in combination, reduce human breast cancer cell adhesion, invasion and migration *in vitro. Breast Cancer Res. Treat.* 2003;80:163-70.

Chen S, Zhang F, Sherman MA. Structure-function studies of aromatase and its inhibitors: a progress report. *J. Steroid Biochem. Mol. Biol.* 2003;86:231-7.

Chie WC, Chang SH, Huang CS, Tzeng SJ, Chen JH, Fan BY, Chang KJ. Prognostic factors for the survival of Taiwanese breast cancer patients. *J. Formos Med. Assoc.* 2002;101:98-103.

Claassen H, Briese V, Manapov F, Nebe B, Schünke M, Kurz B. The phytoestrogens daidzein and genistein enhance the insulin –stimulated sulphate uptake in articular chondrocytes. *Cell Tissue Res.* 2008;333:71-9.

Clarke DB, Barnes KA, Lloyd AS. Determination of unusual soya and non-soya phytoestrogen sources in beer, fish products and other foods. *Food Addit. Contam.* 2004;21:949-62.

Clarkson TB. Soy, soy phytoestrogens and cardiovascular disease. J Nutr. 2002;132:566-69.

Clavel T, Fallani M, Lepage P, Levenez F. Isoflavones and functional food alter the dominant intestinal microbiota in postmenopausal women. *J. Nutr.* 2005;135:2786-92.

Cooper R, Morré DJ, Morré DM. Medicinal benefits of green tea: part II. Review of anticancer properties. *J. Altern. Complement Med.* 2005;11:639-52.

Cotroneo MS, Wang J, Fritz WA. Genistein action in the prepubertal mammary gland in a chemoprevention model. *Carcinogenesis.* 2002;23:1467-74.

Coward L, Barnes S, Setchell KDR, Barnes S. Genistein and daidzein and their ß - glycosides conjugates: Anti tumor isoflavones in soybean foods from American and Asian diets. *J. Agr. Food Chem.* 1993;41:1961-7.

Danbara N, Yuri T, Tsujita-Kyutoku M, Tsukamoto R, Uehara N, Tsubura A. Enterolactone induces apoptosis and inhibits growth of Colo 201 human colon cancer cells both in vitro and in vivo. *Anticancer Res.* 2005;25:2269-76.

Dedhar S, Hannigan GE. Integrin cytoplasmic interactions and bidirectional transmembrane signalling. *Curr. Opin. Cell Biol.* 1996;8:657-69.

Demark-Wahnefried W, Price DT, Polascik TJ, Robertson CN, Paulson DF, Walther PJ. Pilot study of dietary fat restriction and flaxseed supplementation in men with prostate cancer before surgery: Exploring the effects on hormonal levels, prostate-specific antigen, and histopathologic features. *Urology.* 2001;58:47-52.

Dembitsky VM, Maoka T. Allenic and cumulenic lipids. Prog Lipid Res. 2007;46:328-75.

DePasquale JA. Rearrangement of the F-actin cytoskeleton in estradiol-treated MCF-7 breast carcinoma cells. *Histochem. Cell Biol.* 1999;112:341-50.

DePasquale JA. Cell matrix adhesions and localization of the vitronectin receptor in MCF-7 human mammary carcinoma cells. *Histochem. Cell Biol.* 1998;110:485-94.

Dimitrakakis C, Gosselink L, Gaki V, Bredakis N, Keramopoulos A. Phytoestrogen supplementation: a case report of male breast cancer. *Eur. J. Cancer Prev.* 2004;13:481-4

Dong Y, Yang MM, Kwan CY. In vitro inhibition of proliferation of HL-60 cells by tetrandrine and coriolus vesicolor peptide derives from Chinese medicinal herbs. *Life Sci.* 1997;60:135-40.

Dorbritz S. Methods for the extraktion of phytoestrogens from plants e.g. genistein (article in german). Diplomarbeit, Universität Rostock, Fachbereich Chemie, Abteilung Technische Chemie, 2002.

Duncan AM, Phipps WR, Kurzer MS. Phyto-oestrogens. *Best Pract. Res. Clin. Endocrinol. Metab.* 2003;2:253-71.

Duan J, Xu H, Dai S, Wang X, Wu Y, Zhang Y. Phytoestrogen alpha-zearalanol inhibits homocysteine-induced endothelin-1 expression and oxidative stress in human umbilical vein endothelial cells. *Atherosclerosis.* 2008;197:549-55.

Ferguson LR, Chavan RR, Harris PJ. Changing concepts of dietary fiber: implications for carcinogenesis. Nutr Cancer. 2001;39:155-69.

Flouriot G, Brand H, Denger S. Identification of a new isoform of the human estrogen receptor-alpha (hER-alpha) that is encoded by distinct transcripts an that is able to repress hER-alpha activation function 1. *Embo. J.* 2000;19:4699-700.

Fotsis T, Pepper M, Adlercreutz H, Hase T, Montesano R, Schweigerer L. Genistein, a dietary ingested isoflavonoid, inhibits cell proliferation and in vitro angiogenesis. J Nutr. 1995;125:790-7.

Fotsis T, Pepper M, Adlercreutz H, Fleischmann G, Hase T, Montesano R. Genistein, a dietary-derived inhibitor of in vitro angiogenesis. *Proc. Natl. Acad. Sci. USA.* 1993;90:2690-4.

Fournier DB, Erdman JW Jr, Gordon GB. Soy, its components and cancer prevention: a review of the in vitro, animal, human data. *Cancer Epidemiol. Biomarkers Prev.* 1998;7: 1055-65.

Frankenfeld CL, Atkinson C, Thomas Wk, Goode EL, Gonzales A, Jokelo T. Familial correlations, segregation analysis, and nongenetic correlates of soy isoflavone-metabolizing phenotypes. *Exp. Biol. Med.* 2004;229:902-13.

Franz G, Köhler H. Allgemeine Nachweismethoden für Flavonoide in Drogen. In: Drogen und Naturstoffe (Franz G and Köhler H, eds). Springer-Verlag Berlin Heidelberg; 1992;120.

Fuss E. Lignans in plant cell and organ cultures: An overview. *Phytochem. Rev.* 2003;2: 307-20.

Gamet-Payrastre L, Manenti S, Gratcap MP, Tulliez J, Chap H, Payratsre B. Flavonoids and the inhibition of PKC and PI 3-konase. *Gen. Pharmacol.* 1999;32:279-86.

Gaynor ML. Isoflavones and the prevention and treatment of prostate disease: is there a role? *Cleve Clin. J. Med.* 2003;70:203-9.

Gebhardt G. Polymethoxyflavone in Zitrusfrüchten: blutlipidsenkende und antikanzerogene Eigenschaften. *Ernährungsumschau.* 2008;5:290-5.

Gikas PD, Mokbel K. Phytoestrogens and the risk of breast cancer: a review of the literature. *Int. J. Fertil Womens Med.* 2005;50:250-8.

Hanf V, Gonder U. Nutrition and primary prevention of breast cancer: foods, nutrients and breast cancer risk. *Eur. J. Obstet. Gynecol. Reprod. Biol.* 2005;123:139-49.

Hall WL, Vafeiadou K, Hallund J, Bügel S, Koebnick C, Reimann M. Soy-isoflavone-enriched foods and inflammatory biomarkers of cardiovascular disease risk in postmenopausal women: interactions with genotype and equol production. *Am. J. Clin. Nutr.* 2005; 82:1260-628.

Hallund J, Tetens I, Bügel S, Tholstrup T, Bruun JM. The effect of a lignan complex isolated from flaxseed on inflammation markers in healthy postmenopausal women.*Nutr. Metab. Cardiovasc. Dis.* 2008; 18:497-502.

Hansen RK, Bissell MJ. Tissue architecture and breast cancer: the role of extracellular matrix and steroid hormones. *Endocr. Relat. Cancer.* 2000;7:95-113.

Hansen LK, Mooney DJ, Vacanti JP, Ingber DE. Integrin binding and cell spreading on extracellular matrix act at different points in the cell cycle to promote hepatocyte growth. *Mol. Biol. Cell.* 1994;5:967-75.

Harding C, Tetlow L, McMichael Phillifs D, Osundeko O, Potten CS, Bundred NJ. Oestrogenic effects of soy on nipple aspirate Fluid. *Breast Canc. Res. Treatment.* 1997;46:81.

Hau JT, Hung HC, Chen CJ, Hsu WL, Ying C. Effects of the dietary phytoestrogen biochanin A on cell line MCF-7. *J. Nutr. Biochem.* 1999;10:510-7.

Hawrylewicz EJ, Zapata JJ, Blair WH. Soy and experimental cancer: animal studies. *J. Nutr.* 1995;125:698-708.

Hayashi Y, Fukushima S, Kishimoto S, Kawaguchi T, Numata M, Isoda Y. Anticancer effects of fre polyunsaturated fatty acids in a oily lymphographic agent following intrahepatic arterial administration to a rabbit bearing VX-2 tumor. *Cancer Res.* 1992;52:400-5.

Hedelin M, Löf M, Olsson M, Adlercreutz H, Sandin S, Weiderpass E. Dietary phytoestrogens are not associated with risk of overall breast cancer but diets rich in coumestrol are inversely associated with risk of estrogen receptor and progesterone receptor negative breast tumors in Swedish women. *J. Nutr.* 2008;138:938-45.

Hedlung TE, Johannes WU, Miller GJ. Soy isoflavonoid equol modulates the growth of benign and malignant prostatic epithelial cells in vitro. *Prostate* 2003;54:68-78.

Heinonen SM, Wähälä K, Adlercreutz H. Identification of urinary metabolitesof the red clover isoflavones formononetin and biochanin A in human subjects. *Agric. Food Chem.* 2004;52:6802-9.

Helferich WG, Andrade JE, Hoagland MS. Phytoestrogens and breast cancer: a complex story. *Inflammopharmacol.* 2008;26.

Henderson IC, Patek AJ. Are breast cancers in young women qualitatively distinct? *Lancet.* 1997;349:1488.

Ho CK, Chi CW, Yu KJ, Wang SY. Tamoxifen-mediated anti-cellular effect against a chorion carcinoma cell line. *Int. J. Oncol.* 1998;12:1171-6.

Ho KJ, Liao JK. Non-nuclear actions of estrogen: new targets for prevention and treatment of cardiovascular disease. *Mol. Interv.* 2002;2:219-28.

Hussain M, Baneriee M, Sarkar FH, Djuric Z, Pollak MN, Doerge D. Soy isoflavones in the treatment of prostate cancer. *Nutr. Cancer.* 2003;47:111-7.

Ho CK, Chi CW, Yu KJ, Wang SY. Tamoxifen-mediated anti-cellular effect against a chorioncarcinoma cell line. *Int. J. Oncol.* 1998;12:1171-6.

Holmberg L, Iversen OE, Rudenstam CM, Hammar M, Kumpulainen E, Jaskiewicz J. HABITS Study Group: Increased risk of recurrence after hormone replacement therapy in breast cancer survivors. *J. Natl. Cancer Inst.* 2008;100:475-82.

Hynes RO. Integrins: versatility, modulation and signaling in cell adhesion. *Cell.* 1992;69:11-25.

Hynes RO. The dynamic dialogue between cells and matrices: Implications of fibronectin's elasticity. *Proc. Natl. Acad. Sci. USA.* 1999;96:2588-90.

Ingram D, Sanders K, Kolybaba M, Lopez D. Case - control study of phyto-estrogens and breast cancer. *Lancet.* 1997;350:990-4.

Iype T, Jayasree K, Sudhakaran PR. Modulation of alpha2beta1 integrin changes during mammary gland development by beta-oestradiol. *Biochim. Biophys. Acta.* 2001;15:232-41.

Jansen GH, Arts IC, Nielen MW, Muller M, Hollman PC, Keijer J. Uptake and metabolism of enterolactone and enterodiol by human colon epithelial cells. *Arch. Biochem. Biophys.* 2005;435:74-82.

Jeschke U, Richter D-U, Walzel H, Bergemann C, Mylonas I, Sharma S et al. Stimulation of hCG and inhibition of hPL in isolated human trophoblast cells in vitro by glycodelin A. *Arch. Gynecol. Obstet.* 2003;268:162-7.

Jiang SW, Lloyd RV, Jin L, Eberhardt NL. Estrogen receptor expression and growth-promoting function in human chorion carcinoma cells. DNA Cell Biol. 1997;16:969-77.

Jisa E, Jungbauer A. Kinetic analysis of estrogen receptor homo- and heterodimerization in vitro. *J. Steroid. Biochem. Mol. Biol.* 2003;84:141-8.

Jisa E, Graumann K, Jungbauer A. Proteins accompanying the estrogen receptor alpha and beta: a model for studying protein hetero-complexes. *Biocatalysis Biotransformation.* 2001;9:427-42.

Jo EH, Kim SH, Ra JC, Kim SR, Cho SD, Jung JW. Chemopreventive properties of the ethanol extract of chinese licorice (Glycyrrhiza uralensis) root: induction of apoptosis and G1 cell cycle arrest in MCF-7 human breast cancer cells. *Cancer Lett.* 2004;230:239-47.

Jungbauer A, Pfitscher A. Prävention durch polyphenolreiche Ernährung. *Frauenarzt.* 2005;12.

Juan ME, Planas JM, Ruiz-Gutierrez V, Daniel H, Wenzel U. Antiproliferative and apoptosis-inducing effects of maslinic and oleanolic acids, two pentacyclic triterpenes from olives, on HT-29 colon cancer cells. *Br. J. Nutr.* 2008;26:1-8.

Kilkkinen A, Stumpf K, Pietinen P, Valsta LM, Tapanainen H, Adlercreutz H. Determinants of serum enterolactone concentration. *Am. J. Clin. Nutr.* 2001;73:1094-100.

Kleine-Gunk B. Phyto-Östrogene: Die sanfte Alternative während der Wechseljahre. 2008 TRIAS Verlag in MVS Medizinverlage Stuttgart GmbH and Co.KG, Germany.

Klinge CM, Risinger KE, Watts MB. Estrogenic activity in white and red wine extracts. *J. Agricult. Food Chem.* 2003;51:1850-57.

Knight DC, Eden JA. A review of the clinical effects of phytoestrogens: *Obstet. Gynecol.* 1996;87:897-904.

Kreijkamp-Kaspers S, Kok L, Grobbee DE, de Haan EH, Aleman A, Lampe JW. Effect of soy protein containing isoflavones on cognitive function, bone mineral density, and plasma lipids in postmenopausal women: a randomized, controlled trial. *Obstet. Gynecol. Surv.* 2005;60:41-3.

Kuhnle GG, Dellàquila C, Aspinall SM, Runswick SA, Mulligan AA, Bingham SA. Phytoestrogen content of beverages, nuts, seeds, and oils. *J. Agric. Food Chem.* 2008;56:7311-315.

Kulling EK, Watzl W. Phytoestrogens (article in german). Ernährungs-Umschau. 2003;50:234-9.

Kulp KS, Montgomery JL, Nelson DQ, Cutter B, Latham FR, Shattuck DL. Essiac and Flor-Essence herbal tonics stimulate the in vitro growth of human breast cancer cells. *Breast Cancer Res. Treat.* 2006;98:249-59.

Kumar NB, Krischer JP, Allen K, Riccardi D, Besterman-Dahan K, Salup R. Safety of purified isoflavones in men with clinically localized prostate cancer. *Nutr. Cancer.* 2007; 59:169-75.

Kuo WH, Yen AM, Lee PH, Hou MF, Chen SC, Chen KM, Chen TH, Chang KJ. Incidence and risk factors associated with bilateral breast cancer in area with early age diagnosis but low incidence of primary breast cancer: analysis of 10-year longitudinal cohort in Taiwan. *Breast Cancer Res .Treat.* 2006;99:221-8.

Lechner D, Kallay E, Cross HS. Phytoestrogens and colorectal cancer prevention. Vitamin Horm. 2005;70:169-98.

Lee AH, Fraser ML, Meng X, Binns CW. Protective effects of green tea against prostate cancer. *Expert Rev. Anticancer Ther.* 2006;6:507-13.

Lee J, Demissie K, Lu SE, Rhoads GG. Cancer incidence among Korean-American immigrants in the United States and native Koreans in South Korea. *Cancer Control.* 2007;14:78-85.

Lee KH and Xiao Z. Lignans in treatment of cancer and other diseases: *Phytochem. Rev.* 2003;2:341-62.

Lee MK, Sung SH, Lee HS, Kim YC. Lignan and neolignan glycosides from Ulmus davidiana var. Japonica. *Arch. Pharm. Res.* 2001;24:198-201.

L`home R, Brouwers E, Al-Maharik N, Lapcik O. Time-resolved fluoroimmunoassay of plasma and urine O-desmethylangolensin. *J. Steroid Biochem.* 2002;81:353-61.

Lu LJ, Anderson KE, Grady JJ, Nagamani M. Effects of soy consumption for one month on steroid hormones in premenopausal women: implications for breast cancer risk reduction. *Cancer Epidemiol. Biomarkers Prev.* 1996;5:63-70.

Luo W, Birkett NJ, Ugnat AM, Mao Y. Cancer incidence patterns among Chinese immigrant populations in Alberta. *J. Immigr. Health.* 2004;6:41-8.

Luyengi L, Suh N, Fong HH S, Pezzuto JM and Kinghorn AD. A lignan and four terpenoids from Brucea javanica that induce differentiation with cultured HL-60 promyelocytic leukemia cells. *Phytochemistry.* 1996;43:409-12.

Maskarinec G, Noh JJ. The effect of migration on cancer incidence among Japanese in Hawaii. *Ethn. Dis.* 2004;14:431-9.

Martín-Benito D, García-Vallejo MC, Pajares JA, López D. Triterpenes in elms in Spain. *Can. J. Forest Res.* 2005;35:199-205.

Matscheski A, Richter D-U, Hartmann A-M, Effmert U, Jeschke U, Kupka MS. Effects of phytoestrogen extracts isolated from rye, green and yellow pea seeds on hormone production and proliferation of trophoblast tumor cells Jeg3. Horm Res. 2006;65:276-88.

Messina M, Barnes St, Setchell KD. Phyto-estrogens and breast cancer. *Lancet.* 1997;350:971-2.

Messina M. Soy, soy phytoestrogens (isoflavones), and breast cancer. *Am. J. Clin. Nutr.* 1999;70:4395-505.

Michnovicz JJ, Bradlow HL. Induction of estradiol metabolism by dietary indole-3-carbinol in humans. *J. Natl. Cancer Inst.* 1990;82:947-9.

Mothes K. Historical introduction. In: Bell EA, Charlwood BV, editors. Secondary Plant Products. New York: Springer; 1980. p. 1-10.

Mousavi Y, Adlercreutz H. Enterolacton and enterodiol inhibit each other's proliferative effect on MCF-7 breast cancer cells in culture. *J. Steroid Biochem. Mol. Biol.* 1992;41: 615-19.

Muir AD, Westcott ND. Mammalian metabolism of flax lignans. In: Westcott ND, Muir AD, editors. Flax, the genus *Linum*. London, New York: Taylor and Francis Inc; 2003. p. 230-42.

Nahrstedt A. Nutzung pflanzlicher Sekundärstoffe durch Tier und Mensch. Dtsch Apoth Zeit. 1990;130:2155-61.

Nakaya Y, Mawatari K, Takahashi A, Harada N, Hata A, Yasui S. The phytoestrogen ginsensoside Re activates potassium channels of vascular smooth muscle cells through PI3K/Akt and nitric oxide pathways. *J. Med. Invest.* 2007; 54:381-84.

Nebe B, Bohn W, Sanftleben H, Rychly J. Induction of a physical linkage between integrins and the cytoskeleton depends on intracellular calcium in an epithelial cell line. *Exp. Cell Res.* 1996;229:100-10.

Nebe B, Peters A, Duske K, Richter DU, Briese V. Influence of phytoestrogens on the proliferation and expression of adhesion receptors in human mammary epithelial cells in vitro. *Eur. J. Cancer Prev.* 2006;15:405-15.

Nebe B, Rychly J, Knopp A, Bohn W. Mechanical induction of β1-integrin mediated calcium signaling in a hepatocyte cell line. *Exp. Cell Res.* 1995;218:479-84.

Nesbitt PD, Lam Y, Thompson LU. Human metabolism of mammalian lignan precursors in raw and processed flaxseed. *Am. J. Clin. Nutr.* 1999;69:549-55.

Ofir R, Seidman R, Rabinski T, Krup M, Yavelsky V, Weinstein Y. Taxol-induced apoptosis in human SKOV3 ovarian and MCF7 breast carcinoma cells in caspase-3 and caspase-9 independent. *Cell Death Differ.* 2002;9:636-42.

Page DL. The woman at high risk for breast cancer. Importance of hyperplasia. *Surg. Clin. North Am.* 1996;76:221-30.

Pan A, Demark-Wahnefried W, Ye X, Yu Z, Li H, Qi O. Effects of a flaxseed-derived lignan supplement on C-reactive protein, IL-6 and retinol-binding protein 4 in type 2 diabetic patients. *Br. J. Nutr.* 2008;8:1-5.

Park HJ, Della-Fera MA, Hausman DB, Rayalam S, Ambati S, Baile CA. Genistein inhibits differentiation of primary human adipocytes. *J. Nutr. Biochem.* 2008;9.

Patisaul HB. Phytoestrogen action in the adult and developing brain. *J. Neuroendocrinol.* 2005;17:57-64.

Peeters PHM, Keinan-Boker L, van der Schouw YT, Grobbee DE. Phytoestrogens and breast cancer risk. *Breast Canc. Res. Treatm.* 2003;77:171-83.

Pendleton JM, Tan WW, Anai S, Chang M, Hou W, Shiverick KT. Phase II trial of isoflavone in prostate-specific antigen recurrent prostate cancer after previous local therapy. *BMC Cancer.* 2008;8:132.

Pineda MD, White E, Kristal AR. Asian breast cancer survival in the US: a comparison between Asian immingrants, US-born Asian Americans and Caucasians. *Int. J. Epidemiol.* 2001;30:976-82.

Poulsen RC, Kruger MC. Soy phytoestrogens: impact on postmenopausal bone loss and mechanisms of action. *Nutr .Rev.* 2008;66:359-74.

Pommerenke H, Schreiber E, Duerr F, Nebe B, Hahnel C, Rychly J. Stimulation of integrin receptors using a magnetic drag force device induces an intracellular free calcium response. Eur J Cell Biol. 1996;70:157-64.

Qiao X, McConnell KR, Khalil RA. Sex steroids and vascular responses in hypertension and aging. *Gend Med.* 2008;5:46-64.

Rafii F, Davis C, Park M, Heinze TM, Beger RD. Variations in metabolism of the soy isoflavonoid daidzein by human intestinal microfloras from different individuals. *Arch. Microbiol.* 2003;180:11-6.

Rice S, Whitehead SA. Phytoestrogens oestrogen synthesis and breast cancer. *J. Steroid Biochem. Mol. Biol.* 2008;108:186-95.

Rickard-Bon SE and Thompson LU. The role of flaxseed lignans in hormone-dependent and independent cancer. In: Westcott ND, Muir AD, editors. Flax, the genus Linum. London, New York: Taylor and Francis Inc; 2003. p. 181-203.

Rohr U. Soja und Rotklee – Phytoestrogene in der Prävention. Konsensuspapier Phytoestrogene. Österreichische Menopause und Andropause Asutrian Society of Sterility, Fertility and Endocrinology, Vienna, April 17th, 2004.

Rosero AMA, Rosero AE, Portacelli AMA, Garcia GMA. Usefulness of phyto-oestrogens in reduction of blood pressure. Systematic review and meta-analysis. Aten Primaria. 2008;40:177-86.

Roskelley CD, Desprez PY, Bissell MJ. Extracellular matrix-dependent tissue-specific gene expression in mammary epithelial cells requires both physical and biochemical signal transduction. *Proc. Natl. Acad. Sci. USA.* 1994;91:12378-82.

Rowe JW, Seikel MK, Roy DN, Jorgensen E. Chemotaxonomy of Ulmus. *Phytochemistry.* 1972;11:2513-7.

Sacks FM. Dietary phytoestrogens to prevent cardiovascular disease: early promise unfulfilled. *Circulation.* 2005;111:385-7.

Santti R, Makela S, Strauss L, Korkman J, Kostian ML. Phytoestrogens: potential endocrine disruptors in males. *Toxicol. Ind. Health.* 1998;14:223-37.

Schreihofer DA. Transcriptional regulation by phytoestrogens in neuronal cell lines. *Mol. Cell Endocrinol.* 2005;231:13-22.

Selvaraj V, Zakroczymski MA, Naaz A, Mukai M. Estrogenicity of the isoflavone metabolite equol on reproductive and non-reproductive organs in mice. *Biol. Reprod.* 2004;71:966-972.

Setchell KDR, Adlercreutz H. Mammalian lignans and phyto-oestrogens. Recent studies on their formation, metabolism and biological role in health and disease. In: Rowland IR, editor. Role of the Gut Flora in Toxicity and Cancer. London: Academic Press; 1988. p. 315-45.

Setchell KDR, Brown NM, Lydeking-Olsen E. The clinical importance of the metabolite equol – A clue to the effectiveness of soy and its isoflavones. J. Nutr. 2002;132:3577-84.

Setchell KD, Zimmer-Nechemias L, Cai J, Heubi JE. Exposure of infants to phyto-estrogens from soy-based infant formula. *Lancet.* 1997;350:23-7.

Setchell KD, Lydeking-Olsen E. Dietary phytoestrogens and their effect on bone: evidence from in vitro and in vivo, human observational and dietary intervention studies. *Am. J. Clin. Nutr.* 2003;78:593-609.

Schulten H-R, Leinweber P. Thermal stability and composition of mineral bound organic matter in density fractions of soil. *Eur. J. Soil Sci.* 1999;50:237-48.

Sjastaad MD, Nelson WJ. Integrin-mediated calcium signaling and regulation of cell adhesion by intracellular calcium. *Bioessays.* 1997;19:47-55.

Stark A, Madar Z. Phytoestrogens: a review of recent findings. *J. Pedia. Endocrin.* 2002;15:561-72.

Steinmetz KA, Potter JD. Vegetables, fruit and cancer. II. Mechanism. *Cancer Causes Control.* 1991;2:427-42.

Stephens FO: Breast cancer: aetiological factors and associations (a possible protective role of phytoestrogens). *Aust. N. Z. J. Surg.* 1997;67:755-60.

Speranza A, Pellizzaro C, Coradini D. Hyaluronic acid butyric esters in cancer therapy. *Anticancer Drugs.* 2005;16:373-79.

Szewczyk M. Untersuchungen zum Einfluss von Pflanzenextrakten aus der Leinpflanze *Linum usitatissimum* auf die Zellproliferation und Cytotoxizität humaner Karzinomzellen sowie Trophoblasten und Fibroblasten. Diplomarbeit, Universität Rostock, Institut für Biowissenschaften; 2007.

Tai J, Cheung S. In Vitro studies of FlorEssence on human tumor cell lines. *Phytother. Res.* 2005;19:107-12.

Taku K, Umengaki K, Sato Y, Taki Y, Endoh K, Watanabe S. Soy isoflavones lower serum total and LDL cholesterol in humans: a meta-analysis of 11 randomized controlled trials. *Am. J. Clin. Nutr.* 2007;85:1148-56.

Tham DM, Gardner CD, Haskell WL. Clinical review 97. potential health benefits of dietary phytoestrogens: a review of the clinical, epidemiological and mechanistic evidence. *J. Clin. Endocrinol. Metab.* 1998;83:2223-35.

Thompson LU, Boucher BA, Cotterchio M, Kreiger N, Liu Z. Dietary phytoestrogens, including isoflavones, lignans, and coumestrol, in nonvitamin, nonmineral supplements commonly consumed by women in Canada. *Nutr. Cancer.* 2007;59:176-84.

Touillaud MS, Thiebaut AC, Fournier A, Niravong M, Boutron-Ruault MC, Clavel-Chapelon F. Dietary lignan intake and postmenopausal breast cancer risk by estrogen and progesterone receptor status. *J. Natl. Cancer Inst.* 2007;99:475-86.

Thorp AA, Howe PR, Morl TA, Coates AM, Buckley JD, Hodgson J, et al. Soy food consumption does not lower LDL cholesterol in either equol or nonequol producers. *Am. J. Clin. Nutr.* 2008;88:298-304.

Tomar RS, Shiao R. Early life and adult exposure to isoflavones and breast cancer risk. *J. Environ. Sci. Health C Environ. Carcinog. Ecotoxicol. Rev.* 2008;26:113-73.

Tsourounis C. Clinical effects of phytoestrogens. *Clin. Obstet. Gynecol.* 2001;44:836-42.

Valentzis LS, Woodside JV, Cantwell MM, Leathem AJ, Keshtgar MR. Do phytoestrogens reduce the risk of breast cancer recurrence? What clinicians need to know? *Eur. J. Cancer.* 2008;44:1799-806.

Van der Heide D, Kastelijn J, Schroder- van der Elst JP. Flavonoids and thyroid disease. *Biofactors.* 2003;19:113-19.

Van der Schouw YT, Grobbee DE. Menopausal complaints, estrogens, and heart disease risk: an explanation for discrepant findings on the benefits of post-menopausal hormone therapy. *Eur. Heart. J.* 2005;26:1358-61.

Van Kranen HJ, Mortensen A, Sørensen IK, van den Berg-Wijnlands J, Beems R, Nurmi T. Lignan precursors from flaxseed or rye bran do not protect against the development of intestinal neoplasia in Apc^{min} mice. *Nutr. Cancer.* 2003;45:203-10.

Wang C, Kurzer MS. Phytoestrogen concentration determines effects on DNA synthesis in human breast cancer cells. *Nutr. Cancer.* 1997;28:236-47.

Wang C, Kurzer MS. Effects of phytoestrogens on DNA synthesis in MCF-7 cells in the presence of estradiol and growth factors. *Nutr. Cancer.* 1998;31:90-100.

Wang C, Makela T, Hase T, Adlerkreutz H, Kurzer MS. Lignans and flavonoids inhibit aromatase enzyme in human preadipocytes. *J. Steroid Biochem. Mol. Biol.* 1994;50:205-12.

Wang D, Xia MY, Cui Z, Tashiro S-I, Onodera S, Ikejima T. Cytotoxic effects of Manson E and F isolated from Ulmus pupila. *Biol. Pharm. Bull.* 2004;27:1025-30.

Wang LQ. Mammalian phytoestrogens: enterodiol and enterolactone. *J Chromatogr B Analyt Technol. Biomed. Life Sci.* 2002;777:289-309.

Ward H, Chapelais G, Kuhnle GG, Luben R, Khaw KT, Bingham S. Breast cancer risk in relation to urinary and serum biomarkers of phytoestrogen exposure in the European Prospective into Cancer – Norfolk cohort study. *Breast Cancer Res.* 2008; 32.

Wang HS, Hung Y, Su CH, Peng ST, Guo YJ, Lai MC. CD44 cross-linking induces integrin-mediated adhesion and transendothelial migration in breast cancer cell line by up-regulation of LFA-1 (alpha L beta2) and VLA-4 (alpha4beta1). *Exp. Cell. Res.* 2005;304:116-26.

Warri A, Saarinen NM, Makela S, Hilakivi-Clarke L. The role of early life genistein exposures in modifying breast cancer risk. *Br. J. Cancer.* 2008;98:1485-93.

Wattenberg LW. Inhibiton of neoplasis by minor dietary constituents. *Cancer Res.* 1983;43:2448-53.

Waterman E, Lockwood B. Active components and clinical applications of olive oil. *Altern. Med. Rev.* 2007;12:331-42.

Watzl B, Hänsch GM, Pool-Zobel BL. Ernährung und Immunsystem. Ernähr Umsch. 1994;41:368-77.

Watzl B, Leitzmann C. Bioaktive Substanzen in Lebensmitteln. Hippokrates, Stuttgart; 1995.

Weggemanns RM, Trautwein EA. Relation between soy associated isoflavones and LDL and HDL cholesterol concentrations in humans: a meta-analysis. *Eur. J. Clin. Nutr.* 2003;57:940-46.

Westcott ND, Muir AD. Flax seed lignan in disease prevention and health promotion. *Phytochem. Rev.* 2003;2:401-17.

Wiesner S, Legate KR, Fässler R. Integrin-actin interactions. Cell Mol Life Sci. 2005;62:001-19.

Wiseman H, Casey K, Bowey EA, Duffy R, Davies M, Rowland IR. Influence of 10 wk of soy consumption on plasma concentrations and excretion of isoflavonoids and on gut microflora metabolism in healthy adults. *Am. J. Clin. Nutr.* 2004;80:692-9.

Windhövel J, Mohagheghzadeh A, Godt D, Wink M, Wildi E, Alfermann AW. Lignan production in hairy root cultures of Linum species. Proceedings of the International Meeting Phytochemistry and Lignans, Bornheim-Walberberg, 2003; p 103.

Wu AH, Yu MC, Tseng C-C, Pike MC. Epidemiology of soy exposures and breast cancer risk. *Brit. J. Cancer.* 2008;98:9-14.

Wuttke W, Jarry H, Seidlova-Wuttke D. Isoflavones – Safe food additives or dangerous drugs? *Ageing Res. Rev.* 2007;6:150-88.

Yoo YC, Shin BH, Hong JH, Lee J, Chee HY, Song KS. Isolation of fatty acids with anticancer activity from Protaetia brevitarsis larva. *Arch. Pharm. Res.* 2007;30:361-65.

Yuan JP, Wang JH, Liu X. Metabolism of dietary soy isoflavones to equol by human intestinal microflora – implications for health. *Mol. Nutr. Food Res.* 2007;51:765-781.

Yamamoto S, Sobue T, Sasaki S, Kobayashi M, Arai Y, Uehara M. Validity and reproducibility of a self-administered food-frequency questionnaire to assess isoflavone intake in a japanese population in comparison with dietary records and blood and urine isoflavones. *J. Nutr.* 2001;131:2741-7.

Yap SP, Shen P, Butler MS, Gong Y, Loy CJ, Yong EL. New estrogenic prenylflavone from epimedium brevicornum inhibits the growth of breast cancer cells. *Planta Med.* 2005;71:114-9.

Zava DT, Blen M, Duwe G. Estrogenic activity of natural and synthetic estrogens in human breast cancer cells in culture. *Environ. Health Perspect.* 1997;105:637-45.

Zava DT, Duwe G. Estrogenic and antiproliferative properties of genistein and other flavonoids in human breast cancer cells in vitro. *Nutr. Cancer.* 1997;27:31-40.

In: Estrogens: Production, Functions and Applications
Editor: James R. Bartos, pp. 55-93
ISBN: 978-1-60741-086-7

Chapter II

The Role of Estrogens in Cardiovascular Disease: An Update from the NHLBI-Sponsored WISE Study

Smruti Nalawadi, Chrisandra Shufelt, B. Delia Johnson*, Leslee Shaw †, Glenn D. Braunstein, Carl J. Pepine ‡, Ricardo Azziz, Frank Stanczyk ξ, Sarah Berga†, Vera Bittner||, George Sopko #, C. Noel Bairey Merz ¶

The Women's Heart Center, the Heart Institute and the Department of Medicine, Division of Endocrinology and the Department of Obstetrics and Gynecology, Cedars-Sinai Research Institute, Cedars-Sinai Medical Center,
*Department of Epidemiology, Graduate School of Public Health, University of Pittsburgh, Pittsburgh, Pennsylvania, USA
†Emory Program in Cardiovascular Outcomes Research and Epidemiology, Department of Gynecology and Obstetrics, Emory University School of Medicine, Atlanta, Georgia, USA
‡Division of Cardiology, Department of Medicine, University of Florida, Gainesville, Florida, USA
ξUniversity of Southern California, Los Angeles, California, USA
||Division of Cardiology, Department of Medicine, University of Alabama at Birmingham, Birmingham, Alabama, USA
Division of Heart and Vascular Diseases, National Heart, Lung and Blood Institute, National Institutes of Health, Bethesda, Maryland, USA

¶ Address for correspondence: C. Noel Bairey Merz, MD, 444 S. San Vicente Blvd, Suite 600, Los Angeles, California 90048, Phone: (310) 423-9680, Fax: (310) 423-9681, merz@cshs.org.

Abstract

Introduction. Cardiovascular disease (CVD) is the leading killer of women (aged over 18 years) in United States, with an annual mortality rate of over 450,000, and a majority of deaths attributable to heart disease. One in 30 female deaths is due to breast cancer in contrast to one in six deaths from heart disease. Declining ovarian estrogen levels during perimenopause and menopause have been implicated in the development of CVD. The Women's Ischemic Syndrome Evaluation (WISE) is a National Heart, Lung and Blood Institute (NHLBI)-sponsored, multi-center study designed to optimize the symptom evaluation, and diagnostic testing for ischemic heart disease. A specific aim within WISE is to study the influence of reproductive hormones on pathophysiology, symptoms and diagnostic test response of myocardial ischemia. In this chapter we discuss new data on the role of estrogen in CVD obtained from the WISE study.

A synopsis and discussion of new reproductive hormone data from ten WISE publications are organized into four categories: A) Pre- and perimenopause; B) Postmenopause; C) Hormone Therapy; D) Phytoestrogens as Selective Estrogen-Receptor Modulators (SERMs). The chapter begins with a description of the WISE method of determining menopausal status. New data is presented on the topics of hypothalamic hypoestrogenemia (HHE) and coronary artery disease (CAD), including women with diabetes mellitus (DM), polycystic ovary syndrome (PCOS) and CAD, estrogen levels and statin lipid lowering medication, estrogen levels and obesity patterns, past oral contraceptive (OC) use and CAD, estrogen hormone therapy on psychological factors among women of different ethnic backgrounds, and dietary phytoestrogen-rich products relations to blood lipoproteins and coronary microvascular function.

Conclusions. New research from the WISE study suggests that estrogen plays a role in CVD in women. Specific findings include: 1) the use of a simple WISE hormone algorithm can improve the accuracy of menopausal status classification for research purposes; 2) disruption of ovulatory cycling characterized by HHE appears to be associated with angiographic CAD; 3) the presence of DM and HHE predicts a greater burden for angiographic CAD; 4) in postmenopausal women with past OC use is associated with less angiographic CAD; 5) clinical features of PCOS are associated with more angiographic evidence of CAD and worsening CVD event-free survival; 6) blood estrogen levels vary according to central vs. general obesity; 7) there are ethnic differences observed between HT use and psychological health; 8) higher blood levels of the phytoestrogen, daidzein, are associated with beneficial lipoprotein levels in women with low blood estrogen; 9) higher blood level of the phytoestrogen, genistein, are associated with impaired non-endothelial–dependent and endothelial-dependent coronary microvascular function; 10) use of statins, and resultant lower cholesterol levels, are not associated with lower levels of reproductive hormones. New data from WISE study suggests that estrogen plays a role in CVD in women. Ongoing research is directed at further understanding.

Keywords: *Women, Estrogens, Hormones, Cardiovascular Disease.*

Abbreviations and Acronyms

ADO: Adenosine
ACH: Acetylcholine
APV: Averaged peak velocity
BMI: Body mass index
BDI: Beck depression inventory
CVD: Cardiovascular Disease
CRT: Coronary reactivity test
CFR: coronary flow reserve
CAD: Coronary Artery Disease
DM: Diabetes Mellitus
ER: Estrogen receptor
E2: estradiol
E1: estrone
FSH: Follicle-stimulating hormone
HT: Hormone therapy
HHE: Hypothalamic hypoestrogenemia
HDL: High density lipoprotein
hs-CRP: High-sensitive C-reactive protein
HOMA: Homeostasis model assessment
IHD: Ischemic Heart Disease
LH: Luteinizing hormone
LMP: Last menstrual period
NHLBI: National Heart, Lung and Blood Institute
NCEP: National Cholesterol Education Program
NTG: Nitroglycerine
NHANES: National Health and Nutrition Evaluation Survey
OC: Oral Contraceptives.
PCOS: Polycystic ovary syndrome
SERMs: Selective Estrogen-Receptor Modulators
SHBG: Sex hormone binding globulin
STRAW: Stages of reproductive aging workshop
T: Testosterone
TC: Total Cholesterol
VFR: Volumetric flow reserve
WC: Waist Circumference
WISE: Women's Ischemic Syndrome Evaluation

Introduction

Cardiovascular disease (CVD) is the leading killer of women (aged over 18 years) in United States, with an annual mortality rate of over 450,000, and a majority of deaths attributable to heart disease [1]. CVD is a dominant contributor to the nation's morbidity and health care expenditures [1] [2] [3]. One in 30 female deaths is due to breast cancer in contrast to one in six deaths from heart disease [1]. Overall, 32% percent of deaths from CVD occurred prematurely (i.e., before age 75 in women, which is well below the average life expectancy of 77.9 years) [1] [4]. Recently published data on mortality rates show an increase in the CVD mortality in women between the ages of 35 and 44 years compared to decreases in CVD mortality in all other age groups [5].

Long felt to be predominantly a disease of men, starting in 1984 more women than men now die from to CVD annually in the US [6] [7] [8]. The dominance of CVD ascribed to women is not simply due to the greater absolute numbers of older women compared to men, or due to female longevity. The symptoms, pathogenesis, and prognosis [9] for CVD have important differences between women and men and CVD outcomes following onset of disease are more adverse in women [10] [11]. Accurate and timely diagnosis of CHD in women is a major challenge to physicians.

There are several management challenges. Women have a higher frequency of presentation with chest pain, yet have a lower prevalence of epicardial coronary artery stenosis [12]. Chest pain/discomfort characteristic of angina are a less specific diagnostic marker for obstructive CAD in women [13]. On the other hand, women with CAD are often under-diagnosed [14] [15], and their disease is identified [9] [16] [17] in their disease and suffer worse prognosis compared to men [18] [19]. Women also have relatively smaller coronary arteries compared to men, even after correcting for body surface area [20] [21] and plaque erosion with subsequent thrombus formation is twice as likely to be the precipitating event in sudden cardiac death compared to men [9]. Outward coronary artery remodeling is believed to be more common in women than men [22]. Moreover, women with acute coronary syndromes and myocardial infraction are more likely than men to show atypical symptom manifestations, and fewer flow–limiting coronary stenosis at angiography [23] [24]. Finally diabetes, hypertriglyceridemia, and low levels of high-density lipoprotein appear to be the more potent risk factors for CVD in women than in men [25] [26]. This suggests that sex-related differences in disease detection and treatment may influence prognosis. More women are currently identified to be at risk for CVD due to several novel and evolving CVD risk factors such as the metabolic syndrome, low estrogen levels, hyperandrogenism and polycystic ovary syndrome (PCOS), chronic inflammation and endothelial dysfunction [9].

The role that reproductive hormones play in symptom manifestation and diagnostic testing for CVD is largely unknown. The concept that cyclical reproductive hormone fluctuations throughout a woman's reproductive and menopausal phases can affect CVD symptoms and pathophysiology makes biological sense. In postmenopausal women, endogenous estrogen is derived from conversion of androgens of both adrenal and ovarian origin in peripheral tissue, mostly adipose tissue [27] [22]. A variety of relations between reproductive hormones and the coronary vasculature have been postulated, as follows.

These include:

- Women exhibit a higher frequency of chest pain symptoms and abnormal stress testing in the absence of obstructive CAD compared to men. This has been attributed to the fluctuating levels of estrogen and its affect on the vasculature. Experimental data supports an impact of estrogen on coronary artery vasomotor function [28].

- Both genomic and non-genomic effects of endogenous estrogen during premenopause provide protective effects on the vasculature [29] [30] [31].
- Diminished estrogen-mediated nitric oxide production causes vascular constriction, platelet aggregation, and impaired vascular growth [32] [33] [34].
- Declining ovarian estrogen secretion during perimenopause and postmenopause has been implicated in bone loss, susceptibility to fractures, decline in cognitive function, reduced physical functioning, changes in body mass and fat distribution, glucose intolerance, diabetes, and development of CVD risk factors and CAD [35].
- Sex-specific metabolic differences such as hypertension, dyslipidemia and diabetes appear to be exacerbated by hormonal changes at menopause [4] [36] [37] [38] [39] [40] [41] [42] [43] [44] [45] [46] [47] [48]. Also the development of androidal shape and abdominal fat deposition, is associated with an increased CAD risk in women [49].
- Although a number of beneficial estrogen- and estrogen receptor (ER)-mediated effects on cardiovascular system have been investigated, it is not clear how these effects could safely explored into clinical cardiovascular benefits. The results from various clinical trials with hormone therapy (HT) [29] have not shown convincing benefits. Differences in the pharmacokinetics and physiological impact of exogenous versus endogenous hormones, including hepatic first pass effects, and effects of synthetic progestins, basal endogenous hormone status, phyto-estrogens in the diet, and timing of exogenous HT may contribute in preventing the therapeutic benefits of HT on CVD [29].

New findings support the concept of multifactorial and conditional risk markers leading to an increase in the functional expression of atherosclerotic plaque deposition, vascular function, and metabolic alterations resulting in worsening outcomes for women [50] [51]. Vascular endothelial dysfunction, the inability of arteries and arterioles to appropriately dilate when needed, and failure of endothelium to produce appropriate level of nitric oxide, a natural relaxant of vascular smooth muscle [30] [31] may contribute to the atypical symptoms and worsened prognosis for women with symptoms. Diagnostic testing for ischemia in women demonstrates higher levels of test variability compared to men [52] [53] [54] [55]. The long-established CAD management strategies that focus on detection of critical epicardial coronary stenoses often fail to identify women at-risk for future CVD events.

The Women's Ischemia Syndrome Evaluation(WISE) Study

The WISE is a NHLBI-sponsored, multi-center study designed to address ischemic heart disease pathopysiology and diagnosis in women. The primary objectives of the original WISE was: 1) To improve diagnostic testing for IHD in women, including symptom evaluation tools, risk assessment algorithms, and non-invasive imaging techniques; 2) To study pathophysiologic mechanisms and prognosis in women with chest pain and abnormal diagnostic testing for myocardial ischemia in the absence of epicardial coronary artery stenosis; 3) To evaluate the influence of cyclical hormones, menopausal status and reproductive hormone levels on symptoms and diagnostic testing results.

Patient and Methods

The WISE study brought together a variety of leading edge expertise to assess different but complementary innovative diagnostic tests performed by the clinical sites on a large and well defined cohort of women with suspected ischemia. The WISE common core data include demographic and clinical data, symptom and psychosocial variables, WISE core lab quantitative assessment of coronary angiography and ventriculography data, brachial artery reactivity testing, resting/ambulatory electrocardiographic (ECG) monitoring, and a variety of blood determinations. The WISE common core protocol is itemized in Figure 1. Site specific complementary methods include physiologic and functional cardiovascular assessments of myocardial perfusion and metabolism, ventriculography, endothelial vascular function and coronary angiography. Phase I (1996 -7) was a pilot phase and enrolled 256 women. Data from the common core protocol as well as individual site protocols for this phase were examined leading to protocol revisions prior to proceeding on to Phase II. Phase II (1997 – 9) studied an additional 680 women, with a total WISE enrollment of 936 women. Phase III (2000) included patient follow-up, data analysis and a NIH WISE workshop summarizing the findings and potential future research implications.

Study Recruitment and Inclusion/Exclusion Criteria. Women older than 18 years of age who were undergoing a clinically-indicated coronary angiogram as part of their regular medical care for chest pain symptoms or suspected myocardial ischemia were eligible for participation. Women with co-morbidities which compromised one year follow-up such as pregnancy, contraindications to provocative diagnostic testing, cardiomyopathy, New York Heart Association Class IV congestive heart failure, recent myocardial infarction, significant valvular or congenital heart disease, or a language barrier to questionnaire testing were excluded from the study. Women with recent coronary angioplasty or coronary bypass surgery or who underwent these procedures following angiography but prior to their WISE testing were also excluded.

Reproductive Hormone Analysis. Reproductive hormone assays were performed at an established reproductive hormone core laboratory using stored serum samples. Reproductive hormone blood determinations included estradiol (E2), bioavailaible E2, estrone (E1), progesterone, follicle-stimulating hormone ([FSH), luteinizing hormone (LH), androstenedione and total testosterone (T) were quantified. Validated steroid and protein assay were used and the methodology was maintained for the duration of the study. Specific details are described below.

Testosterone. Serum was extracted with hexane-ethyl acetate (3:2) and purified by Celite column partition chromatography before RIA, using ethylene glycol as the stationary phase. Elution off the column was carried out with 40% toluene in isooctane. Sensitivity is 1.5 ng/dl. The intra-assay coefficient of variation (CV) is 7.0% at 14.3 ng/dl and inter-assay CV is

10.4% at 6.1 ng/dl [56]. Normal postmenopausal range is 5–50 ng/dl (to convert nanograms per deciliter to picomoles per liter, multiply by 34.67).

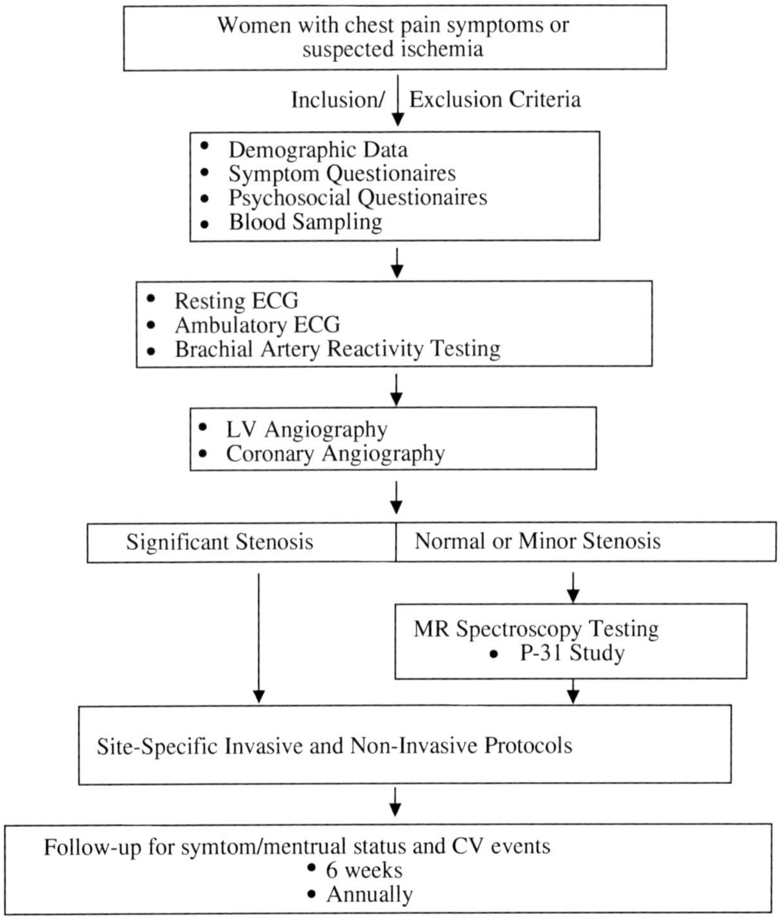

Figure 1. Women's Ischemic Syndrome Evaluation common core testing flow diagram. CV = cardiovascular; ECG = electrocardiography; LV = left ventricular; MR = magnetic resonance; P = phosphorus [120]. Copyright permission obtained.

Androstenedione. Serum was extracted as described for T (above) but eluted off the column with isooctane without toluene. Sensitivity is 30 pg/ml. Intra-assay CV is 6% at 400 pg/ml and inter-assay CV is 7.8% at 130 pg/ml [57]. Normal postmenopausal range is 160-1200 pg/ml (to convert nanograms per deciliter to picomoles per liter, multiply by 3.492).

E2. Serum was extracted as described above and subjected to Celite column chromatography with elution by 40% ethyl acetate in isooctane before RIA. Sensitivity is 4 pg/ml, intra-assay CV is 8.9% at 14 pg/ml and inter-assay CV is 14% at 14 pg/ml [58]. Normal postmenopausal levels are less than 25 pg/ml (to convert picograms per milliliter to picomoles per liter, multiply by 3.67).

Bioavailable E2 (non-sex hormone binding globulin [SHBG] bound). Bioavailable E2 (non-SHBG bound) was determined by a modified ammonium-sulfate precipitation method with a sensitivity of 1.5 pg/ml, intra-assay CV of 6.1%, and inter-assay CV of 7.9% [59]. Normal postmenopausal range is 0.19–14 pg/ml [56] (to convert picograms per milliliter to picomoles per liter, multiply by 3.67).

Estrone. Serum was extracted as described for E2 but eluted off of the column with 15% ethyl acetate in isooctane, with a sensitivity of 5 pg/ml, intra-assay CV of 7.9% at 26 pg/ml and inter-assay CV of 12% at 26 pg/ml [58]. Normal postmenopausal range is 15–60 pg/ml [60] (to convert picograms per milliliter to picomoles per liter, multiply by 3.7).

SHBG. Solid-phase, two-site chemiluminescent immunoassay using the Immulite analyzer (Siemens Diagnostic Products Corp., Los Angeles, CA) with a sensitivity of 0.2 nmol/liter, intra-assay and inter-assay CVs of 4.1–7.7 and 5.8–13%, respectively was used. Normal range is 20–100 nmol/liter (to convert nanomoles per liter to micrograms per deciliter, divide by 34.67).

Calculated free T and free E2. Free (non-protein bound) T and E2 as well as bioavailable E2 were calculated using a validated algorithm, based on equations derived by Sodergard *et al [61],* and Vermeulen *et al [62].* The algorithm uses the measured concentration of total T or E2 and SHBG, an assumed average concentration of albumin as well as the appropriate affinity constants of SHBG and albumin fort or E2. This method has been shown to have high validity [63]. Normal postmenopausal range for free T is 0.6–6.7 pg/ml and for free E2 is 0.06–0.75 pg/ml. Using the regression equation derived from the data in this paper (calculated bioavailable E2 - 1.08 – [measured bioavailable E2], the normal range for calculated bioavailable E2 is 1.26–14.5 pg/ml. The correlation coefficient between the calculated and measured bioavailableE2 was 0.93, and therefore, only the measured bioavailable E2 are reported for this study.

Lipoprotein Assays. Lipoproteins (total cholesterol [TC], low-density lipoprotein [LDL], and high-density lipoprotcin [HDL]), lipid peroxidation, homocysteine, and fasting blood glucose levels were measured following overnight fasting. Lipoprotein determinations were performed at a lipid core laboratory enrolled in the Centers for Disease and Prevention lipid standardization program and previously used in multiple NHBI-sponsored lipid-lowering intervention trials. TC and triglyceride, and HDL cholesterol levels were determined by enzymatic assay. LDL cholesterol was measured using the Friedewald formula [64]. The coefficient variation within assay was for TC, HDL-C and triglycerides were 1, 80%, 1.23%, and 3.90% respectively.

High-Sensitive C-Reactive Protein. C-reactive protein was measured using the high-sensitivity C-reactive protein (Hs-CRP) method on a Hitachi 911 analyzer by a blinded core laboratory using reagents from Denka Seiken. These techniques are previously validated [65].

Phytoestrogen Analysis. Plasma Phytoestrogen levels were determined at WISE Core laboratory for daidzein, dihydrodaizein, glycitein, ethyl phenol, equol, genistein, and 0-desmethylangolensin. Modification of the technique of Coward technique with an high performance liquid chromatography (HPLC) coupled to single and array electrochemical detection was used to run the samples in duplication [66].

Coronary Angiography. Core lab measurements by coronary angiograms included qualitative and quantitative assessments of the presence, severity and complexity of epicardial coronary artery stenosis [51]. The following definitions are used for disease classification and group categorization: normal/minimal disease = <20% stenosis; mild =

20% to 49% stenosis; significant stenosis in any one major epicardial coronary artery = ≥ 50% [67].

Coronary Reactivity Testing. In women with normal or mild stenosis, the left anterior descending coronary artery is studied for coronary reactivity testing (CRT). When appropriate, the artery suspected as causing the abnormal diagnostic test response is studied. After administration of systemic heparin, a 0.014- to 0.018-in. (0.036 to 0.046 cm) Doppler-tipped guide wire is advanced into the target vessel, as previously described [68]. After baseline recordings, adenosine (18 μg diluted in 2 ml saline followed by 5 ml saline flush) is hand-injected as a bolus via the coronary guiding catheter, and recordings are repeated. Time-averaged peak coronary blood flow velocity (APV) is assessed at baseline and after intracoronary adenosine and nitroglycerin (200 μg). A cineangiogram is performed immediately after measurement of coronary blood flow velocity. Quantitative coronary angiography is performed off-line to quantify epicardial coronary cross-sectional area 5.2 mm distal to the guide wire tip. Coronary flow reserve (CFR) is computed as the ratio of post- to pre-adenosine average peak velocity [68]. Volumetric blood flow (VFR) calculations, using coronary lumen diameter measured from the angiograms, is also performed using previously reported techniques [69]. The ratio of flow during each intervention (speech task, intracoronary and intravenous adenosine, intracoronary nitroglycerin) to baseline is used as a standard to define coronary vasomotion in the studied women.

Coronary flow velocity reserve (CFVR) and VFR to adenosine (ADO) and nitroglycerin (NTG) (nonendothelial-dependent responses) and acetylcholine (ACH) (endothelial-dependent response) are assessed. The CRT is performed in the left coronary branch free of obstruction (<50% diameter narrowing). After the boluses of 18 mcg of adenosine were administered, CFR was measured as the increase in flow resulting from dilation of small arteries and arterioles, as well as flow-related of epicardial vessels with intact endothelial function that occurs in response to an increase in microvascular flow. Endothelial-dependent function was assessed using intracoronary infusion of acetylcholine at 10^{-6} M (lower dose) followed by 10^{-4} M (higher dose). NTG was then infused intracoronary to assess nonendothelial-dependent epicardial coronary reactivity. Pulsed-wave Doppler flow spectra were used to record time-averaged APV. Coronary cross-sectional was measured and coronary blood flow was calculated using the standard equation. Epicardial response to ACH also was assessed by measuring coronary diameter at baseline and after ACH infusion using quantitative coronary angiography. For quantitative coronary angiography, angiograms were analyzed by investigators and CAD score was calculated as previously described [70]. CFVR was defined as the ratio of peak coronary APV after each vasoactive agent to baseline coronary APV. VFR was the ratio of peak calculated coronary blood flow after each vasoactive agent to calculated baseline flow. A normal response to ACH was dilation from baseline, whereas an abnormal response was defined as either no dilation or constriction.

Premenopausal Status and Menstrual Phase Status Determination. The study participant's menopause status was determined by WISE reproductive status algorithm. An expert consensus classification was used as the gold standard. The WISE hormone expert committee included two reproductive endocrinologists, two clinical cardiologist, and a nurse who individually examined the complete data (age, education level, body mass index=BMI, ethnicity, current medication use [including lipid-lowering medication], coronary risk factors, physical activity, and functional status level, postmenopausal HT and menopause status, menstrual phase, alcohol intake and cigarette smoking) were also determined for each patient. The WISE Hormonal Status algorithm which classifies women into five categories is shown in Table 1 and Figure 2.

Hormone Therapy. The hormonal status determination developed for WISE used both historical and single sampling blood hormonal characterization. Information regarding exogenous use of hormone therapy (HT), including estrogens, progestins and androgenic agents taken within 24 h of each WISE test was recorded. Women were questioned on the use of HT during their lifetime and specifically in the last three months during their baseline visit. The type of HT therapy used (estrogen alone, combination of estrogen and progestin, other) was recorded as well as the history and duration of menopausal symptoms.

Table 1. WISE Menopausal Status Determination Algorithm

Amenorrheic/definitely postmenopausal	Either had had a bilateral salpingo-oophorectomy or were aged 55 years and older and amenorrheic.
Regular cycling	Women reporting regular menstrual periods during the preceding 12 months were assumed to be premenopausal, and reproductive hormone levels were used to corroborate this assumption
Irregular cycling	Women reporting irregular menstrual periods during the preceding 12 months were equally likely to be premenopausal or perimenopausal and required additional reproductive information, such as hormone levels, age, and last menstrual period, in order to be classified
Amenorrheic without hysterectomy	Among women without a menstrual period during the preceding 12 months, those without a hysterectomy had a high probability of being postmenopausal. If they did not fit the postmenopausal hormone profile, their cases were closely examined for other possible reasons for their amenorrhea and could be pre- or perimenopausal.
Amenorrheic with hysterectomy	For women with hysterectomy, the combination of age and reproductive hormone levels was used for classification

[35]. Copyright permission obtained.

Coronary Risk Factors. Coronary risk factors were defined according to the National Cholesterol Education Program (NCEP) Adult Treatment Panel III [71] [72]. DM was defined as a self-reported history of DM, with the assistance of the site physician or nurse or fasting blood glucose ≥126 mg/dl. BMI ≥25.0 and <30 was defined as overweight and BMI ≥30 was defined as obese [73]. Waist circumference (WC) > 35 inches was considered central obesity [27].

Follow-up. Women were contacted at six weeks and then annually to assess clinical events which included non-fatal myocardial infraction (MI), coronary angioplasty, coronary bypass surgery, cardiac transplantation and hospitalization for unstable angina and to assess symptom status and menstrual status.

Overall WISE Study Results. Experience from Phase I (1996-7), a pilot phase of 256 women showed that the WISE protocol was safe and feasible for identifying symptomatic women with and without significant epicardial coronary artery stenoses. The refined protocols were implemented in the Phase II (1997- 9) an additional cohort of 680 women, with a total of WISE enrollment of 936 women, who were then followed for clinical events in Phase III (2000-2007). The total population patient characteristics are shown below in the Table 2.

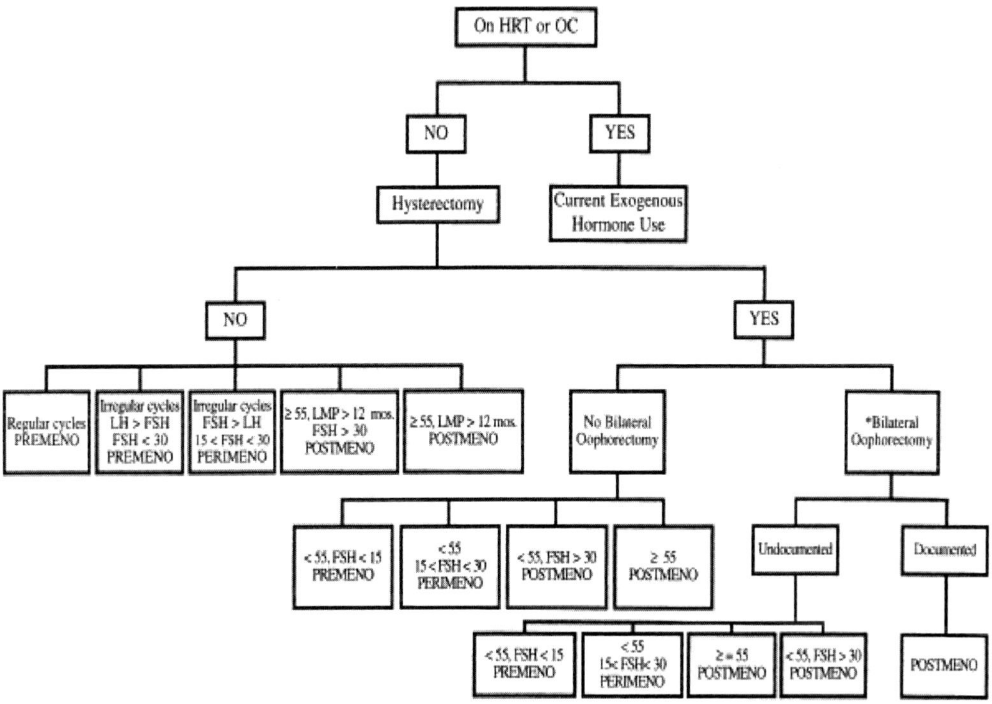

Figure 2. Women's Ischemia Syndrome Evaluation reproductive hormone status characterization diagram. FSH = follicle-stimulating hormone; HT = hormone replacement therapy; LH = luteinizing hormone; LMP = last menstrual period; OC = oral contraceptives; PERIMENO = perimenopausal; POSTMENO = postmenopausal; PREMENO = premenopausal. *>3 months before study entry [120].

Table 2. Baseline Characteristics of the WISE Cohort (N=936)

Characteristic	Means±SD (Range) or %
Demographics:	
Age	58 ± 12 (21-86)
Race (%): White	81
Black	17
Other	2
Education (%): <High School	20
High School Diploma	41
Training Beyond High Sch.	26
College Diploma +	14
Menop Status (%): Premenopausal	17
Perimenopausal	6
Postmenopausal	75
Indeterminate	2
Angiographic CAD:	
CAD (%) ≥50% Stenosis	39
≥70% Stenosis	24
CAD Risk Factors:	
Diabetes (%)*	33
Characteristic	Means±SD (Range) or %
Demographics:	
Obese (BMI ≥30) (%)	41
Ever Smoked (%)	53
History of Hypertension† (%)	81
History of Dyslipidemia‡ (%)	88
Metabolic Syndrome$^{\Delta}$ (%)	47
Low Functional Capacity $^{\Omega}$ (%)	70
Number of Risk Factors (%)Ψ: 0	2
1-2	30
3	30
4	26
5	11
Reproductive History:	
Bilateral Oophorectomy (%)	28
Hysterectomy Only (%)	26
Number of Pregnancies	3.4 ± 2.4 (0-17)

Table 2. (Continued)

Medications:	
Current Lipid Lowering (%)	29
Current Anti-Hypertensive (%)	48
Oral Contraceptives Ever (%)	50
Hormone Therapy Ever (%)	52
CurrentAnti-Depressives or Anti-Anxiety (%)	30

Variable Definitions:

* Self-reported, medication or insulin use, or fasting blood sugar >120.

† Self-reported, use of anti-hypertensive medications, or LDL-C ≥130, Triglycerides ≥ 150, or HDL<50.

‡ Self-reported, use of lipid lowering medications, or systolic blood pressure ≥ 130 or diastolic blood pressure ≥90.

Δ Defined by ATP III criteria

Ω DASI score < 25

Ψ Includes: diabetes, hypertension, dyslipidemia, BMI ≥30, smoking. Possible range = 0-5.

In this chapter, we discuss the new data on the role of reproductive hormones, including estrogen in CVD obtained from the WISE studies. We present a synopsis and discussion of new data from ten WISE studies is organized into four hormone categories: 1) Pre- and perimenopausal; 2) Postmenopausal; 3) Hormone Therapy; 4) Phytoestrogens as Selective Estrogen-Receptor Modulators (SERMs).

A. Pre- and Perimenopause

1) Determination of Menopausal Status in Women

Menopause is an ongoing process characterized by diminution and then cessation of ovarian steroid hormone secretion caused by depletion of oocytes and adjoining follicular apparatus. There have been many investigations examining the link between menopausal status and health status in large populations, but these investigations have been limited by the inaccuracy of methods of determining menopausal status. Methods relying on menstrual history, hysterectomies as surgical menopause, hormone levels exclusively, timing of last menstrual period (LMP), menstrual regularity or menopausal symptoms [74] [75], are all limited by inherent misclassification and poor reliability. Methods such as developed by the Stages of Reproductive Aging Workshop (STRAW) [76] that depend on hormone levels, menstrual regularity, prospective menstrual calendar data, and imaging of the uterus, for staging reproductive aging are often not feasible in population and clinical studies. Precise classification of menopausal status is important to research evaluating the role of reproductive hormones in health and disease.

This section summarizes the development and validation of the WISE Hormonal Status algorithm for determining premenopausal, perimenopausal, and post-menopausal status uses menstrual history, surgical reproductive history and reproductive hormone blood levels obtained at a single clinic visit. The accuracy of the WISE algorithm was compared against self-reported algorithms that are most commonly used in non-gynecological research to determine menopausal status. The two self-reported algorithms are *Menstrual*, based only on reported last menstrual period, and *Historical,* which adds reproductive surgical history. The *Menstrual* menopausal status algorithm is defined as: women who were amenorrheic in the preceding 12 months were classified as postmenopausal, those amenorrheic in the preceding 3 – 12 months were classified as perimenopausal, everybody else as pre-menopausal. *Historical* menopausal status algorithm considered additional questionnaire information including age and surgical history. Thus, if a woman had a hysterectomy, at least one intact ovary, and were <55 years of age, then she was classified as premenopausal. No attempt was made to use this algorithm to classify perimenopausal status [77] because of the inclusion of women with hysterectomies, for whom there was no information about their menstrual cycling.

Methods. 515 WISE study participants, aged 21- 86 years were examined. Women currently on oral contraceptives (OC) and HT were excluded. Women were first determined to be definitely postmenopausal as defined above. Those that were not definitely postmenopausal were then classified by three algorithms: *Menstrual and Historical,* STRAW staging system, and WISE Hormonal Status. The WISE Hormonal Status algorithm which classifies women into five categories is shown in Table 1 and Figure 2, the comparison of the accuracy of the WISE reproductive status algorithm was made with other *Menstrual* and *Historical* methods of menstrual status classifications

Results. The study population consisted of 329 definitely postmenopausal women out of a total of 515. The remaining 186 were classified by the three different algorithms and an expert consensus classification.

The *Menstrual* and *Historical* classifications differed significantly (both $p < 0.0001$) from expert consensus, with 26% - 32% discordant classifications, respectively, compared to 4% discordance for the WISE Hormonal Status algorithm (Figure 3A and 3B). The WISE Hormonal Status algorithm was also more feasible compared to other new algorithms, such as the STRAW staging system [75]. For example, the STRAW staging system could not be applied to 88% of the study participants due to exclusion criteria, such as hysterectomy, abnormal uterine anatomy (e.g., fibroids), cigarette smoking which are prevalent in women of WISE age.

Conclusions. The use of the WISE Hormonal Status algorithm, a relatively simple determination that includes a one-time measurement of reproductive blood hormone levels, is feasible, relatively simple and significantly improves the accuracy of menopausal status classification compared with commonly used self-report algorithms.

Our results suggested that the self-reported algorithms previously used in research may have significantly contributed to the variability in studies linking menopausal status to health and disease outcomes.

2) Hypoestrogenemia of Hypothalamic Origin and Coronary Artery Disease in Premenopausal Women.

Recent studies have shown that the relatively higher gender-specific CAD mortality observed in women [9] [17] [16] is due to increased death rates among relatively young women [78]. In fact, CAD is the leading killer of women in this age group, outpacing even breast cancer [8]. Additional investigation of CAD in premenopausal women is needed. Previous animal and human studies demonstrate that hypoestrogenemia in females [79] [33] [80] is associated with loss of normal coronary artery dilatation or even constriction in response to an endothelial stimulus. Since such responses are observed in early atherosclerosis, we hypothesized that hypothalamic hypoestrogenemia (HHE) is likely to be associated with CAD in young women.

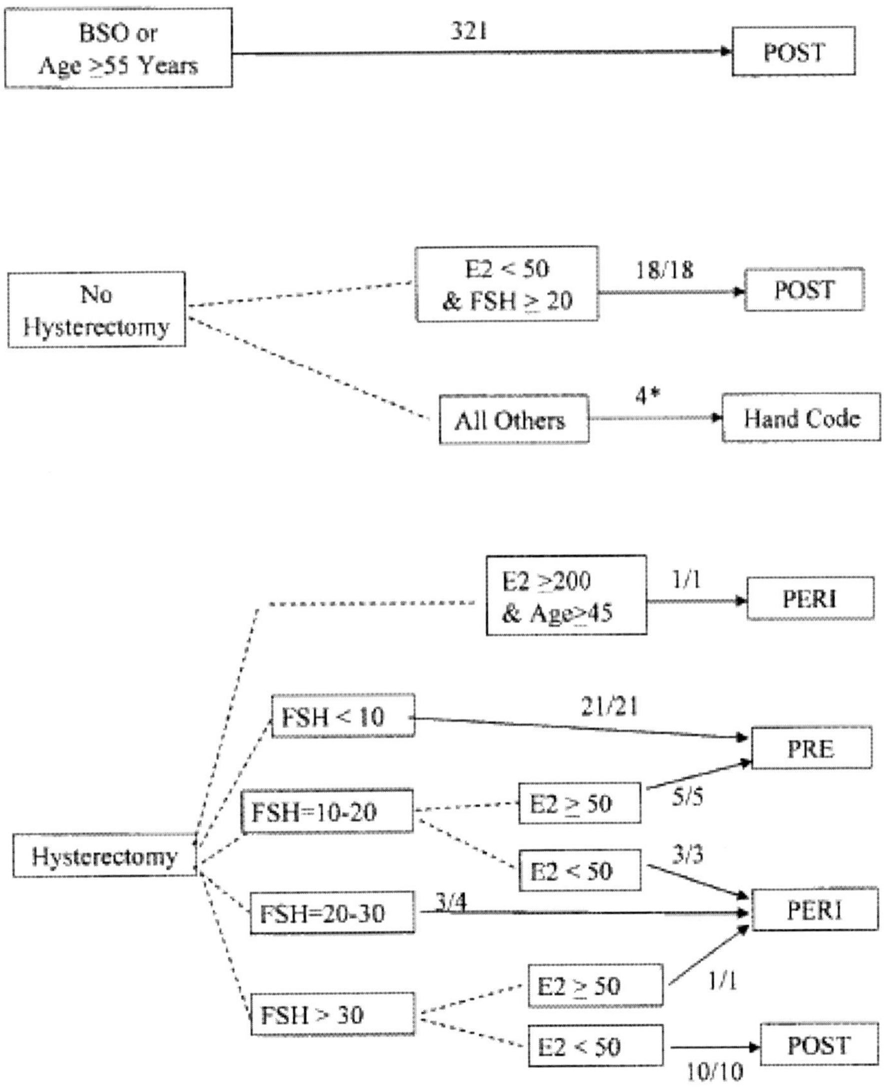

Figure 3A. WISE Hormone algorithm for women who are not currently on hormone therapy (HT) or oral contraceptions (OC). Women with menstrual period < 12 months. PRE = premenopausal; PERI = perimenopausal; POST = postmenpausal; E2 = estradiol; FSH = follicle-stimulating hormone; LMP = time since last menstrual period. Numerator, number of women assigned to status by WISE Hormone algorithm; denominator, number of women assigned to status by expert consensus adjudication [35]. Copyright permission obtained.

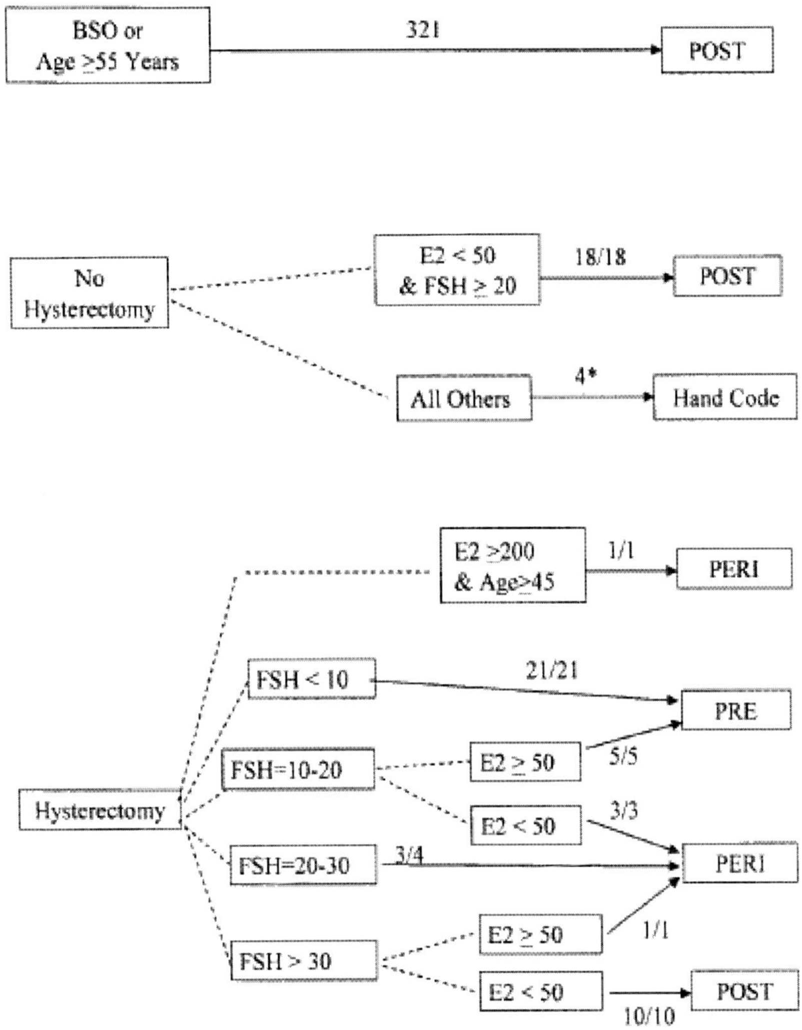

Figure 3B. WISE Hormone algorithm for women who are not currently on HT or OCs for women with no menstrual period < 12 months. Three of the women were either premenopausal or perimenopausal. Their amenorrhea was due to other physical causes (e.g., hypothalamic amenorrhea. Abbreviations as in prior, plus BSO = bilateral salpingo-oopherectomy. Numerator, number of women assigned to status by WISE Hormone algorithm; denominator, number of women assigned to status by expert consensus adjudication [35]. Copyright permission obtained.

Methods. A total of 95 WISE premenopausal women were evaluated. Premenopausal status and menstrual phase were determined using the WISE menstrual status algorithm [35]. Environmental stress was determined by a single question using a five-point scale questionnaire previously demonstrated to predict future adverse cardiac events in patients [81]. Psychological state was assessed using the Beck Depression scale and Spiel Berger trait anxiety scale [51] [82]. If a woman had a history of current use of psychotropic medications, it was considered evidence of more chronic psychological distress. Socioeconomic status assessment included marital/partner status, years of education, and job situation.

Reproductive hormone blood levels and lipoproteins were measured. HHE was defined as E2 <184 pmol/l (50 pg/ml), FSH < 10 IU/L, and LH <10 IU/L.

Results. Premenopausal women with significant angiographic CAD had significantly lower blood levels of E2, bioavailable E2, and FSH (all $p < 0.05$) compared to women without angiographic CAD, even after controlling for age (Figure 4). HHE was significantly more prevalent among the women with CAD than those without CAD (69% vs. 29%, respectively, $p = 0.01$). In a multivariate model, HHE was the most powerful predictor of angiographic CAD (OR 7.4, CI 1.7 to 3.3, $p = 0.008$) among the women with CAD than those without CAD (69% vs. 29%, respectively, $p = 0.01$). In a multivariate model anxiolytic/ sedative/ hypnotic and antidepressant medication use were independent predictors of HHE (OR 4.6, CI 1.3 to 15.7, $p = 0.02$, OR 0.10, CI 0.01 to 0.92, $p = 0.04$, respectively).

Conclusions. The results show a significant association between HHE and CAD in premenopausal women undergoing coronary angiography for suspected myocardial ischemia. Specifically, these findings suggest that low estrogen levels due to disruption of ovarian function are associated with greater coronary angiographic pathology. Notably, traditional CAD risk factors, with the exception of diabetes, were similarly prevalent in the women with and without CAD, suggesting that HHE may be a particularly potent risk factor for premenopausal women. These results suggest that premenopausal women with CAD may be at higher mortality risk due to adverse physiological effects linked with hypoestrogenemia, although the study was unable to evaluate a link with mortality due to the relatively small sample size.

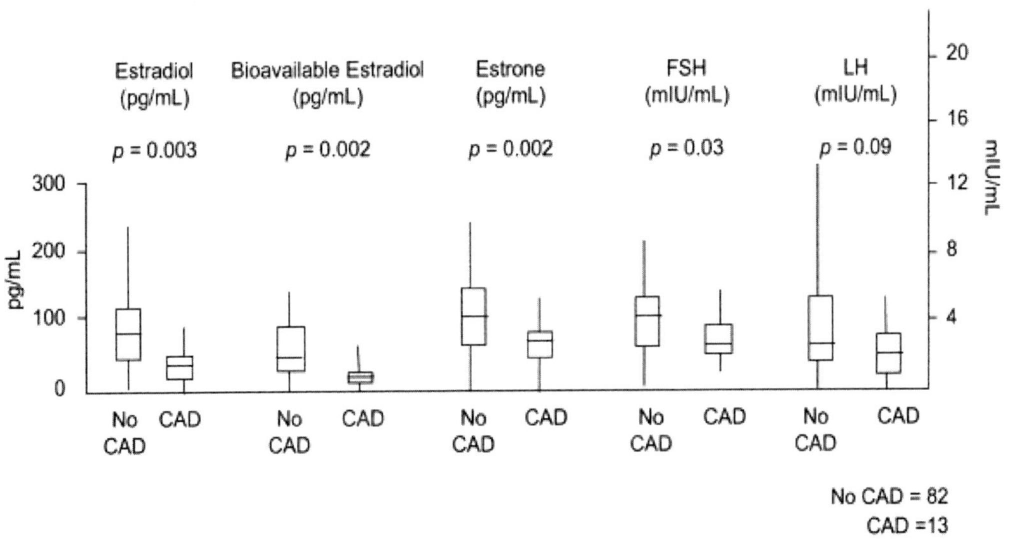

Figure 4. Reproductive hormone levels stratified by angiographic coronary artery disease (CAD) (≥70% luminal diameter stenosis in at least one epicardial coronary artery) (n = 95 women) (to convert bioavailable estradiol (E2), and estrone (E1) from picograms per milliliter to picomoles per liter, divide picomoles per liter by 3.671). The bottom and top of the boxes represent the 25th and 75th percentiles, respectively. The center horizontal line gives the sample median. The central vertical lines (the whiskers) range from the box to the 1.5 interquartile ranges from each side of the box (where an interquartile range is the distance between the 25th and the 75th percentile) [90]. Copyright permission obtained.

3) Cholesterol Lowering Medication, Cholesterol Levels and Reproductive Hormones in Women

Adequate reproductive blood hormone levels are necessary for phenotypic secondary sexual characteristics, reproductive competence, and other various health benefits [18]. Steroid reproductive hormones, such as estrogen, progesterone, and testosterone, are synthesized from a common cholesterol precursor pathway. Statins lower blood cholesterol levels by inhibiting a critical step in cholesterol synthesis. Despite concerns about the safety of lowering cholesterol of statins, these medications have proven to be safe in clinical trials [83]. However, less than 20% of trial participants have been women [84]. In fact, previous studies of statin use and reproductive hormones did not include premenopausal women of childbearing age [85] [86]. This WISE study analyzed the relationship among use of statins, lipoprotein levels, and blood reproductive hormone levels in a large sample of women. In addition, we explored evaluated this association between cholesterol levels and reproductive hormone levels, independent of statin use, particularly among premenopausal women of childbearing age.

Methods. Total of 453 WISE participants (mean ± SD) age, 58 ± 13 years, who were not taking OC or HT were enrolled. Blood lipoprotein levels and serum reproductive hormone levels were measured. Self-reported questionnaire reported during the baseline study visit was used to obtain the history of current medication use, including lipid-lowering medications.

Results. 453 WISE participants were included. The mean ages were 43 ± 6 years in premenopausal women, 49 ± 3 years in perimenopausal women, and 64 ± 10 years in postmenopausal women. The use of statins was statistically significantly associated with lower TC levels (184 ± 45 mg/dl vs. 198 ± 47 mg/dl, $p = 0.002$), higher triglyceride levels (167 ± 101 mg/dL vs. 137 ± 92, $p = 0.003$), and lower LDL cholesterol levels (100 ± 41 mg/dL vs. 119 ± 40mg/dL, $p = 0.001$). No association was found with lower reproductive hormone blood levels in the premenopausal, perimenopausal and postmenopausal women. Further analyses by menopausal status did not demonstrate differences in blood reproductive hormone levels when stratified by use of statins. However, slightly lower progesterone levels in postmenopausal women taking statins was observed relative to postmenopausal women not taking statins, although not significant, ($p=0.12$). Mean E2 levels among premenopausal women with very low LDL cholesterol levels compared with women with higher LDL cholesterol levels was 71± 52 pg/ml vs 88 ± 67 pg/ml, respectively, $p=0.32$ (Table 3), although this difference was not statistically different.

Conclusions. Among women undergoing coronary angiography for suspected myocardial ischemia, use of statins or lower cholesterol levels is not associated with lower blood levels of reproductive hormones. Lower blood lipoprotein levels (as low as LDL <70 mg/d) and statin use were not associated with adverse effects on blood reproductive levels in premenopausal women of child-bearing age.

Table 3. Serum Reproductive Hormone Levels by Very Low LDL Cholesterol Level in Premenopausal Women

Premenopausal	LDL Cholesterol < 70 mg/dL (n=15)	LDL Cholesterol ≥70 mg/dL (n = 99)	P Value*
Biologically available E2 (pg/mL)	43 ± 34	53 ± 38	0.29
E2 (pg/mL)	71 ± 52	88 ± 67	0.32
Estrone (pg/mL)	106 ± 81	104 ± 62	0.93
Progesterone (ng/mL)	1.2 ± 1.3	3.0 ± 4.3	0.12

LDL=low density lipoprotein, * Age-adjusted. LDL = low-density cholesterol [124].

4) Diabetes Mellitus, Hypothalamic Hypoestrogenemia and Coronary Artery Disease in Premenopausal Women

The presence of diabetes mellitus (DM) portends a higher risk of CVD mortality in women compared with men independent of traditional CAD risk factors [36] [87] [88] [89]. In light of the prior WISE findings which showed the potential interaction between estrogen deficiency and DM, and HHE was a potent independent risk factor for angiographic CAD in premenopausal women [90]. We further explored the role of reproductive hormones in CVD events. This analysis assessed the relationship between DM, HHE, angiographic CAD, and major adverse CVD events in premenopausal women enrolled in the WISE study.

Methods. The cross-sectional analysis was limited to 95 premenopausal WISE women not on hormone therapy or OC. All women received annual follow-up for a total median of 5.9 years. Age ranged from 21 to 54 years. A major adverse CVD event was defined as all cause mortality, nonfatal myocardial infarction, congestive heart failure, stroke, or other major vascular event (e.g. peripheral thrombosis, carotid endarterectomy, or transient ischemic attack). Medical records were reviewed for confirmation, dates, and documentation of the occurrence. Reproductive hormone assay and lipoproteins determinations were performed. Angiographic CAD was defined as ≥ 70% luminal diameter stenosis in any ≥ 1 epicardial coronary artery.

Results. From the WISE study subject, 95(18%) women were premenopausal, and were not currently using exogenous hormones and had no previous history of CAD. Overall, 23 (24%) were nonwhite, age ranged from 21 to 54 years, with BMI ranged from 17.7 to 52.2, 30 women were defined as having diabetes, and 19 had self-report history of diabetes, with 12 (63%) of these women using insulin. DM or HHE alone were associated with a higher prevalence and severity of angiographic CAD when stratified for DM and HHE. Among the 95 women in this analysis, 11 (12%) experienced an major adverse CVD event during a median of 5.9 years. Five of the 65 women without DM (6%), and 6 of the 30 women with DM (20%) had an event. DM but not HHE was associated with a higher risk of major adverse CVD event (Figure 5). Results showed no difference in age between diabetics (n=30) and non-diabetics (n=65) (43 ± 6 years). DM was associated with hypertension, HHE, angiographic CAD, and coronary artery severity score (all $p < 0.05$). Diabetics were twice as likely to have HHE (50% vs. 26%; p = 0.02) compared with non-diabetics. Presence of both DM and HHE was associated with significantly higher prevalence (40% vs. 12% or 13%, p = 0.006) and severity of angiographic CAD (CAD severity score 19.9 ± 19.2 vs. 7.7 ± 4.6 or 12.3 ± 18.8; p = 0.008), respectively, compared with either HHE or DM alone.

Conclusions. DM is associated with HHE in premenopausal women undergoing coronary angiography for suspected myocardial ischemia. The extent and severity of angiographic CAD appears to be increased in women with both DM and HHE compared to non-diabetics or with DM or HHE alone. Diabetics had more adverse CVD events, and we expect that the relation between DM and adverse CVD events may have been underestimated by the relatively small sample size. Further prospective research is necessary to better understand casual relations between DM, endogenous hormones, and adverse CVD events in premenopausal women.

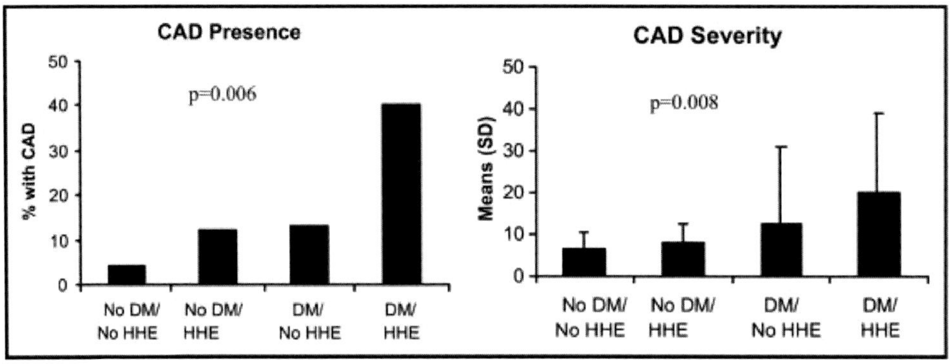

Figure 5. Prevalence of angiographic CAD stratified by diabetes mellitus (DM) and hypothalamic hypoestrogenemia (HHE) status [121]. Copyright permission obtained.

B. Postmenopause:

5) Past OC Use and Angiographic Coronary Artery Disease in Postmenopausal Women

Previous animal models [92] and epidemiological studies [93] have observed increased risk of CAD in premenopausal females after oophrorectomy. The role of endogenous reproductive hormones in CAD has not been extensively studied and convincingly established [94]. We investigated the relationship between CAD measured quantitative by coronary angiography and prior OC use.

Methods. A total of 672 of postmenopausal women enrolled in the WISE study were analyzed in this study. Mean age was 62 ± 10 years. CAD was defined as ≥70% luminal diameter stenosis in at least one epicardial coronary artery. Past OC questionnaire was assessed by WISE reproductive questionnaire.

Results. All women were postmenopausal, and had at least one CAD risk factor. African Americans, Asians, Hispanics, and American Indians represented 18% of the study population. Overall, 39% reported past OC use. Prior OC use was associated with significantly lower CAD severity score (mean ± SD: 11.8 ± 10.3 vs. 18.7 ± 17.3, (p = 0.02, respectively; Figure 6) compared to no prior use of OC use. Duration of the past OC use was not associated with CAD severity score using a threshold of > 3 years (p = 0.88). After adjusting for the coronary risk factors including age, DM, triglycerides, LDL cholesterol, smoking, aspirin use, psychoactive medication, antihypertensive medication, metabolic syndrome, functional status, income, marital status, education, creatinine, hs-CRP, and Beck depression index, the variable of past OC use remained a significant independent negative predictor for CAD ($R = 0.19$, $p = 0.04$).

Conclusions. Our data showed that a history of past use of OC during premenopausal years is associated with less CAD in postmenopausal women.

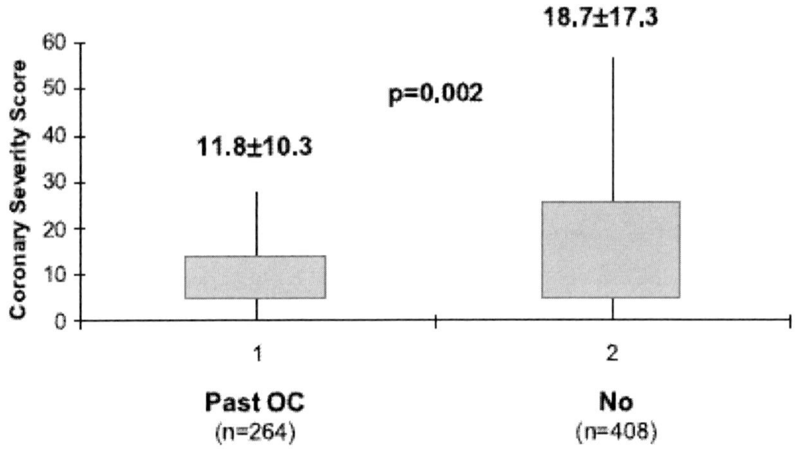

Figure 6. Coronary artery severity score, assessed by quantitative coronary angiography (17), stratified by reported prior OC use [122]. Copyright permission obtained

6) Postmenopausal Women with a History of Irregular Menses and Elevated Androgen Measurements are at High Risk for Worsening Cardiovascular Event-Free Survival

Women with PCOS have greater clustering of CAD risk factors. PCOS is an established disorder associated with androgen excess and may also independently raise CVD risk in women compared to the age-matched men [95] [96] [97]. However, a link between PCOS and CVD is incompletely understood. Our substudy tested the hypothesis that women with features of PCOS have more frequently angiographic CAD and CVD events in a carefully characterized group of postmenopausal women enrolled in the NHLB-sponsored WISE study.

Methods: A total of 390 postmenopausal WISE women were included in this study with and evaluated for defined characteristics of PCOS. Of these, 104 had clinical features of PCOS as defined as biochemical evidence of hyperandrogenemia and history of irregular menses. A pattern of irregular periods was defined as that occurring during a woman's premenopausal years. PCOS as defined as biochemical evidence of hyperandrogenemia (top quartile of androstenedione >701 pg/ml, T ≥30.9 ng/dl, or free T ≥4.5 pg/ml), and history of irregular menses. Insulin resistance was estimated using the homeostasis model assessment (HOMA) index with a threshold of at least 2.5 [61]. Follow-up was complete in more than 95% of surviving patients with prospective annual follow-up accruing through 6 yr.

Results. Women classified as PCOS were more often diabetic ($p < 0.0001$), obese ($p = 0.005$), had the metabolic syndrome ($p < 0.001$), and had angiographic CAD ($p = 0.04$) compared to non-PCOS women. The mean age of menopause was 52.3 years for women compared with 54.3 years for non-PCOS ($p = 0.197$). The insignificant younger age of menopause largely had to do with a greater frequency of bilateral oopherectomy occurring more often in PCOS women (35 vs. 25% for non-PCOS women, $p = 0.052$). PCOS women were more often insulin resistant, as defined by a HOMA of at least 2.5 ($p < 0.0001$). PCOS status remained an independent estimator of angiographic CAD in a subsequent multivariable model that also include covariate adjustment for diabetes and triglycerides ($p = 0.038$). Cumulative 5-yr CVD event- free survival was 79% for PCOS women (Figure 7; n = 104, $p = 0.006$) vs. 89% for women without PCOS (n= 286; $p = 0.06$). PCOS women with elevated hs-CRP had a 12.2–fold higher risk of CVD death or nonfatal MI ($p < 0.0001$) compared to non-PCOS women and lower levels of hs-CRP. PCOS status remained a significant predictor ($p < 0.01$) in prognostic models including DM, WC, hypertension, and angiographic CAD as covariates.

Conclusions. Our data show that subset of women with more angiographic CAD findings and elevated risk of adverse CVD events may be identified by applying a historical definition of PCOS combined with the postmenopausal measurements of hyperandrogenemia. These novel findings suggest a new hypothesis that the prolonged and persistent PCOS status may promote and possibly accelerate angiographic CAD as well as a higher risk of CVD events only as exposure times lengthen substantially (i.e. in the postmenopause). Moreover, it is also possible that PCOS-related protracted hyperandrogenemia may be one of the mechanisms responsible for their adverse CVD risk. Independent adverse relationships between PCOS status and CVD events after menopause may exist via an inflammatory pathway.

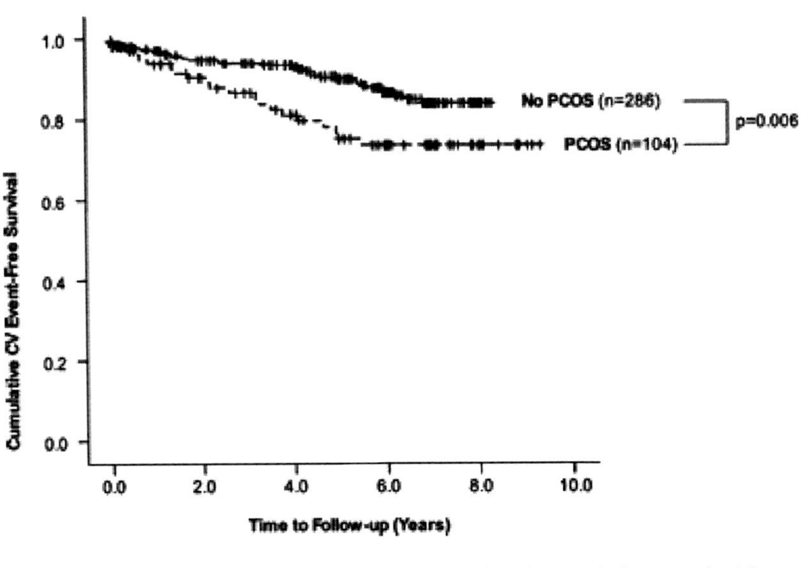

Figure 7. Cumulative unadjusted CV death or myocardial infarction (MI) free survival in post menopausal women with or without clinical features of PCOS (P = 0.006) [19]. Copyright permission obtained.

Our findings suggest that recognition of clinical features of PCOS, in postmenopausal women, may facilitate an opportunity for early risk factor intervention for the prevention of CAD and CVD events.

7) Obesity Distribution and Reproductive Hormone Levels in Women

The recent obesity prevalence figures show that women are more obese than men (33% vs. 28%, respectively), particularly among the older ages [1] [4]. The recent NHANES III data compares individuals of normal weight to the extremes of weigh, both underweight and obese. Compared to normal weight individuals, those who fall into the extremes of weight are associated with excess mortality [48]. Obesity is associated with DM, hypertension [41] [98] [44] and cancer in both men and women [99] [100] and higher incidence of breast cancer and higher mortality in postmenopausal women [101] [102], whereas may be protective in premenopausal women [103]. These data suggest a multi-factorial effect of obesity possibly moderated by reproductive hormones. Our sub-study explored the relations between reproductive hormones and obesity distribution markers, including BMI and waist circumference (WC), in a cohort of postmenopausal women with detailed reproductive status characterization.

Methods. The analysis included 207 WISE postmenopausal women. WC > 35 inches was considered central obesity [104]. Two sets of regression models were used to predict blood estrogen levels. First model measured BMI and WC. In the second model BMI, WC as well as demographic and risk factors were measured.

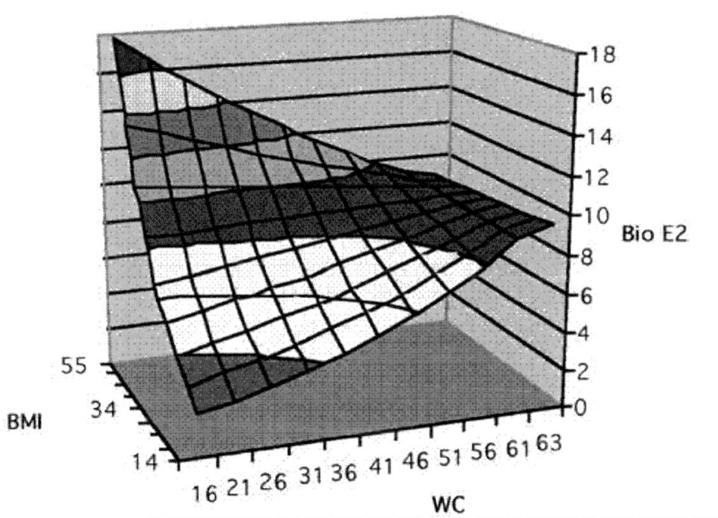

Figure 8. Relationship of bioavailable E2 (Bio E2) with waist circumference (WC) and body mass index (BMI) in postmenopausal women. Units for WC are in inches; units for Bio E2 are in pg/mL. Regression analyses with both BMI and WC in the model show that Bio E2 is significantly positively related to both BMI ($p = 0.03$) and WC ($p = 0.05$) [123]. Copyright permission obtained.

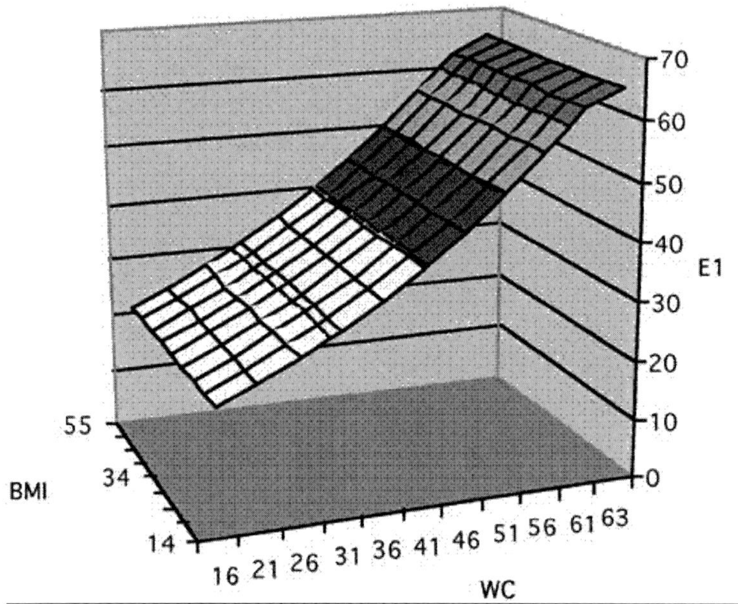

Figure 9. Relationship of estrone (E1) with WC and BMI in postmenopausal women. Units for WC are in inches; units for E1 are in pg/mL. Regression analyses with both BMI and WC in the model show that E1 is significantly positively related to WC ($p = 0.001$), but not to BMI, in postmenopausal women [123]. Copyright permission obtained.

Results. The mean age of 66 years (range 43 - 85 years) and all had at least one risk factor, predominantly HTN and dyslipidemia. Overall, 79 (38%) were overweight and 76 (37%) were obese. African Americans represented 16% of the cohort and were found to have more DM (48.5%) and history of HTN (81.8%) as compared to the Caucasian women. Both BMI and WC were positively related with all three blood estrogen levels at (Figure 8 and Figure 9; $p < 0.01$). The regression models further defined the relationship between BMI and WC with the blood estrogen levels. The highest estrogen levels were seen in obese women with larger WC and higher BMI ($p < 0.01$).

Conclusions. Our results demonstrated the differences in the association and dominance of the obesity pattern (general vs. central) with respect to bioavailable E2 vs. estrone levels respectively in the cohort of WISE postmenopausal women. Among postmenopausal women, there were differences in the obesity measurement and the relationship between the bioavailable E2 and estrone levels. The data also showed that the differing types of obesity have differing associations to diseases, suggesting the further need of prospective investigations in larger populations for evaluating these relationships.

C. Hormone Therapy

8) Hormone Therapy, Ethnicity and Psychosocial Health in Women

The value of HT is currently being debated. Studies of HT efficacy for symptom relief and psychological well-being have used a variety of measures and demonstrated that HT users have better health-related quality of life, including improved SF-36 scores, better emotional well-being, and less hostility [105] [105] [106] [107]. However, the results from the Women's Health Initiative (WHI) showed that after an average of 5.2 years of follow-up, users of conjugated equine estrogen/medroxyprogesterone acetate had similar mortality rates, higher rates of CHD, breast cancer, stroke, and pulmonary embolism, and lower rates of colorectal cancer and hip fractures compared to women who received placebo [108]. These findings in combination with the earlier results from the Heart and Estrogen/Progestin Replacement Study (HERS) trial differs from the prior cohort observational and surrogate end point studies that suggested a range of benefits of HT on CVD [109] [110]. Since few hormone replacement studies included African American women, race may play a role in the effectiveness of HT. We analyze the psychological factors and HT use comparing white and black women and hypothesized that both groups of women would have fewer symptoms of depression (lower Beck Depression Inventory [BDI] scores) and lower hostility (Cook Medley Hostility scores) associated with HT use.

Methods. The substudy population consisted of 463 WISE postmenopausal women were questioned on the use of HT. The BDI depression score which includes items that describe manifestations of depression in relation to general life satisfaction, relations with others, appetite, sleep, and libido was used. Totals score ranged from 0 - 63 and the higher scores indicated more symptoms of depression. The subset of Cook Medley Hostility inventory which is the scales of cynicism, hostile affect, and aggressive responding scores was used. This subset of Cook Medley used in the WISE study has been established to be a better predictor of health outcomes when compared to the complete scale.

Results. A total of the 463 postmenopausal women who had complete demographic and psychosocial data. 222 (48%) indicated that they were taking HT (estrogen, combination of estrogen and progesterone, other) were analyzed. There were no differences in HT use, duration, type of HT or presence of menopausal symptoms by ethnicity.However African-American women exhibiting higher BDI scores and higher total Cook Medley scores when compared to Caucasian women ($p = 0.03$). African-American women reported a higher proportion of household income below $20,000 ($p \leq 0.01$), and reported more CVD risk factors (history of HTN, DM, smoking), and angiographic evidence of CAD than Caucasian women. Higher levels of serum estrogen were seen in both Caucasians and African-American women taking HT in the 3 months prior to their enrollment. HT use was associated with better psychological health in Caucasian women, with fewer symptoms of depression and lower aggression and cynicism scores (Table 4). African-American women with menopausal symptoms who used HT had noticeably lower hostility ($p < 0.01$) and cynicism scores ($p < 0.05$) compared to African-American women who did not use HT. The presence of menopausal symptoms and hysterectomy status were significant independent predictors of HT use for both Caucasian and African-American women ($p = 0.05$). African-American women had higher total Cook-Medley scores and higher scores in all three subscales.

Conclusions. Racial differences in the baseline psychological measurements as well as in the association of HT use and psychological state was observed between WISE African-American and Caucasian women. Fewer symptoms of depression and lower levels of aggression scores were observed within the Caucasian than the African-American HT users. Cynicism scores were lower among both Caucasian and African-American HT users. Both Caucasian and African-American women reported better psychological health in association with HT use.

Table 4. Psychological Characteristics by Race and HRT Status

	White			Black		
Characteristics	No HRT (n = 205)	Use HRT (n = 194)	P value[a]	No HRT (n = 35)	Use HRT (n = 28)	P value[a]
Beck Depression Inventory	10.5 ± 8.2	9.4 ± 7.9	0.03	12.1 ± 8.1	13.9 ± 8.0	0.75
Total Cook Medley score	9.8 ± 5.1	8.7 ± 5.1	0.02	12.4 ± 6.0	10.6 ± 5.5	0.32
Aggression Score	2.9 ± 1.6	2.6 ± 1.7	0.04	3.1 ± 1.7	3.2 ± 1.8	0.69
Hostile affect	1.9 ± 1.3	1.8 ± 1.3	0.32	2.2 ± 1.3	1.7 ± 1.3	0.14
Cynicism	5.1 ± 3.5	4.4 ± 3.1	0.02	7.2 ± 3.5	5.7 ± 3.6	0.11

HRT=hormone replacement therapy, [a] Adjusted for age, education, and CAD risk factor [18]. Copyright permission obtained .

D. Phytoestrogens as Selective Estrogen-Receptor Modulators (SERMS)

9) Phytoestrogens and Lipoproteins in Women

Previous work has suggested that blood lipoprotein levels are beneficially associated with soy protein ingestion [111], attributed to plant estrogens (phytoestrogens). Soy phytoestrogen extracts contain genistein and daidzein in near equal amounts. Acting as Selective Estrogen-receptor Modulators (SERMS), the relative binding affinity of genistein for the estrogen receptor-α and estrogen receptor-β is about 20-40 times and 10-50 higher than daidzein, respectively [112]. The beneficial role and the potential mechanisms of plant estrogens (phytoestrogens) on the blood lipoproteins in humans are controversial. In this WISE substudy we evaluated relationships among blood phytoestrogen levels, lipoprotein levels, estrogen levels and angiographically defined CAD in women.

Methods. A cross-sectional analysis in 483 WISE women were evaluated for blood phytoestrogen levels, lipoprotein levels estrogen levels and angiographic CAD. Among 483 WISE women (mean age of 58 ± 12, range 21 - 86 years), included a population of which 79% were post menopausal, and had a mean BMI of 29.4 ± 6.4 (range 15.0-57.2). Most women had at least one coronary risk factor, and 38% had angiographic CAD. Overall 38% used HT, and 24% used lipid-lowering therapy. African-Americans, Hispanics, and American Indians represented 18% minority population.

Results. A beneficial association was seen among the subgroup of women with low (<184 pmol/liter [<50 pg/ml]) blood E2 levels, including relations between daidzein and triglycerides, $r = -0.16$, $p = 0.002$, HDL cholesterol, $r = 0.10$, $p = 0.06$, TC, $r = -0.09$, $p = 0.07$, and LDL cholesterol, $r = -0.10$, $p = 0.07$. Furthermore, these associations were stronger and extended to beneficial associations with TC and LDL-cholesterol, regardless of age and lipoprotein levels. Higher blood levels of phytoestrogen daidzein were associated with lower triglyceride ($p = 0.05$) levels, and a beneficial TC to HDL-C ratio ($p = 0.02$). No noticeable relationship between the phytoestrogen levels and angiographic CAD was observed, despite controlling for other significant variables, or after exploring interactions.

Conclusions. Higher blood phytoestrogen daidzein levels were associated with beneficial blood lipoprotein levels in women with well defined CAD risk factors among the subset with low estrogen levels. This could be possibly explained as a result of mechanistic action at the estrogen receptor. These results are consistent with the previous studies [112] in which the dietary consumption of phytoestrogen-rich products have shown to result in beneficial blood lipoprotein changes in humans and may operate via higher daidzein levels.

10) Phytoestrogens and Coronary Microvascular Function in Women with Suspected Ischemia

A large number of women consumes soy phytoestrogens, particularly genistein and daidzein, as part of their diet routinely, with the conviction that these more "natural" substances are a better sources of estrogen replacement [113] [114] [115]. Yet there is a lack of evidence-based clinical data to support widespread recommendation of phytoestrogens for women. Postmenopausal HT improves endothelial-dependent dilation in animal models and in humans [116] [117] [118] [119], but the effect of phytoestrogens on endothelial and nonendothelial-dependent microvascular coronary function in women with suspected ischemic heart disease is unknown. This WISE study examined the relationship between blood phytoestrogen levels and coronary reactivity in women with suspected CAD.

Methods. This study included 106 WISE women who underwent extensive evaluation with intra-coronary vasoactive agents. CFVR, and VFR to Adenosine (ADO) and nitroglycerine (NTG) (nonendothelial-dependent responses) and ACH (endothelial-dependent response) were assessed. CFR was measured. Endothelial-dependent function and nonendothelial-dependent epicardial coronary reactivity was assessed. Epicardial coronary response to ACH also was assessed. Blood phytoestrogen and estrogen levels were correlated with CRT measures.

Results. The mean age was 56 ± 9 years, with most women were post menopausal (79%), and 24% having obstructive angiographic CAD, although the diseased vessels were not used for CRT measurements. A negative correlation was seen between blood genistein levels and nonendothelial-dependent coronary flow responses ($r = -0.48$, $p < 0.001$). The highest genistein tertile (>6.1ng/ml) had a CFVR of 2.1 ± 0.5 and VFR_{ado} of 1.0 ± 0.6, and both were significantly ($p=0.0001$) lower compared with the other genistein tertiles combined (Table 5). Similar associations were noted for $CFVR_{ntg}$ and VFR_{ntg} ($p= 0.03$ and $p= 0.01$, respectively). The highest genistein tertile was associated with lower $CFVR_{ach}$ compared with the other tertiles ($p= 0.03$) (Table 6). A multivariable model demonstrated that blood genistein levels were significant independent predictors of coronary flow responses to ADO, however no significant correlations between coronary reactivity variables and daidzein or endogenous estrogen.

Conclusions. This study suggests the presence of a potentially adverse relationship between coronary vasodilator function and increasing blood levels of the phytoestrogen genistein for the first time. In women with suspected myocardial ischemia, an independent association is seen between higher blood levels of genistein and reduced microvascular coronary flow reserve to ADO (nonendothelial-dependent) and ACH (endothelial-dependent) dilation. A similar trend was also observed, though statistically non-significant, with response to NTG. Other endogenous estrogens or blood phytoestrogen levels showed no correlation or interactions with coronary vasodilator function. Reduction in these coronary reactivity variables has been associated with early atherosclerosis. Results of this study support the hypothesis that higher blood genistein levels are associated with diminished coronary microvascular and endothelial function in women referred for coronary angiography.

Table 5. Coronory Flow Velocity Reserve and Volumetric Flow Reserve by Blood Genistein Level Tertiles

	Low genistein (<= 2.49 ng/mL) n=35	Medium genistein (2.5–6.0 ng/mL) n=35	High genistein (_6.1 ng/mL) n = 36	High tertile Vs. others (rank sums)
CFVRADO[a]	2.9 ± 0.9b	2.7 ± 0.7	2.1 ± 0.5	0.0001
VFRADO	2.8 ± 1.1	2.7 ± 0.7	1.9 ± 0.6	0.0001
CFVRNTG	2.4 ± 0.6	2.3 ± 0.6	2.0 ± 0.6	0.03
VFRNTG	3.1 ± 1.1	3.0 ± 1.0	2.4 ± 0.6	0.01
CFVRACH	1.7 ± 0.9	2.0 ± 0.9	1.4 ± 0.4	0.03
VFRACH	1.5 ± 0.7	1.8 ± 0.9	1.4 ± 0.5	0.23

[a]ADO, adenosine; ACH, acetylcholine; CFVR, coronary flow velocity reserve; NTG, nitroglycerin; VFR, volumetric flow reserve [125].

[b]Mean ± SD. Copyright permission obtained.

Table 6. Significant Independent Predictors of Coronary Reactivity to Adenosine (Nonendothelial-dependent flow)

	CFVRADOa		VFRADO	
Predictor	Parameter Estimate	P	Parameter Estimate	P
Blood genistein (log)	-0.41	0.0001	- 0.43	0.0002
Age	-0.02	0.008	-	-
Hypertension history	-0.28	0.06	-0.47	0.02
CAD severity score (log)	-	-	-0.38	0.02
R2	0.34		0.31	

CAD=coronary artery disease, aCFVR, coronary flow velocity reserve; VFR, volumetric flow reserve [125]. Copyright permission obtained.

Summary of New Findings

The new WISE reproductive status algorithm increases the accuracy of the menopausal status classification compared to other previously used self-reported menopausal status determination methods. The new algorithm is relatively simple and inexpensive and has implications for epidemiological and clinical research in women.

Among pre- and perimenopausal women, HHE appears to be associated with angiographic CAD in premenopausal women undergoing coronary angiography for suspected myocardial ischemia. The findings suggest that centrally-mediated estrogen deficiency with the disruption of ovarian function is associated with a higher risk for CAD in premenopausal women with previous coronary risk factors. The strong independent association between HHE and DM in the cohort of women also supports the hypothesis that estrogen deficiency of hypothalamic origin, rather than the androgen deficiency like in PCOS, may provide a mechanistic link between DM and CAD in premenopausal women. Furthermore, in premenopausal women the burden of angiographic CAD is increased by HHE and DM, collectively predicting the CVD.

Lower blood lipoproteins levels and use of cholesterol lowering medications like statins were not associated with adverse effects on cholesterol derived blood reproductive hormones like E2, estrone and progesterone levels in premenopausal women of child bearing age.

In postmenopausal women, an in-depth look at risk factors demonstrates that comparatively higher levels of endogenous estrogen levels are seen in both general and central pattern of obesity. These findings are consistent with existing literature, however the observed differences in the relationship between estrone and bioavailaible E2 and their predominance in central and obesity patterns respectively, adds to our knowledge regarding epidemiological relationships between obesity and disease seen in postmenopausal women. Further prospective studies in larger general populations are needed to evaluate the clinical implications and refine the mechanism responsible for these results.

Clinical features of PCOS was an independent predictor of angiographic CAD and future adverse CVD events. Within this cohort, the higher prevalence of DM which was seen in postmenopausal women with clinical features of PCOS was also associated with an elevated CVD risk. Furthermore, PCOS in combination with the elevated hs-CRP substantially increased the risk of adverse CVD events, suggesting an inflammatory mechanistic pathway relating PCOS to CVD in these women. This inflammatory process may contribute to the initiation and rapid progression of CAD from subclinical state to more advanced clinical angiographic CAD state.

Both Caucasian and African-American women who report HT use have better psychological health, however African-American women who report suffering from menopausal symptoms have more symptoms of depression than Caucasian women. Similar to previous studies, the WISE demonstrates more adverse CVD events associated with higher Cook-Medley scores, and substantiates a poorer survival time specifically in African-American women with higher Cook-Medley score. However the results should be interpreted with caution because of limited sample size. Prospective studies in larger populations of African-American women are needed to further validate these data.

The most commonly used sources of phytoestrogens are soy-based foods and supplements. Many women consume soy phytoestrogens as part of their daily diet, and basic research suggests that phytoestrogens can act as natural SERMs. The long term use of these soy phytoestrogens is likely to have risks and benefits, as evidenced by the association between relatively higher phytoestrogen genistein blood levels with decreased coronary vasodilatation in women. High genistein levels proved to be independently associated with the reduced coronary vasodilatation. However, other blood phytoestrogen levels and endogenous estrogen levels showed no association with measures of coronary vasodilatation. Whereas in another WISE study, blood phytoestrogen daidzein levels were positively linked with blood lipoprotein levels and especially more benefit was seen in women with lower blood estrogen levels. To verify and determine the complex and comprehensive affects of phytoestrogens on CVD, further studies are needed.

These new data from WISE study suggests that estrogen plays a role CVD in women. Ongoing research is directed at further understating.

Acknowledgements

This work was supported by contracts from the National Heart, Lung and Blood Institutes, nos. N01-HV-68161, N01-HV-68162, N01-HV-68163, N01-HV-68164, a GCRC grant MO1-RR00425 from the National Center for Research Resources, and grants from the Gustavus and Louis Pfeiffer Research Foundation, Denville, New Jersey, the Women's Guild of Cedars-Sinai Medical Center, Los Angeles, California, the Edythe L. Broad Women's Heart Research Fellowship, Cedars-Sinai Medical Center, Los Angeles, California, and the Barbra Streisand Women's Cardiovascular Research and Education Program, Cedars-Sinai Medical Center, Los Angeles, California

References

[1] Thom T, Haase N, Rosamond W, Howard VJ, Rumsfeld J, Manolio T, Zheng ZJ, Flegal K, O'Donnell C, Kittner S, Lloyd-Jones D, Goff DC, Jr., Hong Y, Adams R, Friday G, Furie K, Gorelick P, Kissela B, Marler J, Meigs J, Roger V, Sidney S, Sorlie P, Steinberger J, Wasserthiel-Smoller S, Wilson M, Wolf P. Heart disease and stroke statistics--2006 update: a report from the American Heart Association Statistics Committee and Stroke Statistics Subcommittee. Circulation 113(6): e85-151, 2006.

[2] Shaw LJ, Merz CN, Bittner V, Kip K, Johnson BD, Reis SE, Kelsey SF, Olson M, Mankad S, Sharaf BL, Rogers WJ, Pohost GM, Sopko G, Pepine CJ. Importance of socioeconomic status as a predictor of cardiovascular outcome and costs of care in women with suspected myocardial ischemia. Results from the National Institutes of Health, National Heart, Lung and Blood Institute-sponsored Women's Ischemia Syndrome Evaluation (WISE). J Womens Health (Larchmt) 17(7): 1081-92, 2008.

[3] Hoerger TJ, Downs KE, Lakshmanan MC, Lindrooth RC, Plouffe L, Jr., Wendling B, West SL, Ohsfeldt RL. Healthcare use among U.S. women aged 45 and older: total

costs and costs for selected postmenopausal health risks. J Womens Health Gend Based Med 8(8): 1077-89, 1999.

[4] Lloyd-Jones D, Adams R, Carnethon M, De Simone G, Ferguson TB, Flegal K, Ford E, Furie K, Go A, Greenlund K, Haase N, Hailpern S, Ho M, Howard V, Kissela B, Kittner S, Lackland D, Lisabeth L, Marelli A, McDermott M, Meigs J, Mozaffarian D, Nichol G, O'Donnell C, Roger V, Rosamond W, Sacco R, Sorlie P, Stafford R, Steinberger J, Thom T, Wasserthiel-Smoller S, Wong N, Wylie-Rosett J, Hong Y. Heart Disease and Stroke Statistics--2009 Update. A Report From the American Heart Association Statistics Committee and Stroke Statistics Subcommittee. Circulation 2008.

[5] DeStefano F MR, Anda RF, Casper MI, Eaker ED. Trends in nonfatal coronary heart disease in United States, 1980 through 1989. Archives of Internal Medicine 153(2489-94, 1993.

[6] Hani Jneid MGCF, MD; Christopher P. Cannon, MD; Adrian F. Hernandez, MD; Igor F. Palacios, MD; Andrew O. Maree, MD; Quinn Wells, MD; Biykem Bozkurt, MD; Kenneth A. LaBresh, MD; Li Liang, PhD; Yuling Hong, MD, PhD; L. Kristin Newby, MD, MHS; Gerald Fletcher, MD; Eric Peterson, MD, MPH; Laura Wexler, MD, for the Get With the Guidelines Steering Committee and Investigators Sex Differences in Medical Care and Early Death After Acute Myocardial Infraction. Circulation 118(2803-2810., 2008.

[7] Hochman JS TJ, Thompson TD, Weaver WD, White HD, Van de Werf F, Aylward P, Topol EJ, Califf RM. Global Use of Strategies to Open Occluded Coronary Arteries in Acute Coronary Syndromes IIb Investigators. Sex, clinical presentation, and outcome in patients with acute coronary syndromes. N Engl J Med 341(226 –232., 1999.

[8] Vaccarino V PL, Every NR, Barron HV, Krumholz HM. Sex differences in mortality after myocardial infarction: is there evidence for an increased risk for women? N Eng J Med 341(4): 217-25, 1999.

[9] Bellasi A, Raggi P, Merz CN, Shaw LJ. New insights into ischemic heart disease in women. Cleve Clin J Med 74(8): 585-94, 2007.

[10] Champney KP, Frederick PD, Bueno H, Parashar S, Foody J, Bairey Merz CN, Canto JG, Lichtman JH, Vaccarino V. The Joint Contribution of Sex, Age and Type of Myocardial Infarction on Hospital Mortality Following Acute Myocardial Infarction. Heart 2009.

[11] Tillmanns H, Waas W, Voss R, Grempels E, Holschermann H, Haberbosch W, Waldecker B. Gender differences in the outcome of cardiac interventions. Herz 30(5): 375-89, 2005.

[12] Associates PIoCat. National Heart, lung and Blood Institute Coronary Artery Surgery Study (CASS). Circulation 63(1): 1-81, 1981.

[13] Kennedy JW, Killip T, Fisher LD, Alderman EL, Gillespie MJ, Mock MB. The clinical spectrum of coronary artery disease and its surgical and medical management, 1974-1979. The Coronary Artery Surgery study. Circulation 66(5 Pt 2): III16-23, 1982.

[14] Tobin JN, Wassertheil-Smoller S, Wexler JP, Steingart RM, Budner N, Lense L, Wachspress J. Sex bias in considering coronary bypass surgery. Ann Intern Med 107(1): 19-25, 1987.

[15] Shaw LJ, Miller DD, Romeis JC, Kargl D, Younis LT, Chaitman BR. Gender differences in the noninvasive evaluation and management of patients with suspected coronary artery disease. Ann Intern Med 120(7): 559-66, 1994.

[16] Srichaiveth B, Ruengsakulrach P, Visudharom K, Sanguanwong S, Tangsubutr W, Insamian P. Impact of gender on treatment and clinical outcomes in acute ST elevation myocardial infarction patients in Thailand. J Med Assoc Thai 90 Suppl 1(65-73, 2007.

[17] Colleen Gorman Koch MD MS, Yi-shin Weng ScD, Sharon X. Zhou MD, MS, Joseph S. Savino MD, Joseph P. Mathew MD, Ping H. Hsu PhD, Lawrence J. Saidman MD, Dennis T. Mangano PhD, MD, Investigators of the Ischemia Research and Education Foundation (IREF) and Multicenter Study of Perioperative Ischemia (McSPI) Research Group. Prevalence of risk factors, and not gender per se, determines short- and long-term survival after coronary artery bypass surgery. Journal of Cardiothoracic and Vascular Anesthesia 17(5): 585-593 2003.

[18] Olson MB, Bairey Merz CN, Shaw LJ, Mankad S, Reis SE, Pohost GM, Smith KM, McGorray SP, Cornell CE, Kelsey SF. Hormone replacement, race, and psychological health in women: a report from the NHLBI-Sponsored WISE Study. J Womens Health (Larchmt) 13(3): 325-32, 2004.

[19] Shaw LJ, Bairey Merz CN, Azziz R, Stanczyk FZ, Sopko G, Braunstein GD, Kelsey SF, Kip KE, Cooper-Dehoff RM, Johnson BD, Vaccarino V, Reis SE, Bittner V, Hodgson TK, Rogers W, Pepine CJ. Postmenopausal women with a history of irregular menses and elevated androgen measurements at high risk for worsening cardiovascular event-free survival: results from the National Institutes of Health--National Heart, Lung, and Blood Institute sponsored Women's Ischemia Syndrome Evaluation. J Clin Endocrinol Metab 93(4): 1276-84, 2008.

[20] Dodge JT, Jr., Brown BG, Bolson EL, Dodge HT. Lumen diameter of normal human coronary arteries. Influence of age, sex, anatomic variation, and left ventricular hypertrophy or dilation. Circulation 86(1): 232-46, 1992.

[21] Sheifer SE, Canos MR, Weinfurt KP, Arora UK, Mendelsohn FO, Gersh BJ, Weissman NJ. Sex differences in coronary artery size assessed by intravascular ultrasound. Am Heart J 139(4): 649-53, 2000.

[22] Burke AP, Farb A, Malcom GT, Liang Y, Smialek J, Virmani R. Effect of risk factors on the mechanism of acute thrombosis and sudden coronary death in women. Circulation 97(21): 2110-6, 1998.

[23] Shaw LJ, Lewis JF, Hlatky MA, Hsueh WA, Kelsey SF, Klein R, Manolio TA, Sharrett AR, Tracy RP. Women's Ischemic Syndrome Evaluation: current status and future research directions: report of the National Heart, Lung and Blood Institute workshop: October 2-4, 2002: Section 5: gender-related risk factors for ischemic heart disease. Circulation 109(6): e56-8, 2004.

[24] Pepine CJ, Balaban RS, Bonow RO, Diamond GA, Johnson BD, Johnson PA, Mosca L, Nissen SE, Pohost GM. Women's Ischemic Syndrome Evaluation: current status and future research directions: report of the National Heart, Lung and Blood Institute workshop: October 2-4, 2002: Section 1: diagnosis of stable ischemia and ischemic heart disease. Circulation 109(6): e44-6, 2004.

[25] Barrett-Connor EL. Obesity, atherosclerosis, and coronary artery disease. Ann Intern Med 103(6 (Pt 2)): 1010-9, 1985.

[26] Manson JE, Stampfer MJ, Hennekens CH, Willett WC. Body weight and longevity. A reassessment. JAMA 257(3): 353-8, 1987.

[27] The National Heart, Lung and Blood Institute Expert Panel on the identification, evaluation, and treatment of Overweight and Obesity in Adults. Executive Summary of the Clinical Guidelines on the Identification, Evaluation, and Treatment of Overweight and Obesity in Adults. Journal of the American Dietetic Association 98(10): 1178-1191, 1998.

[28] Shufelt CL, Bairey Merz CN. Contraceptive hormone use and cardiovascular disease. J Am Coll Cardiol 53(3): 221-31, 2009.

[29] Regitz-Zagrosek V. Therapeutic implications of the gender-specific aspects of cardiovascular disease. Nat Rev Drug Discov 5(5): 425-38, 2006.

[30] Bonetti PO, Lerman LO, Lerman A. Endothelial dysfunction: a marker of atherosclerotic risk. Arterioscler Thromb Vasc Biol 23(2): 168-75, 2003.

[31] Halcox JP, Schenke WH, Zalos G, Mincemoyer R, Prasad A, Waclawiw MA, Nour KR, Quyyumi AA. Prognostic value of coronary vascular endothelial dysfunction. Circulation 106(6): 653-8, 2002.

[32] Zhang F, Ram JL, Standley PR, Sowers JR. 17 beta-E2 attenuates voltage-dependent Ca2+ currents in A7r5 vascular smooth muscle cell line. Am J Physiol 266(4 Pt 1): C975-80, 1994.

[33] Williams JK, Adams MR, Klopfenstein HS. Estrogen modulates responses of atherosclerotic coronary arteries. Circulation 81(5): 1680-7, 1990.

[34] Horwitz KB, Horwitz LD. Canine vascular tissues are targets for androgens, estrogens, progestins, and glucocorticoids. J Clin Invest 69(4): 750-8, 1982.

[35] Johnson BD, Merz CN, Braunstein GD, Berga SL, Bittner V, Hodgson TK, Gierach GL, Reis SE, Vido DA, Sharaf BL, Smith KM, Sopko G, Kelsey SF. Determination of menopausal status in women: the NHLBI-sponsored Women's Ischemia Syndrome Evaluation (WISE) Study. J Womens Health (Larchmt) 13(8): 872-87, 2004.

[36] Barrett-Connor EL, Cohn BA, Wingard DL, Edelstein SL. Why is diabetes mellitus a stronger risk factor for fatal ischemic heart disease in women than in men? The Rancho Bernardo Study. JAMA 265(5): 627-31, 1991.

[37] Kanaya AM, Grady D, Barrett-Connor E. Explaining the sex difference in coronary heart disease mortality among patients with type 2 diabetes mellitus: a meta-analysis. Arch Intern Med 162(15): 1737-45, 2002.

[38] Hu FB, Stampfer MJ, Solomon CG, Liu S, Willett WC, Speizer FE, Nathan DM, Manson JE. The impact of diabetes mellitus on mortality from all causes and coronary heart disease in women: 20 years of follow-up. Arch Intern Med 161(14): 1717-23, 2001.

[39] Barzilay JI, Kronmal RA, Gottdiener JS, Smith NL, Burke GL, Tracy R, Savage PJ, Carlson M. The association of fasting glucose levels with congestive heart failure in diabetic adults > or =65 years: the Cardiovascular Health Study. J Am Coll Cardiol 43(12): 2236-41, 2004.

[40] Poehlman ET. Menopause, energy expenditure, and body composition. Acta Obstet Gynecol Scand 81(7): 603-11, 2002.

[41] Carey VJ, Walters EE, Colditz GA, Solomon CG, Willett WC, Rosner BA, Speizer FE, Manson JE. Body fat distribution and risk of non-insulin-dependent diabetes mellitus in women. The Nurses' Health Study. Am J Epidemiol 145(7): 614-9, 1997.

[42] Folsom AR, Prineas RJ, Kaye SA, Munger RG. Incidence of hypertension and stroke in relation to body fat distribution and other risk factors in older women. Stroke 21(5): 701-6, 1990.

[43] Lamon-Fava S, Wilson PW, Schaefer EJ. Impact of body mass index on coronary heart disease risk factors in men and women. The Framingham Offspring Study. Arterioscler Thromb Vasc Biol 16(12): 1509-15, 1996.

[44] Rexrode KM, Carey VJ, Hennekens CH, Walters EE, Colditz GA, Stampfer MJ, Willett WC, Manson JE. Abdominal adiposity and coronary heart disease in women. JAMA 280(21): 1843-8, 1998.

[45] Onat A, Avci GS, Barlan MM, Uyarel H, Uzunlar B, Sansoy V. Measures of abdominal obesity assessed for visceral adiposity and relation to coronary risk. Int J Obes Relat Metab Disord 28(8): 1018-25, 2004.

[46] Lawlor DA, Smith GD, Ebrahim S. Association between childhood socioeconomic status and coronary heart disease risk among postmenopausal women: findings from the British Women's Heart and Health Study. Am J Public Health 94(8): 1386-92, 2004.

[47] Wessel TR, Arant CB, Olson MB, Johnson BD, Reis SE, Sharaf BL, Shaw LJ, Handberg E, Sopko G, Kelsey SF, Pepine CJ, Merz NB. Relationship of physical fitness vs. body mass index with coronary artery disease and cardiovascular events in women. JAMA 292(10): 1179-87, 2004.

[48] Flegal KM, Graubard BI, Williamson DF, Gail MH. Excess deaths associated with underweight, overweight, and obesity. JAMA 293(15): 1861-7, 2005.

[49] Wajchenberg BL. Subcutaneous and visceral adipose tissue: their relation to the metabolic syndrome. Endocr Rev 21(6): 697-738, 2000.

[50] Talbott EO, Guzick DS, Sutton-Tyrrell K, McHugh-Pemu KP, Zborowski JV, Remsberg KE, Kuller LH. Evidence for association between polycystic ovary syndrome and premature carotid atherosclerosis in middle-aged women. Arterioscler Thromb Vasc Biol 20(11): 2414-21, 2000.

[51] Phillips GB. Is atherosclerotic cardiovascular disease an endocrinological disorder? The estrogen-androgen paradox. J Clin Endocrinol Metab 90(5): 2708-11, 2005.

[52] Detrano R, Froelicher VF. Exercise testing: uses and limitations considering recent studies. Prog Cardiovasc Dis 31(3): 173-204, 1988.

[53] Fleischmann KE, Hunink MG, Kuntz KM, Douglas PS. Exercise echocardiography or exercise SPECT imaging? A meta-analysis of diagnostic test performance. JAMA 280(10): 913-20, 1998.

[54] Kwok Y, Kim C, Grady D, Segal M, Redberg R. Meta-analysis of exercise testing to detect coronary artery disease in women. Am J Cardiol 83(5): 660-6, 1999.

[55] Redberg RF, Shaw LJ. Diagnosis of coronary artery disease in women. Prog Cardiovasc Dis 46(3): 239-58, 2003.

[56] Goebelsmann U, Arce JJ, Thorneycroft IH, Mishell DR, Jr. Serum testosterone concentrations in women throughout the menstrual cycle and following HCG administration. Am J Obstet Gynecol 119(4): 445-52, 1974.

[57] Goebelsmann U, Horton R, Mestman JH, Arce JJ, Nagata Y, Nakamura RM, Thorneycroft IH, Mishell DR, Jr. Male pseudohermaphroditism due to testicular 17 -hydroxysteroid dehydrogenase deficiency. J Clin Endocrinol Metab 36(5): 867-79, 1973.

[58] Anderson DC, Hopper BR, Lasley BL, Yen SS. A simple method for the assay of eight steroids in small volumes of plasma. Steroids 28(2): 179-96, 1976.

[59] Tremblay RR, Dube JY. Plasma concentrations of free and non-TeBG bound testosterone in women on oral contraceptives. Contraception 10(6): 599-605, 1974.

[60] Oh JY, Barrett-Connor E, Wedick NM, Wingard DL. Endogenous sex hormones and the development of type 2 diabetes in older men and women: the Rancho Bernardo study. Diabetes Care 25(1): 55-60, 2002.

[61] Sodergard R, Backstrom T, Shanbhag V, Carstensen H. Calculation of free and bound fractions of testosterone and E2-17 beta to human plasma proteins at body temperature. J Steroid Biochem 16(6): 801-10, 1982.

[62] Vermeulen A, Verdonck L, Kaufman JM. A critical evaluation of simple methods for the estimation of free testosterone in serum. J Clin Endocrinol Metab 84(10): 3666-72, 1999.

[63] Rinaldi S, Geay A, Dechaud H, Biessy C, Zeleniuch-Jacquotte A, Akhmedkhanov A, Shore RE, Riboli E, Toniolo P, Kaaks R. Validity of free testosterone and free E2 determinations in serum samples from postmenopausal women by theoretical calculations. Cancer Epidemiol Biomarkers Prev 11(10 Pt 1): 1065-71, 2002.

[64] Barrett-Connor E, Goodman-Gruen D. Prospective study of endogenous sex hormones and fatal cardiovascular disease in postmenopausal women. BMJ 311(7014): 1193-6, 1995.

[65] Ridker PM, Rifai N, Rose L, Buring JE, Cook NR. Comparison of C-reactive protein and low-density lipoprotein cholesterol levels in the prediction of first cardiovascular events. N Engl J Med 347(20): 1557-65, 2002.

[66] Coward L, Kirk M, Albin N, Barnes S. Analysis of plasma isoflavones by reversed-phase HPLC-multiple reaction ion monitoring-mass spectrometry. Clin Chim Acta 247(1-2): 121-42, 1996.

[67] R. Victory CDS, M.P. Diamond, S.G. McNeeley, D. Vista-Deck and S. Hendrix. Adverse cardiovascular disease outcomes are reduced in women with a history of oral contraceptive use: Results from the Women's Health Initiative Database. Fertility and Sterility 91(1): 1-304, 2009.

[68] Reis SE, Gloth ST, Blumenthal RS, Resar JR, Zacur HA, Gerstenblith G, Brinker JA. Ethinyl E2 acutely attenuates abnormal coronary vasomotor responses to acetylcholine in postmenopausal women. Circulation 89(1): 52-60, 1994.

[69] Doucette JW, Corl PD, Payne HM, Flynn AE, Goto M, Nassi M, Segal J. Validation of a Doppler guide wire for intravascular measurement of coronary artery flow velocity. Circulation 85(5): 1899-911, 1992.

[70] Sharaf BL, Pepine CJ, Kerensky RA, Reis SE, Reichek N, Rogers WJ, Sopko G, Kelsey SF, Holubkov R, Olson M, Miele NJ, Williams DO, Merz CN. Detailed angiographic analysis of women with suspected ischemic chest pain (pilot phase data from the NHLBI-sponsored Women's Ischemia Syndrome Evaluation [WISE] Study Angiographic Core Laboratory). Am J Cardiol 87(8): 937-41; A3, 2001.

[71] Burden and Disparities Today: http://www.cdc.gov/dhdsp/library/ action_plan/ 2008_update/burden.htm: 2008 Public Health Action Plan Update: Celebrating Our First Five Year; August 8, 2008

[72] Peter WF Wilson, Estimation of cardiovascular risk in an individual patient without known cardiovascular disease. http://www.uptodate.com/patients/content/ topic.do?topicKey=~/AV/AsQkzr. Januarry 23, 2008

[73] Physical status: the use and interpretation of anthropometry. Report of a WHO Expert Committee. World Health Organ Tech Rep Ser 854(1-452, 1995.

[74] Mitchell ES, Woods NF, Mariella A. Three stages of the menopausal transition from the Seattle Midlife Women's Health Study: toward a more precise definition. Menopause 7(5): 334-49, 2000.

[75] Brambilla DJ, McKinlay SM, Johannes CB. Defining the perimenopause for application in epidemiologic investigations. Am J Epidemiol 140(12): 1091-5, 1994.

[76] Soules MR, Sherman S, Parrott E, Rebar R, Santoro N, Utian W, Woods N. Executive summary: Stages of Reproductive Aging Workshop (STRAW). Fertil Steril 76(5): 874-8, 2001.

[77] Szklo M, Cerhan J, Diez-Roux AV, Chambless L, Cooper L, Folsom AR, Fried LP, Knopman D, Nieto FJ. Estrogen replacement therapy and cognitive functioning in the Atherosclerosis Risk in Communities (ARIC) Study. Am J Epidemiol 144(11): 1048-57, 1996.

[78] Ford ES, Capewell S. Coronary heart disease mortality among young adults in the U.S. from 1980 through 2002: concealed leveling of mortality rates. J Am Coll Cardiol 50(22): 2128-32, 2007.

[79] Kaplan JR, Adams MR, Clarkson TB, Koritnik DR. Psychosocial influences on female 'protection' among cynomolgus macaques. Atherosclerosis 53(3): 283-95, 1984.

[80] Kaplan JR, Manuck SB, Anthony MS, Clarkson TB. Premenopausal social status and hormone exposure predict postmenopausal atherosclerosis in female monkeys. Obstet Gynecol 99(3): 381-8, 2002.

[81] Rosengren A, Tibblin G, Wilhelmsen L. Self-perceived psychological stress and incidence of coronary artery disease in middle-aged men. Am J Cardiol 68(11): 1171-5, 1991.

[82] Beck AT, Ward CH, Mendelson M, Mock J, Erbaugh J. An inventory for measuring depression. Arch Gen Psychiatry 4(561-71, 1961.

[83] Collins R, Keech A, Peto R, Sleight P, Kjekshus J, Wilhelmsen L, MacMahon S, Shaw J, Simes J, Braunwald E, et al. Cholesterol and total mortality: need for larger trials. BMJ 304(6843): 1689, 1992.

[84] Scott M. Grundy; James I. Cleeman; C. Noel Bairey Merz; H. Bryan Brewer JLTC, Donald B. Hunninghake*; Richard C. Pasternak; Sidney C. Smith JNJS, Program ftCCotNCE. Implications of Recent Clinical Trials for the National Cholesterol

Education Program Adult Treatment Panel III Guidelines. Circulation 110(227-239, 2004.
[85] Ide H, Fujiya S, Aanuma Y, Agishi Y. Effects of simvastatin, an HMG-CoA reductase inhibitor, on plasma lipids and steroid hormones. Clin Ther 12(5): 410-20, 1990.
[86] Ushiroyama T, Ikeda A, Ueki M. Beneficial effects of pravastatin in peri- and postmenopausal hyperlipidemic women: a 5-year study on serum lipid and sex hormone levels. Maturitas 37(3): 201-8, 2001.
[87] Barrett-Connor E, Wingard DL. Sex differential in ischemic heart disease mortality in diabetics: a prospective population-based study. Am J Epidemiol 118(4): 489-96, 1983.
[88] Kannel WB. Metabolic risk factors for coronary heart disease in women: perspective from the Framingham Study. Am Heart J 114(2): 413-9, 1987.
[89] Bairey Merz CN, Johnson BD, Braunstein GD, Pepine CJ, Reis SE, Paul-Labrador M, Hale G, Sharaf BL, Bittner V, Sopko G, Kelsey SF. Phytoestrogens and lipoproteins in women. J Clin Endocrinol Metab 91(6): 2209-13, 2006.
[90] Bairey Merz CN, Johnson BD, Sharaf BL, Bittner V, Berga SL, Braunstein GD, Hodgson TK, Matthews KA, Pepine CJ, Reis SE, Reichek N, Rogers WJ, Pohost GM, Kelsey SF, Sopko G. Hypoestrogenemia of hypothalamic origin and coronary artery disease in premenopausal women: a report from the NHLBI-sponsored WISE study. J Am Coll Cardiol 41(3): 413-9, 2003.
[91] Sheehan MT. Polycystic ovarian syndrome: diagnosis and management. Clin Med Res 2(1): 13-27, 2004.
[92] Adams MR, Kaplan JR, Manuck SB, Koritnik DR, Parks JS, Wolfe MS, Clarkson TB. Inhibition of coronary artery atherosclerosis by 17-beta E2 in ovariectomized monkeys. Lack of an effect of added progesterone. Arteriosclerosis 10(6): 1051-7, 1990.
[93] Colditz GA, Willett WC, Stampfer MJ, Rosner B, Speizer FE, Hennekens CH. Menopause and the risk of coronary heart disease in women. N Engl J Med 316(18): 1105-10, 1987.
[94] Barrett-Connor E, Bush TL. Estrogen and coronary heart disease in women. JAMA 265(14): 1861-7, 1991.
[95] Christian RC, Dumesic DA, Behrenbeck T, Oberg AL, Sheedy PF, 2nd, Fitzpatrick LA. Prevalence and predictors of coronary artery calcification in women with polycystic ovary syndrome. J Clin Endocrinol Metab 88(6): 2562-8, 2003.
[96] Guzick DS. Cardiovascular risk in PCOS. J Clin Endocrinol Metab 89(8): 3694-5, 2004.
[97] Legro RS. Polycystic ovary syndrome and cardiovascular disease: a premature association? Endocr Rev 24(3): 302-12, 2003.
[98] Brown CD, Higgins M, Donato KA, Rohde FC, Garrison R, Obarzanek E, Ernst ND, Horan M. Body mass index and the prevalence of hypertension and dyslipidemia. Obes Res 8(9): 605-19, 2000.
[99] Folsom AR, Kushi LH, Anderson KE, Mink PJ, Olson JE, Hong CP, Sellers TA, Lazovich D, Prineas RJ. Associations of general and abdominal obesity with multiple health outcomes in older women: the Iowa Women's Health Study. Arch Intern Med 160(14): 2117-28, 2000.
[100] Calle EE, Thun MJ. Obesity and cancer. Oncogene 23(38): 6365-78, 2004.

[101] Petrelli JM, Calle EE, Rodriguez C, Thun MJ. Body mass index, height, and postmenopausal breast cancer mortality in a prospective cohort of US women. Cancer Causes Control 13(4): 325-32, 2002.

[102] Key TJ, Appleby PN, Reeves GK, Roddam A, Dorgan JF, Longcope C, Stanczyk FZ, Stephenson HE, Jr., Falk RT, Miller R, Schatzkin A, Allen DS, Fentiman IS, Wang DY, Dowsett M, Thomas HV, Hankinson SE, Toniolo P, Akhmedkhanov A, Koenig K, Shore RE, Zeleniuch-Jacquotte A, Berrino F, Muti P, Micheli A, Krogh V, Sieri S, Pala V, Venturelli E, Secreto G, Barrett-Connor E, Laughlin GA, Kabuto M, Akiba S, Stevens RG, Neriishi K, Land CE, Cauley JA, Kuller LH, Cummings SR, Helzlsouer KJ, Alberg AJ, Bush TL, Comstock GW, Gordon GB, Miller SR. Body mass index, serum sex hormones, and breast cancer risk in postmenopausal women. J Natl Cancer Inst 95(16): 1218-26, 2003.

[103] van den Brandt PA, Spiegelman D, Yaun SS, Adami HO, Beeson L, Folsom AR, Fraser G, Goldbohm RA, Graham S, Kushi L, Marshall JR, Miller AB, Rohan T, Smith-Warner SA, Speizer FE, Willett WC, Wolk A, Hunter DJ. Pooled analysis of prospective cohort studies on height, weight, and breast cancer risk. Am J Epidemiol 152(6): 514-27, 2000.

[104] Expert Panel on the identification E, and Treatment of Overweight and Obesity in Adults. Clinical Guidelines on the Identification, Evaluation, and Treattment of Overweight and Obesity in Adults. The evidence Report NIH Publication No. 98-4083(1998, September.

[105] Tosteson AN, Gabriel SE, Kneeland TS, Moncur MM, Manganiello PD, Schiff I, Ettinger B, Melton LJ, 3rd. Has the impact of hormone replacement therapy on health-related quality of life been undervalued? J Womens Health Gend Based Med 9(2): 119-30, 2000.

[106] Wiklund I, Karlberg J, Mattsson LA. Quality of life of postmenopausal women on a regimen of transdermal E2 therapy: a double-blind placebo-controlled study. Am J Obstet Gynecol 168(3 Pt 1): 824-30, 1993.

[107] Adamson DL, Webb CM, Collins P. Esterified estrogens combined with methyltestosterone improve emotional well-being in postmenopausal women with chest pain and normal coronary angiograms. Menopause 8(4): 233-8, 2001.

[108] Rossouw JE, Anderson GL, Prentice RL, LaCroix AZ, Kooperberg C, Stefanick ML, Jackson RD, Beresford SA, Howard BV, Johnson KC, Kotchen JM, Ockene J. Risks and benefits of estrogen plus progestin in healthy postmenopausal women: principal results From the Women's Health Initiative randomized controlled trial. JAMA 288(3): 321-33, 2002.

[109] Barrett-Connor E, Grady D. Hormone replacement therapy, heart disease, and other considerations. Annu Rev Public Health 19(55-72, 1998.

[110] Grodstein F, Manson JE, Colditz GA, Willett WC, Speizer FE, Stampfer MJ. A prospective, observational study of postmenopausal hormone therapy and primary prevention of cardiovascular disease. Ann Intern Med 133(12): 933-41, 2000.

[111] Anderson JW, Johnstone BM, Cook-Newell ME. Meta-analysis of the effects of soy protein intake on serum lipids. N Engl J Med 333(5): 276-82, 1995.

[112] Honore EK, Williams JK, Anthony MS, Clarkson TB. Soy isoflavones enhance coronary vascular reactivity in atherosclerotic female macaques. Fertil Steril 67(1): 148-54, 1997.
[113] Clarkson TB, Anthony MS. Phytoestrogens and coronary heart disease. Baillieres Clin Endocrinol Metab 12(4): 589-604, 1998.
[114] Tikkanen MJ, Adlercreutz H. Dietary soy-derived isoflavone phytoestrogens. Could they have a role in coronary heart disease prevention? Biochem Pharmacol 60(1): 1-5, 2000.
[115] Glazier MG, Bowman MA. A review of the evidence for the use of phytoestrogens as a replacement for traditional estrogen replacement therapy. Arch Intern Med 161(9): 1161-72, 2001.
[116] Saitta A, Altavilla D, Cucinotta D, Morabito N, Frisina N, Corrado F, D'Anna R, Lasco A, Squadrito G, Gaudio A, Cancellieri F, Arcoraci V, Squadrito F. Randomized, double-blind, placebo-controlled study on effects of raloxifene and hormone replacement therapy on plasma no concentrations, endothelin-1 levels, and endothelium-dependent vasodilation in postmenopausal women. Arterioscler Thromb Vasc Biol 21(9): 1512-9, 2001.
[117] Higashi Y, Sanada M, Sasaki S, Nakagawa K, Goto C, Matsuura H, Ohama K, Chayama K, Oshima T. Effect of estrogen replacement therapy on endothelial function in peripheral resistance arteries in normotensive and hypertensive postmenopausal women. Hypertension 37(2 Part 2): 651-7, 2001.
[118] Herrington DM, Braden GA, Williams JK, Morgan TM. Endothelial-dependent coronary vasomotor responsiveness in postmenopausal women with and without estrogen replacement therapy. Am J Cardiol 73(13): 951-2, 1994.
[119] Guzic-Salobir B, Keber I, Seljeflot I, Arnesen H, Vrabic L. Combined hormone replacement therapy improves endothelial function in healthy postmenopausal women. J Intern Med 250(6): 508-15, 2001.
[120] Merz CN, Kelsey SF, Pepine CJ, Reichek N, Reis SE, Rogers WJ, Sharaf BL, Sopko G. The Women's Ischemia Syndrome Evaluation (WISE) study: protocol design, methodology and feasibility report. J Am Coll Cardiol 33(6): 1453-61, 1999.
[121] Ahmed B, Bairey Merz CN, Johnson BD, Bittner V, Berga SL, Braunstein GD, Hodgson TK, Smith K, Shaw L, Kelsey SF, Sopko G. Diabetes mellitus, hypothalamic hypoestrogenemia, and coronary artery disease in premenopausal women (from the National Heart, Lung, and Blood Institute sponsored WISE study). Am J Cardiol 102(2): 150-4, 2008.
[122] Merz CN, Johnson BD, Berga S, Braunstein G, Reis SE, Bittner V. Past oral contraceptive use and angiographic coronary artery disease in postmenopausal women: data from the National Heart, Lung, and Blood Institute-sponsored Women's Ischemia Syndrome Evaluation. Fertil Steril 85(5): 1425-31, 2006.
[123] Olson MB, Shaw LJ, Kaizar EE, Kelsey SF, Bittner V, Reis SE, Smith K, Braunstein GD, Berga SL, Johnson BD, Bairey Merz CN. Obesity distribution and reproductive hormone levels in women: a report from the NHLBI-sponsored WISE Study. J Womens Health (Larchmt) 15(7): 836-42, 2006.

[124] Bairey Merz CN, Olson MB, Johnson BD, Bittner V, Hodgson TK, Berga SL, Braunstein GD, Pepine CJ, Reis SE, Sopko G, Kelsey SF. Cholesterol-lowering medication, cholesterol level, and reproductive hormones in women: the Women's Ischemia Syndrome Evaluation (WISE). Am J Med 113(9): 723-7, 2002.

[125] Pepine CJ, von Mering GO, Kerensky RA, Johnson BD, McGorray SP, Kelsey SF, Pohost G, Rogers WJ, Reis SE, Sopko G, Bairey Merz CN. Phytoestrogens and coronary microvascular function in women with suspected myocardial ischemia: a report from the Women's Ischemia Syndrome Evaluation (WISE) Study. J Womens Health (Larchmt) 16(4): 481-8, 2007.

In: Estrogens: Production, Functions and Applications ISBN: 978-1-60741-086-7
Editor: James R. Bartos, pp. 95-119

Chapter III

Inhibitory Effect of Estrogens on the Progression of Liver Disease

Ichiro Shimizu[1]
Department of Gastroenterolog, Seirei Yokohama Hospital,
215 Iwai-cho, Hodogaya-ku, Yokohama, Kanagawa 240-8521, Japan

Abstract

Chronic infections with hepatitis C virus (HCV) and hepatitis B virus (HBV) appear to progress more rapidly in males than in females. Nonalcoholic fatty liver disease (NAFLD), cirrhosis and hepatocellular carcinoma (HCC) are predominately diseases of men and postmenopausal women. Female sex hormone, estrogen is a potent endogenous antioxidant. Estrogen suppresses hepatic fibrosis, or the collagen deposition, in animal models, and attenuates induction of redox sensitive transcription factors, and hepatocyte apoptosis by inhibiting the generation of reactive oxygen species in primary cultures. Hepatic steatosis is observed in aromatase-deficient mice, and it is shown to decrease in animals after estrogen treatment. In addition, estrogen has salutary effects on various hepatic stresses including ischemia/reperfusion, hemorrhagic shock-resuscitation, and hepatectomy. Variant estrogen receptors are expressed to a greater extent in male patients with chronic liver disease than in females. Better knowledge of the basic mechanisms underlying the sex-associated differences during the progression of liver disease may open up new avenues for the prevention and treatment of chronic liver disease.

1 Correspondence to: Ichiro Shimizu, MD, AGAF, Department of Gastroenterology, Seirei Yokohama Hospital, 215 Iwai-cho, Hodogaya-ku, Yokohama, Kanagawa 240-8521, Japan, Phone: 81-45-715-3111, Fax: 81-45-715-3387; E-mail: ichiro.Shimizu@me4.seikyou.ne.jp; shimizui@clin.med.tokushima-u.ac.jp

Introduction

Clinical observations and death statistics support the view that chronic hepatitis B and C appear to progress more rapidly in males than in females [1, 2], and that cirrhosis is largely a disease of men and postmenopausal women, with the exception of classically autoimmune liver diseases, such as primary biliary cirrhosis and chronic autoimmune hepatitis [3]. The most clearly established risk factors for hepatocellular carcinoma (HCC) are chronic infection with either hepatitis B virus (HBV) or hepatitis C virus (HCV), cirrhosis, male sex, older age, and alcohol abuse [4]. Liver injury in chronic hepatitis B is predominantly caused by the cellular immune response to the HBV, and the balance between HBV and the immune response changes over time [5], while the high frequency of chronicity in HCV infection and evidence of high rates of HCV mutations could be due to either an ineffective immune response or immunological escape by HCV. According to a report of the International Agency for Research on Cancer [6], the male:female ratio of the age-standardized incidence per 100,000 of liver cancer worldwide is 2.9 : 1, and in Asia (particularly in China, Japan, and Taiwan), the incidence of liver cancer is high and it accounts for half of all liver cancer cases in the world [7]. In the Asian-Pacific region including China and Taiwan, and sub-Saharan Africa, HBV is hyperendemic, whereas in Japan, Western Europe and the USA, HBV infection is also much less common, but HCV infection is more prevalent, and it has been recognized to be a major causative factor of HCC.

Moreover, there is a growing concern regarding the development of nonalcoholic fatty liver disease (NAFLD) in clinical hepatology. Fatty liver, which is histologically called hepatic steatosis, results from the deposition of triglycerides via the accumulation of free fatty acids in hepatocytes. Although in most cases, fatty liver does not progress to more severe liver diseases, approximately 15-20% of patients have histological signs of fibrosis and necroinflammation, thus indicating the presence of nonalcoholic steatohepatitis (NASH). These patients are at higher risk for developing cirrhosis, terminal liver failure, and HCC [8]. Oxidative stress, proinflammatory cytokines, and other proinflammatory mediators as well as lipotoxicity may each play a role in transition of hepatic steatosis to NASH [9]. Earlier impressions that NAFLD/NASH was a female-predominate condition have been dispelled; it actually appears to be more prevalent in men [10-12].

Differences in social circumstances and lifestyles of men and women may be involved in the basic mechanisms underlying the sex-associated differences of these chronic liver diseases. In general, men have a greater risk of exposure to hepatitis viruses as well as greater opportunity for drinking. The incidence of alcoholic liver disease increases in a dose-dependent manner proportionally to the cumulative alcoholic intake. Environmental facor may result in a higher preponderance of nutritional and exercise-associated problems in men. However, some mechanisms related to sex-associated differences may be based on biological factors, including estrogen-related female sex hormones, such as estradiol, rather than simply gender differences in social environmental and lifestyles. Hepatic estrogen receptors (ERs) mediate estrogen action in the liver. The present review summarizes the current knowledge of the biological functions of estrogens and ER status as it relates to fibrogenesis and carcinogenesis in the liver.

HBV/HCV Infection in Females

During the early phase of chronic HBV infection, patients are positive for HBV e antigen (HBeAg), a surrogate marker of active HBV replication, and have frequent acute flares characterized by substantial increases in the serum aminotransferase levels as the result of specific, T-lymphocyte-mediated cellular responses to viral antigens and apoptosis of hepatocytes. Some acute flares may be followed by seroconversion from HBeAg to its antibody (anti-HBe) and clinical remission [13, 14], but a few progress to cirrhosis and HCC, particularly in elderly men [15, 16]. Positivity for HBeAg is associated with a higher inflammatory activity in the liver and an increased risk of HCC [17]. HBeAg to anti-HBe seroconversion occur more frequently in female subjects than in males [18]. Generally, females produce more vigorous cellular and humoral immune reactions, and suffer a higher incidence of autoimmune disease than males [19]. The prevalence of the HBV surface antigen (HBsAg) was reported to be higher in men as compared with women throughout the world [20]. In the follow-up study of up to 19 years in HBsAg carriers in Okinawa, Japan, clearance of HBsAg was seen more frequently in women (7.8%) than in men (5.8%) [21]. The underlying mechanism by which females seem more likely to develop HBsAg clearance and HBeAg seroconversion remains vague. However, estradiol has been reported to induce the production of interferon (INF)-γ in lymphocytes [22], and augment an antigen-specific primary antibody response in human peripheral blood mononuclear cells (PBMCs) [23]. IFN-γ is a potent cytokine with immunomodulatory and antiproliferative properties. Therefore, female subjects, particularly before menopause, could produce antibodies against HBsAg and HBeAg at a higher frequency than males with chronic HBV infection.

Furthermore, immunization is the most effective way to prevent the transmission of HBV. After appropriate immunization with HBV vaccine, approximately 90% of healthy adults and 95% of infants, children, and adolescents develop a protective serum level of the antibody to HBsAg (anti-HBs). The predictors associated with a nonresponse to HBV vaccination, however, include male sex as well as older age and obesity [24]. In Taiwan, chronic HBsAg carrier rates declined more obviously for females (4.4%) than for males (10.7%) who were born to HBsAg carrier mothers, vaccinated against HBV at birth, and followed up for over 18 years [25].

An analysis of first-time blood donors in Japan showed that the antibody to HCV (anti-HCV) was equally detected in men and women [26]. A report, however, based on the data of anti-HCV-positive residents in Egypt, demonstrated that the rate of HCV-RNA clearance in the blood was significantly higher in women (44.6%) than in men (33.7%) [27]. The sustained virological response (SVR) rate to combination therapy with pegylated interferon and ribavirin in USA patients with chronic hepatitis C was significantly higher in women than in men [28], whereas in Japanese patients given such combination therapy the SVR rate showed no sex differences in those under 50 years of age, and was significantly higher in men (51%) than in women (20%) in those aged over 50 years [29].

"Female Paradox" In Alcoholic Liver Disease

In a study on the gender difference in Japanese patients hospitalized in Tokushima, Japan, the prevalence of alcoholic cirrhosis was 9-fold higher in men than women (Figrue 1). However, females are more vulnerable to alcohol because of their smaller volumes of distribution and reduced gastric alcohol dehydrogenase (ADH) activity [30], suggesting that chronic alcohol consumption may induce more rapid and more severe liver injury in females than males. In studies using animals, the stimulation of Kupffer cells by estrogen increased sensitivity to endotoxin after ethanol [31]. The estrogen addition to ethanol ingestion enhanced production of tumor necrosis factor (TNF)-α in Kupffer cells via elevation of the blood endotoxin level and hepatic endotoxin receptor (CD14) expression, resulting in increased inflammatory activity in the liver [32]. The administration of ethanol induced the hepatic activity of cytochrome P450 2E1 (CYP2E1), a pro-oxidant enzyme, in female rats, and the ethanol-induced CYP2E1 activity was reduced by the treatment with anti-estrogen [33].

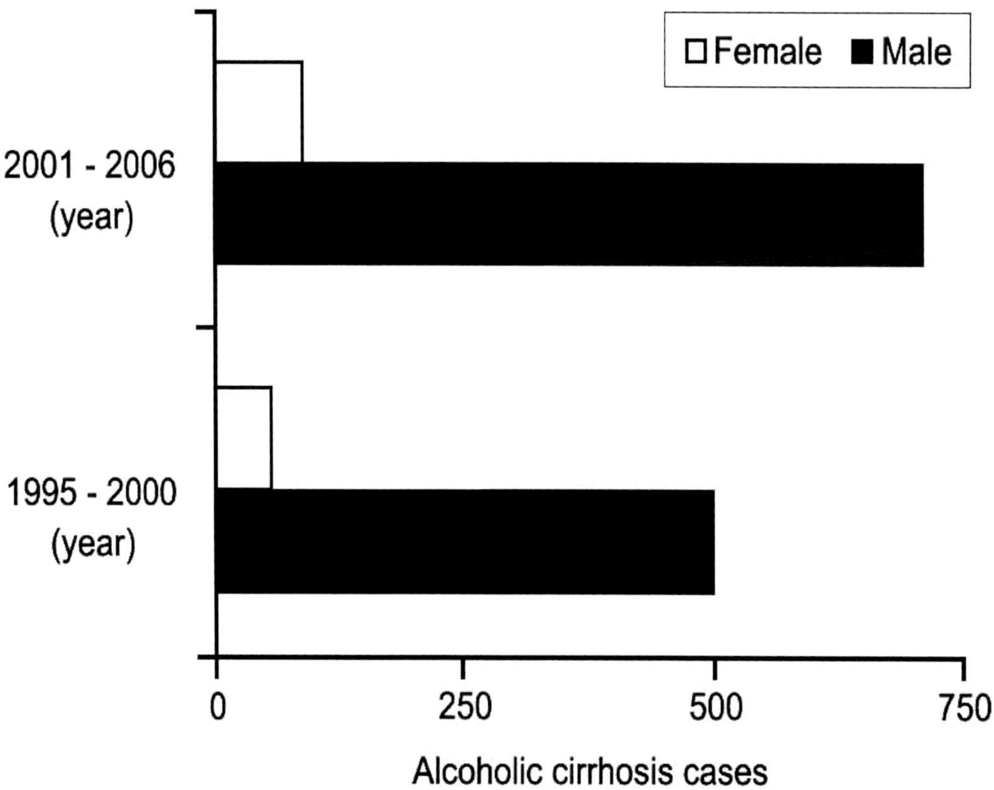

Figure 1. Male-to-female ratio in Japanese patients with alcoholic cirrhosis Male-to-female ratio in alcoholic cirrhosis was examined from 1995 to 2000 and from 2001 to 2006 in 1,353 Japanese patients (mean age 59.6 years, 89.2% males) hospitalized in Tokushima, Japan. The subjects were seronegative for HBsAg and anti-HCV.

The "female paradox" observed in patients with alcoholic liver disease (that is, more rapid liver disease progression in females than males) compared with chronic HBV/HCV infection (slower liver disease progression in females than males) warrants further evaluation [34].

NAFLD in Females

NAFLD has a very high prevalence in much of Asia-Pacific (including Australia and New Zealand), the Middle East, Europe, and the USA. Increased echogenicity ("bright" scan) with ultrasonography or increased radiolucency with computerized tomography (compared with kidney) provide supportive evidence of fatty liver. In most regions, ultrasonographic surveys of the general population indicate that almost one-quarter of the adult population has hepatic steatosis [35, 36]. Fatty liver is more common in males than females, particularly in Asians [37]. In support of sex differences in fatty liver among Asians, the prevalence of ultrasonographic fatty liver was examined by sex and age in 3,229 Japanese adults from 2005 to 2006 in a health checkup center in Tokushima. Fatty liver was 2.5-fold more prevalent in males (31.5%) than in females (12.4%). Although fatty liver was more prevalent in females over the age of 70 years, the biggest difference in the prevalence of fatty liver between females and males was found in individuals of less than 50 years old [7]. Furthermore, among 3,175 Shanghai adults, the peak prevalence of fatty liver in males occurred earlier (40-49 years) than in females (over 50 years) [38].

Central obesity (visceral fat accumulation) is a more important factor for hepatic steatosis than body mass index, which reflects total body fat accumulation, or subcutaneous fat accumulation. It should be noted that regional fat distribution differs between men and women. After correction for total body fat mass, men generally have larger visceral fat areas than women [39], and it has been suggested that this is an important correlate of the sex differences in NAFLD/NASH.

Oxidative Stress in Liver Injury and Hepatic Stellate Cell Activation

Damage to the parenchymal cell membranes could produce reactive oxygen species (ROS) derived from lipid peroxidative processes, which constitute a general feature of a sustained inflammatory response and liver injury, once antioxidant mechanisms have been depleted. Cells are well equipped to neutralize the effects of ROS, by virtue of a series of antioxidant protective systems, including superoxide dismutase (SOD), glutathione peroxidase, glutathione (GSH), and thioredoxin. Although a single liver injury eventually results in an almost complete resolution, the persistence of the original insult causes a prolonged activation of tissue repair mechanisms, thereby leading to hepatic fibrosis rather than to effective tissue repair. Hepatic fibrosis, or the collagen deposition, is associated with inflammation and cell death, which is a consequence of severe liver damage that occurs in many patients with chronic liver disease, regardless of the etiology such as HBV/HCV infection, alcohol abuse, and iron overload [40]. In other words, collagen production predominates over hepatocellular regeneration. When hepatocytes are continuously damaged and replicated, the frequencies of genetic alteration also probably increase along with hepatic fibrosis, leading to the development of cirrhosis and HCC. Collagens are mainly produced by cells known as hepatic stellate cells (HSCs). HSCs are located in the space of Disse in close contact with hepatocytes and sinusoidal endothelial cells (Figrue 2). In the injured liver, HSCs are regarded as the primary target cells for inflammatory and peroxidative stimuli and they are transformed into myofibroblast-like cells. These HSCs are referred to as activated cells and this activation is accompanied by a loss of cellular retinoid, and the synthesis of α-smooth muscle actin (SMA), and large quantities of the major components of the extracellular matrix, including collagen types I and III.

Transgenic mice expressing HBsAg exhibit the generation of oxidative stress and DNA damage, thus leading to the enhancement of hepatic fibrogenesis and carcinogenesis [41, 42]. In addition, HBV X (HBx) protein alters the mitochondrial transmembrane potential and enhances ROS production in the liver [43].

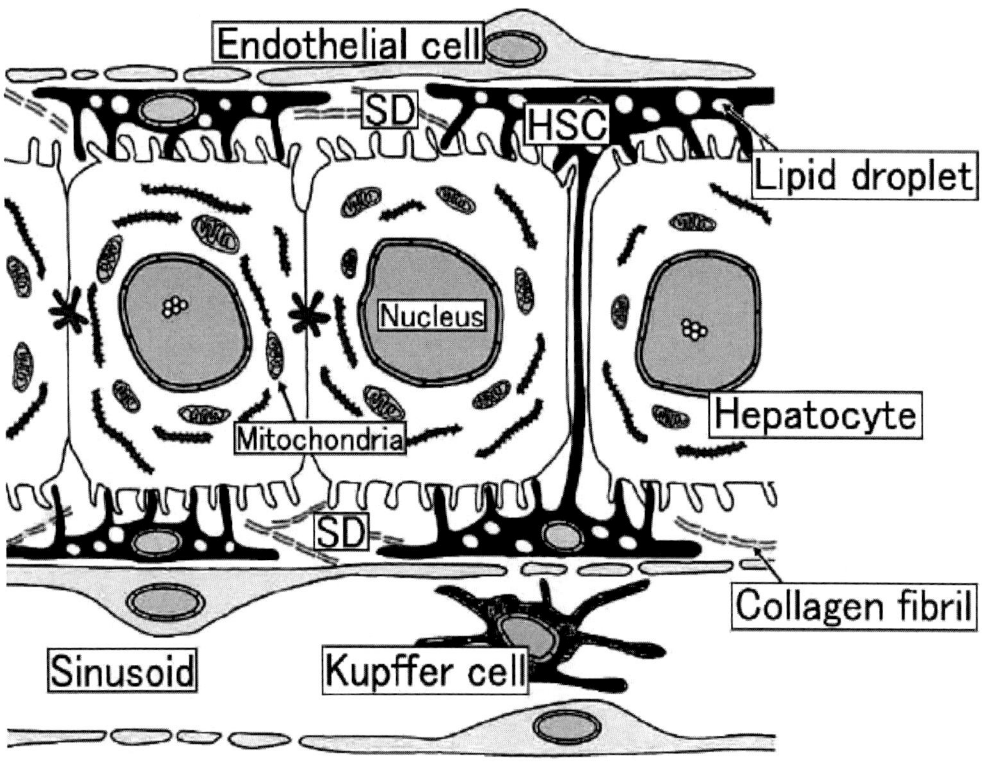

Figure 2. Schema of the sinusoidal wall of the liver. Kupffer cells rest on fenestrated endothelial cells. HSCs are located in the space of Disse (SD) in close contact with endothelial cells and hepatocytes, functioning as the primary retinoid storage area. Retinoids are occupied in the cytoplasmic space by numerous lipid droplets (Lipid droplet). Collagen fibrils course through the SD.

A primary source of ROS production in hepatocytes and HSCs is mitochondrial NADH/NADPH oxidase. Hydrogen peroxide is more stable and membrane permeable in comparison to other ROS, thus leading to the hypothesis that it induces the activation of several signaling pathways including the extracellular signal-regulated kinase (ERK), c-Jun

N-terminal kinase/stress-activated protein kinase (JNK), and p38 mitogen-activated protein kinase (MAPK) cascades, acting as a second messenger to: (1) induce the gene expression of redox sensitive transcription factors, such as activator protein (AP)-1 and nuclear factor (NF)-κB [44], (2) stimulate apoptosis [45], and (3) modulate cell proliferation [46]. AP-1 and NF-κB induce the expression of multiple genes involved in inflammation and oxidative stress response, cell death and fibrogenesis, including proinflammatory cytokines such as TNF-α and growth factors such as platelet-derived growth factor and transforming growth factor (TGF)-β. During TNF-α-induced apoptosis, hydrogen peroxide is an important mediator of cell death [47]. TGF-β is a major fibrogenic cytokine, acting as a paracrine and autocrine (from HSCs) mediator, which triggers and induces the activation of HSCs in vivo. Hydrogen peroxide is converted into the hydroxyl radical, a harmful and highly reactive ROS, in the presence of transition metals such as iron. The hydroxyl radical is able to induce DNA cleavage and lipid peroxidation in the structure of membrane phospholipids, leading to cell death. Malondialdehyde (MDA) and 4-hydroxynonenal (HNE), end products of lipid peroxidation, are discharged from injured hepatocytes into the space of Disse (Figrue 3). Paracrine stimuli derived from hepatocytes undergoing oxidative stress induce HSC proliferation and collagen synthesis, and that HSCs are activated by MDA and HNE as well as ROS [48, 49].

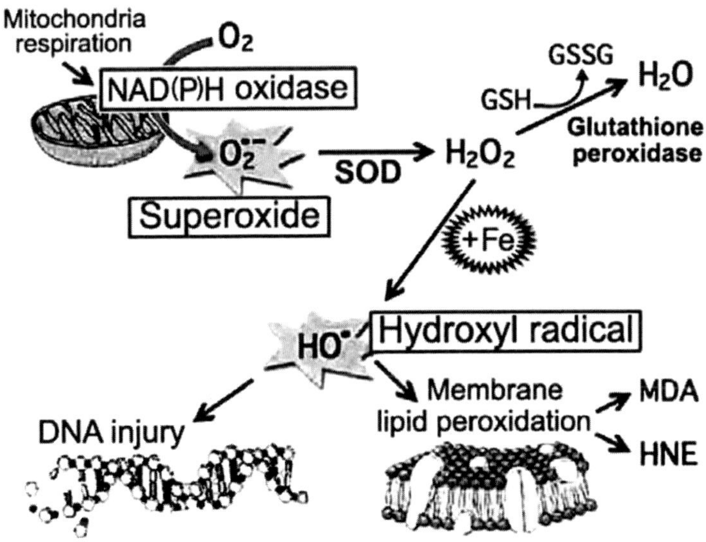

Figure 3. Oxidative stress and hepatocyte injury

A primary source of ROS production is mitochondrial NADH/NADPH oxidase. Hydrogen peroxide (H2O2) is converted to a highly reactive ROS, the hydroxyl radical, in the presence of iron (+ Fe). The hydroxyl radical induces DNA cleavage and lipid peroxidation in the structure of membrane phospholipids, leading to cell death and discharge of end products of lipid peroxidation, malondialdehyde (MDA) and 4-hydroxynonenal (HNE). Cells have comprehensive antioxidant protective systems, including SOD, glutathione peroxidase and GSH. Upon oxidation, GSH forms glutathione disulfide (GSSG).

It has become evidence that structural and non-structural (NS) proteins of HCV are involved in the generation of ROS in an infected liver. HCV core protein has been associated with increased ROS, decreased intracellular and/or mitochondrial GSH content, and increased levels of lipid peroxidation products [50]. NS3 protein of HCV has been found to activate NADPH oxidase in Kupffer cells to increase generation of ROS and other reactive species, which can exert oxidative stress on nearby cells [51].

Increased lipid peroxidation and its product accumulation are also commonly observed in alcoholic liver disease and NAFLD based on studies of human alcohol-related liver injury and animal models of diet-induced hepatic steatosis and drug-induced steatohepatitis [52-54]. In the progression of fatty liver disease, lipid peroxidation products are generated because of impaired oxidation of the accumulated fatty acids. Key mediators of impaired β-oxidation include an increased activity of CYP2E1 and a reduced electron transport in hepatocyte mitochondria. Such mitochondrial defects could possibly have a genetic basis [55] and are likely worsened by aging and environmental factors [56, 57] such as high saturated fats. Free fatty acids and adipocytokines such as leptin, adiponectin, and TNF-α, which are released by adipocytes in visceral fat tissue and flow directly into the liver via the portal vein [58], are involved in the development of metabolic syndrome and NAFLD. Visceral fat accumulation is an independent predictor of a fatty liver, and it arises through enlarged adipocytes (Figrue 4). Mitochondrial abnormalities have been described in the livers of patients with NASH [59]. Kupffer cell production of proinflammatory mediators such as TNF-α and ROS, which results in HSC activation with disordered collagen production (Figrue 5), are also thought to play an important role in NASH-associated cryptogenic cirrhosis. In addition, cell injury may occur when the capacity of hepatocytes to safely store fat is overwhelmed by continued uptake [60], local synthesis, or impaired egress of fatty acids [61]; these fatty acids then become toxic to the cell in a pathobiological process termed lipotoxicity. Lipotoxicity can cause cell death by the direct effects of lipid mediators on apoptosis. The fatty liver is predisposed to forms of injury that involve oxidative stress. Oxidative stress, TNF-α, other cytokines and chemokines are all present in NASH, but the ways in which they initiate or perpetuate steatohepatitis remain uncertain.

In the injured liver, activated Kupffer cells produce TNF-α and ROS as well as TGF-β. HSCs are also able to produce ROS through the activation of NADH/NADPH oxidase by ROS stimuli from outside the cell [62]. Exogenous TGF-β increases the ROS production by HSCs, whereas the addition of ROS induces TGF-β production and secretion by these cells [63]. This so-called autocrine loop of ROS by HSCs is regarded as mechanism corresponding to the autocrine loop of TGF-β which HSCs produce in response to this cytokine with an increased collagen expression in the injured liver [64] (Figrue 5).

Estrogens and Oxidative Stress in Hepatocytes

Estradiol and its derivatives are strong endogenous antioxidants that reduce lipid peroxide levels in the liver and serum [65, 66]. Our studies show that estradiol suppresses iron compound (ferric nitrilotriacetate)-induced ROS generation, lipid peroxidation, the activation of AP-1 and NF-κB, and the loss of SOD and glutathione peroxidase activities in cultured rat hepatocytes [67, 68].

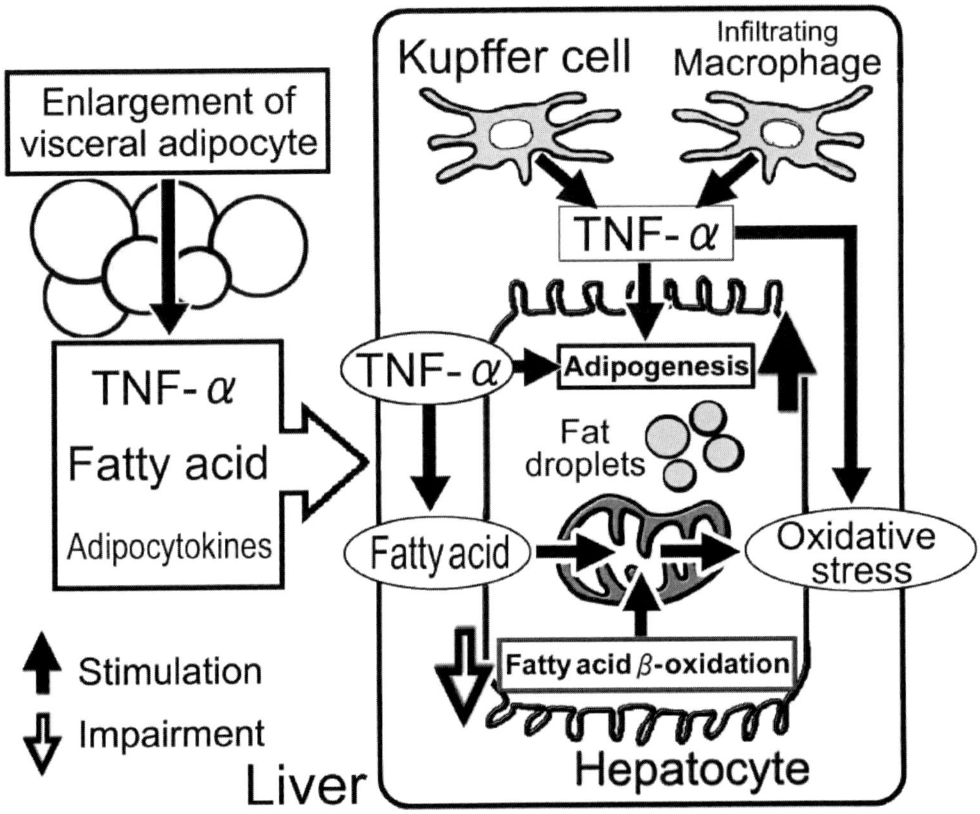

Figure 4. Working hypothesis regarding the disrupted balance between adipogenesis (increased) and fatty acid β-oxidation (impaired) in inducing hepatic steatosis . Hepatic steatosis is characterized by lipid deposition in hepatocytes. Enlargement of visceral adipocytes is an important factor for hepatic steatosis, which is principally induced by the increased adipogenesis and impaired fatty acid β-oxidation.

Estradiol is also found to inhibit iron compound ($FeSO_4$)-induced lipid peroxidation in isolated rat liver mitochondria [67]. These findings suggest that the inhibitory effect of estradiol on AP-1 and NF-κB activation may be caused by scavenging ROS and/or reducing the intracellular production of ROS via antioxidant enzyme induction.

Many of the actions of estradiol are mediated through the ER subtypes ERα and ERβ. In addition to the action of ER as a classical estrogen response element, ERα and ERβ also mediate gene transcription from an AP-1 enhancer element. Paech *et al.* reported that ERα and ERβ from an AP-1 site signaled in opposite ways when combined with estradiol: with ERα, estradiol activated transcription, whereas with ERβ, estradiol inhibited transcription [69]. A high level of expression of ERβ and a low level of ER α expression is seen in human and rat hepatocytes [68, 70, 71].

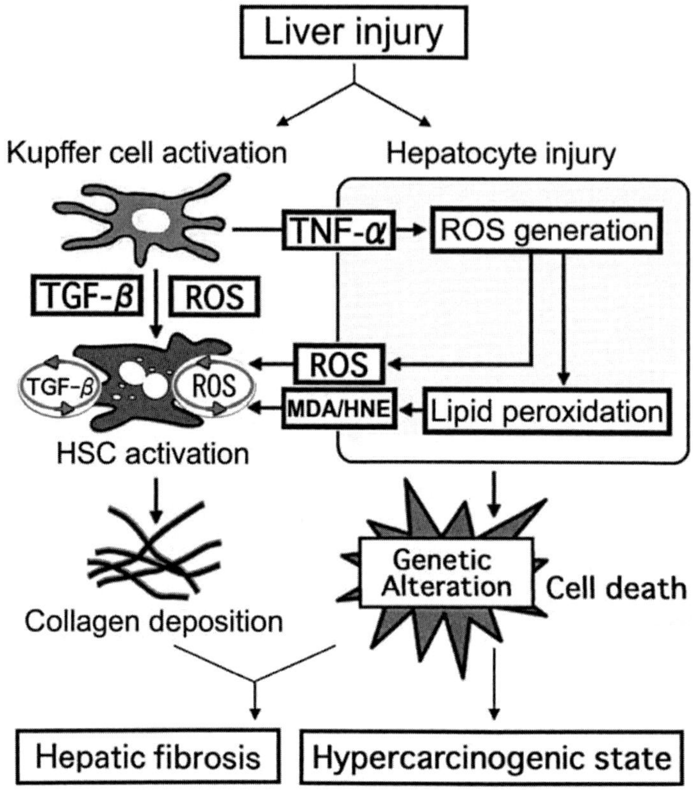

Figure 5. Hepatic fibrosis and hypercarcinogenic state associated with oxidative stress in hepatocytes and HSCs. In inflammatory and oxidative liver injury, activated Kupffer cells produce proinflammatory mediators including TNF-α and ROS. HSCs are activated by MDA and HNE as well as ROS. HSCs produce ROS and TGF-β in response to ROS and TGF-β thus creating a fibrogenic autocrine loop with an increased collagen expression in the injured liver. When hepatocytes are continuously damaged and replicated, the frequencies of genetic alteration also probably increase along with hepatic fibrosis, leading to the development of cirrhosis and HCC.

In addition, estradiol prevents early apoptosis induced by iron compound in cultured rat hepatocytes via the up-regulation of the Bcl-2 expression [68]. The overexpression of Bcl-2 is known to suppress lipid peroxidation and to prevent apoptosis, leading to an increase in cellular longevity. These findings suggest that estradiol may protect hepatocytes from oxidative damage, inflammatory cell injury and cell death by the suppression of AP-1 and NF-κB activation and the induction of Bcl-2 expression.

Estrogens and Hepatic Fibrosis

During ongoing HBV replication irrespective of the HBeAg seroconversion status, hepatic fibrosis eventually reaches the stage of cirrhosis. The rate of progression to cirrhosis in HBsAg-positive patients for 1-16 years was 24% in men and 8% in women [72], although, in a study of 1506 asymptomatic HBV carriers, the cirrhosis incidence rate was 0.7% annually [73]. Using multivariate analysis with patients with chronic HBV infection, Iloeje et al. in Taiwan [74] and Zarski et al. in France [75] have reported that independent predictors for cirrhosis include a male sex and an age of older than 50 years. McMahon also demonstrated that male sex and old age are the most important factors associated with progression of the disease in chronic hepatitis B [76]. However, patients infected with HBV genotype C is shown to have delayed HBeAg seroconversion, longer periods of viremia, a greater risk of progressive disease, and a correspondingly higher rate of cirrhosis and HCC [77]. Genotypes C and B are prevalent in Asia, whereas genotypes A and D prevail in Western countries. In addition, the significance of an older age as a risk factor may reflect the prolonged duration of the underlying liver disease in conjunction with the accumulation of exposure to environmental risk factors such as aflatoxin in highly endemic areas [78]. An increasing prevalence of HBeAg-negative chronic hepatitis B has recently been observed in many countries [79, 80]. The HBeAg-negative chronic hepatitis B patients are usually males and older than those with HBeAg-positive chronic hepatitis B [80]. Moreover, the age at acute infection plays an important role in the development of chronicity. Neonatal infection, common in areas of high or intermittent HBV prevalence, is associated with high rates of chronicity, while infection at an adult age, is only occasionally observed. On the other hand, hepatic fibrosis eventually reaches the stage of cirrhosis in 15-25% of cases for an average of 20-30 years during chronic HCV infection. Using multivariate analysis with patients with chronic hepatics C, Poynard et al. reported that the male gender was associated with advanced fibrosis, which was independent of age at the time of an HCV infection and of alcohol consumption, and that the progression of fibrosis began to accelerate at 50 years of age, irrespective of the duration of the virus infection [2]. Kage et al. also reported that patients $\geq$ 50 years of age have a progression rate of hepatic fibrosis twice as high as those less than 50 years of age [81]. In addition, a preliminary report concluded that concomitant administration of estradiol resulted in a reduction in serum liver enzyme levels and hepatic iron concentration (HIC) in a young male patient with chronic hepatitis C and irradiation-induced testicular dysfunction, in whom testosterone replacement therapy was initiated at puberty [82]. Judging from these findings together with the average menopausal age of 50 years, both factors of a "female sex" and an "age of younger than 50 years", characteristic of premenopausal women could possibly play a protective role against the progression of chronic liver injury leading to cirrhosis [7, 83].

In studies using animals, estradiol treatment results in the suppression of early apoptosis and hepatic fibrosis. This is accompanied by a reduced collagen content and lower levels of procollagen type I and III mRNA and α-SMA expression as well as induced Bcl-2 expression in the liver of the hepatic fibrosis models in male rats [84-86]. In addition, treatment with a neutralizing antibody against rat estradiol in males and an ovarectomy in females leads to enhanced fibrogenesis [84]. In addition, rat HSCs possess functional ERβ, but not ERα, to respond directly to estradiol exposure, and estradiol attenuates the production of collagen type I, α-SMA expression and cell proliferation in cultured rat HSCs [70, 84, 85]. A recent report indicates that estradiol inhibits ROS generation and antioxidant enzyme loss via the suppression of NADH/NADPH oxidase activity, and blocks hydrogen peroxide-induced TGF-β expression, HSC proliferation and transformation, and the activation of MAPK pathways (ERK, JNK, and p38 MAPK) and transcription factors (AP-1 and NF-κB) in cultured rat HSCs [64]. These findings suggest that, by suppressing NADH/NADPH oxidase activity, estradiol prevents the autocrine loop of ROS and TGF-β by HSCs and HSC activation, and estradiol acts as cytoprotective action against hepatocyte injury.

Females and Hepatic Steatosis

Chronic hepatitis B and C are both frequently associated with hepatic steatosis. The frequency of hepatic steatosis in chronic hepatitis B ranges from 27 to 51%, while in chronic hepatitis C it is between 31 and 72% [87-90]. Hepatic steatosis is a characteristic feature of chronic HBV and HCV infections. It is suggested that hepatic steatosis may reflect a direct cytopathic effect of HCV and may play a role in the progression of the disease. In support of these proposals, a transgenic mouse model, which expressed the HCV core gene, develops progressive hepatic steatosis and HCC [91, 92]. It is conceivable that following hepatocyte injury, hepatic steatosis leads to an increase in lipid peroxidation, which might contribute to HSC activation by releasing soluble mediators [93], and thereby inducing hepatic fibrosis.

In contrast to HCV, there is little information on the correlation between HBV-associated hepatic steatosis and hepatic fibrosis. Furthermore, the molecular mechanism by which HBV mediates hepatic steatosis has not yet been clearly studied. Although a cross-sectional study in Australia failed to confirm the impact of hepatic steatosis on hepatic fibrosis in chronic hepatitis B, but not C [94], another cross-sectional analysis in Taiwanese adults revealed that HBV carrier status, ultrasonographic fatty liver and male sex are independently associated with liver damage evaluated by a conventional marker, serum alanine aminotransferase (ALT) level [95]. Recently Kim *et al.* reported that HBx protein induces hepatic lipid accumulation mediated by sterol regulatory element binding protein 1 and peroxisome proliferator-activated receptor γ, leading to hepatic steatosis [96]. Increasing evidence indicates that hepatic lipid accumulation is related to hepatic fibrosis, inflammation, apoptosis, and cancer [97, 98].

Recent findings have shown that visceral fat accumulation can be an independent predictor of a fatty liver, even in patients with a normal body mass index, and it is much more harmful than the subcutaneous accumulation of adipose tissue [99, 100]. Human adipose tissue contains ERα and ERβ. Low estrogen levels in women with menopause are somehow associated with a loss in subcutaneous fat and a gain in visceral fat [101]. It has been reported that women treated with estrogen have a lower visceral accumulation of adipose tissue in comparison to controls [102]. Estrogen treatment of male-to-female transsexuals can increase the amount of subcutaneous adipose tissue; thus, estrogen changes the male type of visceral fat distribution into a female type of fat accumulation [103].

An experimental animal study showed that hepatic steatosis spontaneously becomes evident in an aromatase-deficient mouse, which lacks the intrinsic ability to produce estrogen and is impaired with respect to hepatocellular fatty acid β-oxidation. Estradiol replacement reduces hepatic steatosis and restores the impairment in mitochondrial and peroxisomal fatty acid β-oxidation to a wild-type level [104]. Our preliminary study also demonstrated that estradiol stimulated mRNA expression of adiponectin in matured adipocytes 3T3-L1 and inhibited TNF-α-induced fatty acid uptake into cultured rat hepatocytes [105]. Adiponectin inhibits the enlargement of visceral adipocytes and cellular fat accumulation. In addition, tamoxifen is a well known antiestrogen used in the hormone treatment of ER positive breast cancer, and it has been shown to be associated with an increased risk of developing fatty liver and NASH in such patients [106, 107]. Therefore, the greater progression of liver injury with steatosis regardless of the etiology in the male sex may be due, at least in part, to the decreased production of estradiol.

Menopause and Proinflammatory Cytokines

In inflammatory and oxidative liver injury, the accumulation of leukocytes and macrophages including Kupffer cells to sites of inflammation and injury is thought to be mediated by chemokines, such as macrophage chemotactic protein (MCP)-1 and interleukin (IL)-8. These monocytes and macrophages are in turn able to release proinflammatory cytokines such as TNF-α, IL-1β and IL-6, leading to persistent liver injury. There is large body of evidence indicating that the decline in ovarian function with menopause is associated with spontaneous increases in TNF-α, IL-1β and IL-6 [108]. Estradiol, at physiological concentrations, has been shown to inhibit the spontaneous secretion of these proinflammatory cytokines in whole blood cultures [109] or PBMCs [110]. The spontaneous production of TNF-α and IL-1β by PBMCs is higher in patients with chronic hepatitis C than in healthy subjects [111]. Endotoxin-stimulated TNF-α production by PBMCs is also higher in HBsAg carriers with elevated ALT levels than in HBsAg carriers with normal ALT levels [112]. Moreover, TNF-α production by hepatocytes from patients with chronic HBV infection is reported to be transcriptionally up-regulated by HBx protein [113, 114]. Estradiol is able to attenuate IL-1β in ER expressing HepG2 cells [115], to inhibit secretion of IL-6 from Kupffer cells exposed to necrotic hepatocytes [116], and to ameliorate the burn-induced increase in serum TNF-α levels in rats [117]. In vivo treatment with estradiol transdermally in postmenopausal women decreases spontaneous IL-6 production by PBMCs after 12 months of the therapy [110]. Recent studies have also showed the inhibitory effects of estradiol on the unstimulated and hydrogen peroxide-stimulated production of TNF-α, IL-1β, IL-8, and MCP-1 in PBMCs from patients with chronic hepatitis C and in murine peritoneal macrophages [118, 119]. These findings suggest that estradiol may exert a hepatoprotective action against inflammation and oxidative stress, at least in part, by preventing macrophage accumulation and inhibiting proinflammatory cytokine production.

However, macrophages seem to respond differently to endotoxin in comparison to Kupffer cells as far as the signaling pathways are concerned [120]. Estrogen has been reported to increase the sensitivity of Kupffer cells to endotoxin [31], while estradiol augments increases in the serum levels of TNF-α after endotoxin treatment in animals [121].

Females and HCC

Both indirect and direct carcinogenic mechanisms are involved in the pathogenesis of HCC induced by chronic liver inflammation including HBV and HCV infections, alcoholic hepatitis, and steatohepatitis. HBV/HCV infection may induce HCC indirectly by causing chronic necroinflammatory liver disease [17]. When HBV/HCV replication is sustained, hepatocytes are continuously damaged and regenerated. HCV multiplication is particularly sustained throughout the course of a typical infection. Chronic necroinflammation may induce a malignant transformation by producing mutagenic ROS during the inflammatory process along with hepatic fibrosis, leading to the development of cirrhosis and HCC (Figrue 5). As indicated previously, a transgenic mouse model, expressing the HCV core gene, develops progressive HCC and hepatic steatosis [91, 92]. The active replication of HBV may also initiate malignant transformation through a direct carcinogenic mechanism by increasing the probability of insertion of viral DNA in or near proto-oncogenes, tumor-suppressor genes, or their regulatory elements in cellular DNA [122]. The integration of viral DNA may increase the production of transactivator protein HBx antigen, which may induce the malignant transformation of hepatocytes, and bind to the p53 tumor-suppressor gene and disrupt its functions [17, 123].

In chronic liver disease without regard for its etiology, both ROS and lipid peroxidation products damage DNA. The combination of DNA damage and increased cell proliferation causes gene mutations. It is generally accepted that multiple genetic alteration, which is induced by mutations, is important in carcinogenesis. As these mutations accumulate over the years, accompanied by constant apoptotic pressure, cells that resist apoptosis or escape the control of the cell cycle may be selected for, finally allowing the development of HCC [124].

Like the risk factors for hepatic fibrosis, male sex and age older than 50 years are important risk factors for HCC [125]. Conversely, premenopausal women without either factors of a male sex and an older age are least vulnerable to HCC. The age-specific male-to-female ratios were examined among Japanese HCC patients with HBV (n=901) and HCV (n=1199) infection in Tokushima. When these HCC patients were divided into two age groups, based on whether they were younger or older than the menopausal age of 50 years, the younger groups with HBV (10.5%) and HCV (15.0%) infection had a significant lower proportion of females than the older groups with HBV (32.8%) and HCV (30.0%) infection [7, 126]. The ER levels in cirrhotic livers obtained from premenopausal females were higher than in the male cirrhotic livers. Logistic regression identified an age greater than the menopausal age, male gender, a decreased ER level, and an increase in lipid peroxidation products as variables that were independently associated with the development of HCC in HCV-related cirrhotics [126]. Moreover, variant ERs have been reported to be expressed in HCC patients and, to a greater extent, in male patients with chronic liver disease than in female patients, even at an early stage of chronic liver disease [127, 128]. The occurrence of variant ERs leads to the loss of estrogen responsiveness. Experimentally induced carcinomas using carcinogens, as well as the appearance of spontaneous neoplasms, occur at a higher incidence in male rats and mice. A previous report shows the suppressive effect of estradiol on chemical hepatocarcinogenesis in rats induced with dimethylnitrosamine (DEN)-2-acetylaminofluorene (AAF)-partial hepatectomy (PH) [129] (Figrue 6). Recently Naugler *et al.* reported that suppression of IL-6 secretion from Kupffer cells by estradiol through ER resulted in an inhibition of DEN-induced hepatocarcinogenesis [116]. Taken together, these lines of evidence suggest that both estradiol production and the ER status may therefore play a role in the biological defense against hepatocarcinogenesis.

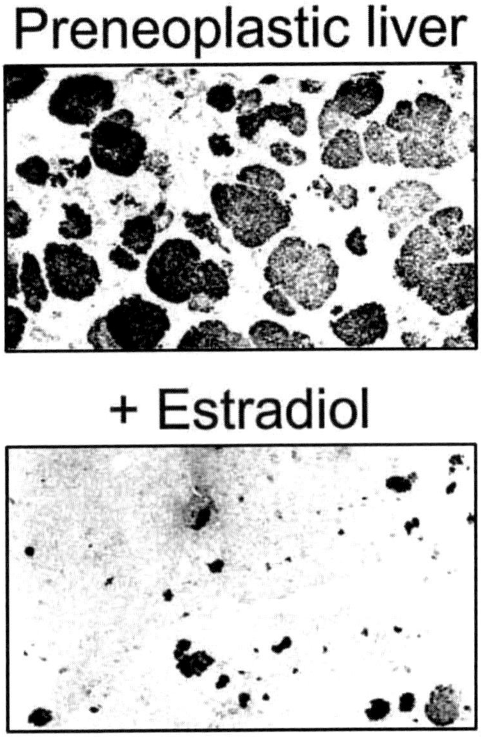

Figure 6. Estrogens and preneoplastic liver. Preneoplastic liver lesions were evaluated by means of an immunohistochemical analysis of glutathione-S-transferase placental form (GST-P) expression. GST-P-positive liver foci were induced using the DEN-AAF-PH model (Preneoplastic liver) in male rats with estradiol (+ Estradiol).

Conclusion

Sex-associated differences are not limited to chronic liver disease and they are of potential interest in cases of other chronic fibrogenic disorders as well. The predominance of atherosclerosis and the higher renal fibrosis progression rate in men are excellent lines of evidence that point to the role of estrogen in the wound healing/fibrogenic process [130]. It has been reported that estradiol inhibits the proliferation of vascular smooth muscle cells (VSMCs) [131]. VSMCs are anatomically analogous to HSCs, and are reported to express ERβ at a higher level after vascular injury with no significant changes in ERα expression [132]. Several studies have documented the antifibrogenic effect of estrogen on VSMCs [133, 134]. Moreover, renal mesangial cells are also the HSC analog and have similar properties including a prominent role in fibrogenesis. The cell proliferation and collagen synthesis in mesangial cells have been shown to be modulated by estradiol [135].

The present review indicates that estradiol may have beneficial properties on the progression of chronic liver disease. However, it should be noted that the administration of estradiol *per se* in women poses some potential risks, including an increased risk of developing breast cancer and endometrial abnormalities [136, 137]. In addition, estradiol and ER subtypes have been reported to play a role in the modulation of cholangiocyte proliferation [138], which is a typical hallmark for influencing cholestatic liver disease progression.

Being male or female is an important basic human variable that affects health and liver disease throughout the life span. A better understanding the biological mechanisms underlying the sex-associated differences during hepatic fibrogenesis and carcinogenesis would provide valuable information to design care of health and liver disease more effectively for individuals, both males and females.

References

[1] McMahon, B. J. Alberts, S. R. Wainwright, R. B. Bulkow, L. and Lanier, A. P. (1990). Hepatitis B-related sequelae: prospective study in 1400 hepatitis B surface antigen-positive Alaska native carriers. *Arch. Intern. Med.*, 150, 1051-1054.

[2] Poynard, T. Ratziu, V. Charlotte, F. Goodman, Z. McHutchison, J. and Albrecht, J. (2001). Rates and risk factors of liver fibrosis progression in patients with chronic hepatitis C. *J. Hepatol.*, 34, 730-739.

[3] Shimizu, I. (2003). Impact of estrogens on the progression of liver disease. *Liver Int.*, 23, 63-69.

[4] Kao, J. H. and Chen, D. S. (2002). Recent research progress in hepatocellular carcinoma. *J. Formos. Med. Assoc.*, 101, 239-248.

[5] Chisari, F. V. and Ferrari, C. (1995). Hepatitis B virus immunopathogenesis. *Annu. Rev. Immunol.*, 13, 29-60.

[6] Parkin, D. M. Whelan, S. L. Ferlay, J. Teppo, L. and Thomas, D. B. (2002). Cancer incidence in five continents Vol. VIII, Lyon, France: IARC Scientific Publications.

[7] Shimizu, I. Kohno, N. Tamaki, K. Shono, M. Huang, H. W. He, J. H. and Yao, D. F. (2007). Female hepatology: favorable role of estrogen in chronic liver disease with hepatitis B virus infection. *World J. Gastroenterol.*, 13, 4295-4305.

[8] Harrison, S. A. Kadakia, S. Lang, K. A. and Schenker, S. (2002). Nonalcoholic steatohepatitis: what we know in the new millennium. *Am. J. Gastroenterol.,* 97, 2714-2724.

[9] Farrell, G. C. and Larter, C. Z. (2006). Nonalcoholic fatty liver disease: from steatosis to cirrhosis. *Hepatology*, 43, S99-S112.

[10] Weltman, M. D. Farrell, G. C. Hall, P. Ingelman-Sundberg, M. and Liddle, C. (1998). Hepatic cytochrome P450 2E1 is increased in patients with nonalcoholic steatohepatitis. *Hepatology*, 27, 128-133.

[11] Clark, J. M. Brancati, F. L. and Diehl, A. M. (2002). Nonalcoholic fatty liver disease. *Gastroenterology*, 122, 1649-1657.

[12] Browning, J. D. Szczepaniak, L. S. Dobbins, R. Nuremberg, P. Horton, J. D. Cohen, J. C. Grundy, S. M. and Hobbs, H. H. (2004). Prevalence of hepatic steatosis in an urban population in the United States: impact of ethnicity. *Hepatology*, 40, 1387-1395.

[13] Brunetto, M. R. Oliveri, F. Coco, B. Leandro, G. Colombatto, P. Gorin, J. M. and Bonino, F. (2002). Outcome of anti-HBe positive chronic hepatitis B in alpha-

interferon treated and untreated patients: a long term cohort study. *J. Hepatol.*, 36, 263-270.

[14] Hsu, Y. S. Chien, R. N. Yeh, C. T. Sheen, I. S. Chiou, H. Y. Chu, C. M. and Liaw, Y. F. (2002). Long-term outcome after spontaneous HBeAg seroconversion in patients with chronic hepatitis *B. Hepatology*, 35, 1522-1527.

[15] Bortolotti, F. Jara, P. Crivellaro, C. Hierro, L. Cadrobbi, P. Frauca, E. Camarena, C. De, L., V Diaz, C. De, M. L. and Noventa, F. (1998). Outcome of chronic hepatitis B in Caucasian children during a 20-year observation period. *J. Hepatol.*, 29, 184-190.

[16] Chan, H. L. Hui, A. Y. Wong, M. L. Tse, A. M. Hung, L. C. Wong, V. W. and Sung, J. J. (2004). Genotype C hepatitis B virus infection is associated with an increased risk of hepatocellular carcinoma. *Gut,* 53, 1494-1498.

[17] Yang, H. I. Lu, S. N. Liaw, Y. F. You, S. L. Sun, C. A. Wang, L. Y. Hsiao, C. K. Chen, P. J. Chen, D. S. and Chen, C. J. (2002). Hepatitis B e antigen and the risk of hepatocellular carcinoma. *N. Engl. J. Med.*, 347, 168-174.

[18] Zacharakis, G. H. Koskinas, J. Kotsiou, S. Papoutselis, M. Tzara, F. Vafeiadis, N. Archimandritis, A. J. and Papoutselis, K. (2005). Natural history of chronic HBV infection: a cohort study with up to 12 years follow-up in North Greece (part of the Interreg I-II/EC-project). *J. Med. Virol.*, 77, 173-179.

[19] Grossman, C. J. (1985). Interactions between the gonadal steroids and the immune system. *Science*, 227, 257-261.

[20] Blumberg, B. S. Sutnick, A. I. London, W. T. and Melartin, L. (1972). Sex distribution of Australia antigen. *Arch. Intern. Med.*, 130, 227-231.

[21] Furusyo, N. Hayashi, J. Sawayama, Y. Kishihara, Y. and Kashiwagi, S. (1999). Hepatitis B surface antigen disappearance and hepatitis B surface antigen subtype: a prospective, long-term, follow-up study of Japanese residents of Okinawa, Japan with chronic hepatitis B virus infection. *Am. J. Trop. Med. Hyg.*, 60, 616-622.

[22] Fox, H. S. Bond, B. L. and Parslow, T. G. (1991). Estrogen regulates the IFN-gamma promoter. *J. Immunol.*, 146, 4362-4367.

[23] Clerici, E. Bergamasco, E. Ferrario, E. and Villa, M. L. (1991). Influence of sex steroids on the antigen-specific primary antibody response in vitro. *J. Clin. Lab. Immunol.*, 34, 71-78.

[24] Sjogren, M. H. (2005). Prevention of hepatitis B in nonresponders to initial hepatitis B virus vaccination. *Am. J. Med.* 118 Suppl 10A, 34S-39S.

[25] Su, F. H. Chen, J. D. Cheng, S. H. Lin, C. H. Liu, Y. H. and Chu, F. Y. (2007). Seroprevalence of Hepatitis-B infection amongst Taiwanese university students 18 years following the commencement of a national Hepatitis-B vaccination program. *J. Med. Virol.*, 79, 138-143.

[26] Tanaka, J. Kumagai, J. Katayama, K. Komiya, Y. Mizui, M. Yamanaka, R. Suzuki, K. Miyakawa, Y. and Yoshizawa, H. (2004). Sex- and age-specific carriers of hepatitis B and C viruses in Japan estimated by the prevalence in the 3,485,648 first-time blood donors during 1995-2000. *Intervirology*, 47, 32-40.

[27] Bakr, I. Rekacewicz, C. El, H. M. Ismail, S. El, D. M. El-Kafrawy, S. Esmat, G. Hamid, M. A. Mohamed, M. K. and Fontanet, A. (2006). Higher clearance of hepatitis C virus infection in females compared with males. *Gut*, 55, 1183-1187.

[28] Conjeevaram, H. S. Fried, M. W. Jeffers, L. J. Terrault, N. A. Wiley-Lucas, T. E. Afdhal, N. Brown, R. S. Belle, S. H. Hoofnagle, J. H. Kleiner, D. E. and Howell, C. D. (2006). Peginterferon and ribavirin treatment in African American and Caucasian American patients with hepatitis C genotype 1. *Gastroenterology*, 131, 470-477.

[29] Nagoshi, S. (2008). Sex- or gender-specific medicine in hepatology. Hepatol Res, 38, 219-224.

[30] Lieber, C. S. (1995). Medical disorders of alcoholism. *N. Engl. J. Med.,* 333, 1058-1065.

[31] Ikejima, K. Enomoto, N. Iimuro, Y. Ikejima, A. Fang, D. Xu, J. Forman, D. T. Brenner, D. A. and Thurman, R. G. (1998). Estrogen increases sensitivity of hepatic Kupffer cells to endotoxin. *Am. J. Physiol.*, 274, G669-G676.

[32] Yin, M. Ikejima, K. Wheeler, M. D. Bradford, B. U. Seabra, V. Forman, D. T. Sato, N. and Thurman, R. G. (2000). Estrogen is involved in early alcohol-induced liver injury in a rat enteral feeding model. *Hepatology*, 31, 117-123.

[33] Jarvelainen, H. A. Lukkari, T. A. Heinaro, S. Sippel, H. and Lindros, K. O. (2001). The antiestrogen toremifene protects against alcoholic liver injury in female rats. *J. Hepatol.*, 35, 46-52.

[34] Poynard, T. Mathurin, P. Lai, C. L. Guyader, D. Poupon, R. Tainturier, M. H. Myers, R. P. Muntenau, M. Ratziu, V. Manns, M. Vogel, A. Capron, F. Chedid, A. and Bedossa, P. (2003). A comparison of fibrosis progression in chronic liver diseases. *J. Hepatol.*, 38, 257-265.

[35] Sanyal, A. J. (2002). AGA technical review on nonalcoholic fatty liver disease. *Gastroenterology,* 123, 1705-1725.

[36] Clark, J. M. and Diehl, A. M. (2003). Defining nonalcoholic fatty liver disease: implications for epidemiologic studies. *Gastroenterology*, 124, 248-250.

[37] Weston, S. R. Leyden, W. Murphy, R. Bass, N. M. Bell, B. P. Manos, M. M. and Terrault, N. A. (2005). Racial and ethnic distribution of nonalcoholic fatty liver in persons with newly diagnosed chronic liver disease. *Hepatology*, 41, 372-379.

[38] Fan, J. G. Zhu, J. Li, X. J. Chen, L. Li, L. Dai, F. Li, F. and Chen, S. Y. (2005). Prevalence of and risk factors for fatty liver in a general population of Shanghai, China. *J. Hepatol.*, 43, 508-514.

[39] Elbers, J. M. Asscheman, H. Seidell, J. C. and Gooren, L. J. (1999). Effects of sex steroid hormones on regional fat depots as assessed by magnetic resonance imaging in transsexuals. *Am. J. Physiol.*, 276, E317-E325.

[40] Poli, G. (2000). Pathogenesis of liver fibrosis: role of oxidative stress. *Mol. Aspects Med.,* 21, 49-98.

[41] Hagen, T. M. Huang, S. Curnutte, J. Fowler, P. Martinez, V. Wehr, C. M. Ames, B. N. and Chisari, F. V. (1994). Extensive oxidative DNA damage in hepatocytes of transgenic mice with chronic active hepatitis destined to develop hepatocellular carcinoma. *Proc. Natl. Acad. Sci. U S A*, 91, 12808-12812.

[42] Nakamoto, Y. Suda, T. Momoi, T. and Kaneko, S. (2004). Different procarcinogenic potentials of lymphocyte subsets in a transgenic mouse model of chronic hepatitis B. *Cancer Res.*, 64, 3326-3333.

[43] Waris, G. Huh, K. W. and Siddiqui, A. (2001). Mitochondrially associated hepatitis B virus X protein constitutively activates transcription factors STAT-3 and NF-kappa B via oxidative stress. *Mol. Cell. Biol.*, 21, 7721-7730.

[44] Pinkus, R. Weiner, L. M. and Daniel, V. (1996). Role of oxidants and antioxidants in the induction of AP-1, NF-kappaB, and glutathione S-transferase gene expression. *J. Biol. Chem.*, 271, 13422-13429.

[45] Clement, M. V. and Pervaiz, S. (1999). Reactive oxygen intermediates regulate cellular response to apoptotic stimuli: an hypothesis. *Free Radic. Res.*, 30, 247-252.

[46] Lundberg, A. S. Hahn, W. C. Gupta, P. and Weinberg, R. A. (2000). Genes involved in senescence and immortalization. *Curr. Opin. Cell Biol.*, 12, 705-709.

[47] Bohler, T. Waiser, J. Hepburn, H. Gaedeke, J. Lehmann, C. Hambach, P. Budde, K. and Neumayer, H. H. (2000). TNF-alpha and IL-1alpha induce apoptosis in subconfluent rat mesangial cells. Evidence for the involvement of hydrogen peroxide and lipid peroxidation as second messengers. *Cytokine*, 12, 986-991.

[48] Lee, K. S. Buck, M. Houglum, K. and Chojkier, M. (1995). Activation of hepatic stellate cells by TGF alpha and collagen type I is mediated by oxidative stress through c-myb expression. *J. Clin. Invest.*, 96, 2461-2468.

[49] Parola, M. Pinzani, M. Casini, A. Albano, E. Poli, G. Gentilini, P. and Dianzani, M. U. (1993). Stimulation of lipid peroxidation or 4-hydroxynonenal treatment increases procollagen (I) gene expression in human liver fat-storing cells. *Biochem. Biophys. Res. Commun.*, 194, 1044-1050.

[50] Moriya, K. Nakagawa, K. Santa, T. Shintani, Y. Fujie, H. Miyoshi, H. Tsutsumi, T. Miyazawa, T. Ishibashi, K. Horie, T. Imai, K. Todoroki, T. Kimura, S. and Koike, K. (2001). Oxidative stress in the absence of inflammation in a mouse model for hepatitis C virus-associated hepatocarcinogenesis. *Cancer Res.*, 61, 4365-4370.

[51] Thoren, F. Romero, A. Lindh, M. Dahlgren, C. and Hellstrand, K. (2004). A hepatitis C virus-encoded, nonstructural protein (NS3) triggers dysfunction and apoptosis in lymphocytes: role of NADPH oxidase-derived oxygen radicals. *J. Leukoc. Biol.,* 76, 1180-1186.

[52] Letteron, P. Duchatelle, V. Berson, A. Fromenty, B. Fisch, C. Degott, C. Benhamou, J. P. and Pessayre, D. (1993). Increased ethane exhalation, an in vivo index of lipid peroxidation, in alcohol-abusers. *Gut,* 34, 409-414.

[53] Letteron, P. Fromenty, B. Terris, B. Degott, C. and Pessayre, D. (1996). Acute and chronic hepatic steatosis lead to in vivo lipid peroxidation in mice. *J. Hepatol.*, 24, 200-208.

[54] Berson, A. De, B., V Letteron, P. Robin, M. A. Moreau, C. El Kahwaji, J. Verthier, N. Feldmann, G. Fromenty, B. and Pessayre, D. (1998). Steatohepatitis-inducing drugs cause mitochondrial dysfunction and lipid peroxidation in rat hepatocytes. *Gastroenterology,* 114, 764-774.

[55] Petersen, K. F. Dufour, S. Befroy, D. Garcia, R. and Shulman, G. I. (2004). Impaired mitochondrial activity in the insulin-resistant offspring of patients with type 2 diabetes. *N. Engl. J. Med.*, 350, 664-671.

[56] Petersen, K. F. Befroy, D. Dufour, S. Dziura, J. Ariyan, C. Rothman, D. L. DiPietro, L. Cline, G. W. and Shulman, G. I. (2003). Mitochondrial dysfunction in the elderly: possible role in insulin resistance. *Science,* 300, 1140-1142.

[57] Lowell, B. B. and Shulman, G. I. (2005). Mitochondrial dysfunction and type 2 diabetes. *Science*, 307, 384-387.

[58] Czaja, M. J. (2004). Liver injury in the setting of steatosis: crosstalk between adipokine and cytokine. *Hepatology*, 40, 19-22.

[59] Sanyal, A. J. Campbell-Sargent, C. Mirshahi, F. Rizzo, W. B. Contos, M. J. Sterling, R. K. Luketic, V. A. Shiffman, M. L. and Clore, J. N. (2001). Nonalcoholic steatohepatitis: association of insulin resistance and mitochondrial abnormalities. *Gastroenterology,* 120, 1183-1192.

[60] Donnelly, K. L. Smith, C. I. Schwarzenberg, S. J. Jessurun, J. Boldt, M. D. and Parks, E. J. (2005). Sources of fatty acids stored in liver and secreted via lipoproteins in patients with nonalcoholic fatty liver disease. *J. Clin. Invest.,* 115, 1343-1351.

[61] Larter, C. Z. and Farrell, G. C. (2006). Insulin resistance, adiponectin, cytokines in NASH: Which is the best target to treat? *J. Hepatol.*, 44, 253-261.

[62] Cui, X. Shimizu, I. Lu, G. Itonaga, M. Inoue, H. Shono, M. Tamaki, K. Fukuno, H. Ueno, H. and Ito, S. (2003). Inhibitory effect of a soluble transforming growth factor b type II receptor on the activation of rat hepatic stellate cells in primary culture [see comments]. *J. Hepatol.*, 39, 731-737.

[63] De Bleser, P. J. Xu, G. Rombouts, K. Rogiers, V. and Geerts, A. (1999). Glutathione levels discriminate between oxidative stress and transforming growth factor-beta signaling in activated rat hepatic stellate cells. *J. Biol. Chem.*, 274, 33881-33887.

[64] Itagaki, T. Shimizu, I. Cheng, X. Yuan, Y. Oshio, A. Tamaki, K. Fukuno, H. Honda, H. Okamura, Y. and Ito, S. (2005). Opposing effects of oestradiol and progesterone on intracellular pathways and activation processes in the oxidative stress induced activation of cultured rat hepatic stellate cells. *Gut,* 54, 1782-1789.

[65] Yoshino, K. Komura, S. Watanabe, I. Nakagawa, Y. and Yagi, K. (1987). Effect of estrogens on serum and liver lipid peroxide levels in mice. *J. Clin. Biochem. Nutr.*, 3, 233-239.

[66] Lacort, M. Leal, A. M. Liza, M. Martin, C. Martinez, R. and Ruiz-Larrea, M. B. (1995). Protective effect of estrogens and catecholestrogens against peroxidative membrane damage in vitro. *Lipids*, 30, 141-146.

[67] Omoya, T. Shimizu, I. Zhou, Y. Okamura, Y. Inoue, H. Lu, G. Itonaga, M. Honda, H. Nomura, M. and Ito, S. (2001). Effects of idoxifene and estradiol on NF-κB activation in cultured rat hepatocytes undergoing oxidative stress. *Liver*, 21, 183-191.

[68] Inoue, H. Shimizu, I. Lu, G. Itonaga, M. Cui, X. Okamura, Y. Shono, M. Honda, H. Inoue, S. Muramatsu, M. and Ito, S. (2003). Idoxifene and estradiol enhance antiapoptotic activity through the estrogen receptor-beta in cultured rat hepatocytes. *Dig. Dis. Sci.*, 48, 570-580.

[69] Paech, K. Webb, P. Kuiper, G. G. Nilsson, S. Gustafsson, J. Kushner, P. J. and Scanlan, T. S. (1997). Differential ligand activation of estrogen receptors ERalpha and ERbeta at AP1 sites. *Science*, 277, 1508-1510.

[70] Zhou, Y. Shimizu, I. Lu, G. Itonaga, M. Okamura, Y. Shono, M. Honda, H. Inoue, S. Muramatsu, M. and Ito, S. (2001). Hepatic stellate cells contain the functional estrogen receptor beta but not the estrogen receptor alpha in male and female rats. *Biochem. Biophys. Res. Commun.*, 286, 1059-1065.

[71] Cheng, X. Shimizu, I. Yuan, Y. Wei, M. Shen, M. Huang, H. Urata, M. Sannomiya, K. Fukuno, H. Hashimoto-Tamaoki, T. and Ito, S. (2006). Combined effects of estradiol and progesterone on tumor necrosis factor alpha-induced apoptosis in human hepatoma HuH-7 cells. *Life Sci.*, 79, 1988-1994.

[72] Fattovich, G. Brollo, L. Giustina, G. Noventa, F. Pontisso, P. Alberti, A. Realdi, G. and Ruol, A. (1991). Natural history and prognostic factors for chronic hepatitis type B. *Gut*, 32, 294-298.

[73] Yu, M. W. Hsu, F. C. Sheen, I. S. Chu, C. M. Lin, D. Y. Chen, C. J. and Liaw, Y. F. (1997). Prospective study of hepatocellular carcinoma and liver cirrhosis in asymptomatic chronic hepatitis B virus carriers. *Am. J. Epidemiol.*, 145, 1039-1047.

[74] Iloeje, U. H. Yang, H. I. Su, J. Jen, C. L. You, S. L. and Chen, C. J. (2006). Predicting cirrhosis risk based on the level of circulating hepatitis B viral load. Gastroenterology, 130, 678-686.

[75] Zarski, J. P. Marcellin, P. Leroy, V. Trepo, C. Samuel, D. Ganne-Carrie, N. Barange, K. Canva, V. Doffoel, M. and Cales, P. (2006). Characteristics of patients with chronic hepatitis B in France: predominant frequency of HBe antigen negative cases. *J. Hepatol.,* 45, 355-360.

[76] McMahon, B. J. (2004). The natural history of chronic hepatitis B virus infection. *Semin. Liver Dis.*, 24 Suppl 1, 17-21.

[77] Fung, S. K. and Lok, A. S. (2004). Hepatitis B virus genotypes: do they play a role in the outcome of HBV infection? *Hepatology*, 40, 790-792.

[78] Kensler, T. W. Egner, P. A. Wang, J. B. Zhu, Y. R. Zhang, B. C. Lu, P. X. Chen, J. G. Qian, G. S. Kuang, S. Y. Jackson, P. E. Gange, S. J. Jacobson, L. P. Munoz, A. and Groopman, J. D. (2004). Chemoprevention of hepatocellular carcinoma in aflatoxin endemic areas. *Gastroenterology*, 127, S310-S318.

[79] Funk, M. L. Rosenberg, D. M. and Lok, A. S. (2002). World-wide epidemiology of HBeAg-negative chronic hepatitis B and associated precore and core promoter variants. *J. Viral. Hepat*., 9, 52-61.

[80] Hadziyannis, S. J. and Papatheodoridis, G. V. (2006). Hepatitis B e antigen-negative chronic hepatitis B: natural history and treatment. *Semin. Liver Dis.* 26, 130-141.

[81] Kage, M. Shimamatu, K. Nakashima, E. Kojiro, M. Inoue, O. and Yano, M. (1997). Long-term evolution of fibrosis from chronic hepatitis to cirrhosis in patients with hepatitis C: morphometric analysis of repeated biopsies. *Hepatology*, 25, 1028-1031.

[82] Shimizu, I. Omoya, T. Kondo, Y. Kusaka, Y. Tsutsui, A. Shibata, H. Honda, H. Sano, N. and Ito, S. (2001). Estrogen therapy in a male patient with chronic hepatitis C and irradiation-induced testicular dysfunction. *Intern. Med.*, 40, 100-104.

[83] Shimizu, I. and Ito, S. (2007). Protection of estrogens against the progression of chronic liver disease. *Hepatol. Res.*, 37, 239-247.

[84] Yasuda, M. Shimizu, I. Shiba, M. and Ito, S. (1999). Suppressive effects of estradiol on dimethylnitrosamine-induced fibrosis of the liver in rats [see comments]. *Hepatology*, 29, 719-727.

[85] Shimizu, I. Mizobuchi, Y. Shiba, M. Ma, Y.-R. Horie, T. Liu, F. and Ito, S. (1999). Inhibitory effect of estradiol on activation of rat hepatic stellate cells in vivo and in vitro. *Gut*, 44, 127-136.

[86] Lu, G. Shimizu, I. Cui, X. Itonaga, M. Tamaki, K. Fukuno, H. Inoue, H. Honda, H. and Ito, S. (2004). Antioxidant and antiapoptotic activities of idoxifene and estradiol in hepatic fibrosis in rats. *Life Sci.*, 74, 897-907.

[87] Scheuer, P. J. Ashrafzadeh, P. Sherlock, S. Brown, D. and Dusheiko, G. M. (1992). The pathology of hepatitis C. *Hepatology*, 15, 567-571.

[88] Bach, N. Thung, S. N. and Schaffner, F. (1992). The histological features of chronic hepatitis C and autoimmune chronic hepatitis: a comparative analysis. *Hepatology*, 15, 572-577.

[89] Lefkowitch, J. H. Schiff, E. R. Davis, G. L. Perrillo, R. P. Lindsay, K. Bodenheimer, H. C., Jr. Balart, L. A. Ortego, T. J. Payne, J. Dienstag, J. L. and . (1993). Pathological diagnosis of chronic hepatitis C: a multicenter comparative study with chronic hepatitis B. The Hepatitis Interventional Therapy Group. *Gastroenterology*, 104, 595-603.

[90] Czaja, A. J. and Carpenter, H. A. (1993). Sensitivity, specificity, and predictability of biopsy interpretations in chronic hepatitis. *Gastroenterology*, 105, 1824-1832.

[91] Moriya, K. Yotsuyanagi, H. Shintani, Y. Fujie, H. Ishibashi, K. Matsuura, Y. Miyamura, T. and Koike, K. (1997). Hepatitis C virus core protein induces hepatic steatosis in transgenic mice. *J. Gen. Virol.*, 78 (Pt 7), 1527-1531.

[92] Moriya, K. Fujie, H. Shintani, Y. Yotsuyanagi, H. Tsutsumi, T. Ishibashi, K. Matsuura, Y. Kimura, S. Miyamura, T. and Koike, K. (1998). The core protein of hepatitis C virus induces hepatocellular carcinoma in transgenic mice. *Nat. Med.*, 4, 1065-1067.

[93] Gressner, A. M. Lotfi, S. Gressner, G. and Lahme, B. (1992). Identification and partial characterization of a hepatocyte-derived factor promoting proliferation of cultured fat-storing cells (parasinusoidal lipocytes). *Hepatology*, 16, 1250-1266.

[94] Gordon, A. McLean, C. A. Pedersen, J. S. Bailey, M. J. and Roberts, S. K. (2005). Hepatic steatosis in chronic hepatitis B and C: predictors, distribution and effect on fibrosis. *J. Hepatol.*, 43, 38-44.

[95] Lin, Y. C. Hsiao, S. T. and Chen, J. D. (2007). Sonographic fatty liver and hepatitis B virus carrier status: synergistic effect on liver damage in Taiwanese adults. *World J. Gastroenterol.*, 13, 1805-1810.

[96] Kim, K. H. Shin, H. J. Kim, K. Choi, H. M. Rhee, S. H. Moon, H. B. Kim, H. H. Yang, U. S. Yu, D. Y. and Cheong, J. (2007). Hepatitis B virus X protein induces hepatic steatosis via transcriptional activation of SREBP1 and PPARgamma. *Gastroenterology*, 132, 1955-1967.

[97] Ohata, K. Hamasaki, K. Toriyama, K. Matsumoto, K. Saeki, A. Yanagi, K. Abiru, S. Nakagawa, Y. Shigeno, M. Miyazoe, S. Ichikawa, T. Ishikawa, H. Nakao, K. and Eguchi, K. (2003). Hepatic steatosis is a risk factor for hepatocellular carcinoma in patients with chronic hepatitis C virus infection. *Cancer*, 97, 3036-3043.

[98] Powell, E. E. Jonsson, J. R. and Clouston, A. D. (2005). Steatosis: co-factor in other liver diseases. *Hepatology*, 42, 5-13.

[99] Bellentani, S. Saccoccio, G. Masutti, F. Croce, L. S. Brandi, G. Sasso, F. Cristanini, G. and Tiribelli, C. (2000). Prevalence of and risk factors for hepatic steatosis in Northern Italy. *Ann. Intern. Med.,* 132, 112-117.

[100] Omagari, K. Kadokawa, Y. Masuda, J. Egawa, I. Sawa, T. Hazama, H. Ohba, K. Isomoto, H. Mizuta, Y. Hayashida, K. Murase, K. Kadota, T. Murata, I. and Kohno, S. (2002). Fatty liver in non-alcoholic non-overweight Japanese adults: incidence and clinical characteristics. *J. Gastroenterol. Hepatol.,* 17, 1098-1105.

[101] Toth, M. J. Tchernof, A. Sites, C. K. and Poehlman, E. T. (2000). Effect of menopausal status on body composition and abdominal fat distribution. *Int. J. Obes. Relat. Metab. Disord.*, 24, 226-231.

[102] Haarbo, J. Marslew, U. Gotfredsen, A. and Christiansen, C. (1991). Postmenopausal hormone replacement therapy prevents central distribution of body fat after menopause. *Metabolism*, 40, 1323-1326.

[103] Elbers, J. M. Asscheman, H. Seidell, J. C. and Gooren, L. J. (1999). Effects of sex steroid hormones on regional fat depots as assessed by magnetic resonance imaging in transsexuals. *Am. J. Physiol.*, 276, E317-E325.

[104] Nemoto, Y. Toda, K. Ono, M. Fujikawa-Adachi, K. Saibara, T. Onishi, S. Enzan, H. Okada, T. and Shizuta, Y. (2000). Altered expression of fatty acid-metabolizing enzymes in aromatase- deficient mice. *J. Clin. Invest.*, 105, 1819-1825.

[105] Takenaka, H. Shimizu, I. Huang, H. He, J. Urata, M. Sannomiya, K. Tamaki, K. Honda, H. Shono, M. and Ito, S. (2007). Impact of estradiol on the sex-associated difference of fatty liver. *Gastroenterology*, 132, A-819.

[106] Van, H. M. Rahier, J. and Horsmans, Y. (1996). Tamoxifen-induced steatohepatitis. *Ann. Intern. Med.,* 124, 855-856.

[107] Oien, K. A. Moffat, D. Curry, G. W. Dickson, J. Habeshaw, T. Mills, P. R. and MacSween, R. N. (1999). Cirrhosis with steatohepatitis after adjuvant tamoxifen. *Lancet*, 353, 36-37.

[108] Pfeilschifter, J. Koditz, R. Pfohl, M. and Schatz, H. (2002). Changes in Proinflammatory Cytokine Activity after Menopause. *Endocr. Rev.*, 23, 90-119.

[109] Rogers, A. and Eastell, R. (2001). The effect of 17beta-estradiol on production of cytokines in cultures of peripheral blood. *Bone*, 29, 30-34.

[110] Rachon, D. Mysliwska, J. Suchecka-Rachon, K. Wieckiewicz, J. and Mysliwski, A. (2002). Effects of oestrogen deprivation on interleukin-6 production by peripheral blood mononuclear cells of postmenopausal women. *J. Endocrinol.*, 172, 387-395.

[111] Kishihara, Y. Hayashi, J. Yoshimura, E. Yamaji, K. Nakashima, K. and Kashiwagi, S. (1996). IL-1 beta and TNF-alpha produced by peripheral blood mononuclear cells before and during interferon therapy in patients with chronic hepatitis *C. Dig. Dis. Sci.,* 41, 315-321.

[112] Hsu, H. Y. Chang, M. H. Ni, Y. H. and Lee, P. I. (1999). Cytokine release of peripheral blood mononuclear cells in children with chronic hepatitis B virus infection. *J. Pediatr. Gastroenterol. Nutr.,* 29, 540-545.

[113] Gonzalez-Amaro, R. Garcia-Monzon, C. Garcia-Buey, L. Moreno-Otero, R. Alonso, J. L. Yague, E. Pivel, J. P. Lopez-Cabrera, M. Fernandez-Ruiz, E. and Sanchez-Madrid, F. (1994). Induction of tumor necrosis factor alpha production by human hepatocytes in chronic viral hepatitis. *J. Exp. Med.*, 179, 841-848.

[114] Lara-Pezzi, E. Majano, P. L. Gomez-Gonzalo, M. Garcia-Monzon, C. Moreno-Otero, R. Levrero, M. and Lopez-Cabrera, M. (1998). The hepatitis B virus X protein up-regulates tumor necrosis factor alpha gene expression in hepatocytes. *Hepatology*, 28, 1013-1021.

[115] Kilbourne, E. J. and Scicchitano, M. S. (1999). The activation of plasminogen activator inhibitor-1 expression by IL-1beta is attenuated by estrogen in hepatoblastoma HepG2 cells expressing estrogen receptor alpha. *Thromb. Haemost.*, 81, 423-427.

[116] Naugler, W. E. Sakurai, T. Kim, S. Maeda, S. Kim, K. Elsharkawy, A. M. and Karin, M. (2007). Gender disparity in liver cancer due to sex differences in MyD88-dependent IL-6 production. *Science,* 317, 121-124.

[117] Ozveri, E. S. Bozkurt, A. Haklar, G. Cetinel, S. Arbak, S. Yegen, C. and Yegen, B. C. (2001). Estrogens ameliorate remote organ inflammation induced by burn injury in rats. *Inflamm. Res.*, 50, 585-591.

[118] Huang, H. He, J. Yuan, Y. Aoyagi, E. Takenaka, H. Itagaki, T. Sannomiya, K. Tamaki, K. Harada, N. Shono, M. Shimizu, I. and Takayama, T. (2008). Opposing effects of estradiol and progesterone on the oxidative stress-induced production of chemokine and proinflammatory cytokines in murine peritoneal macrophages. *J. Med. Invest.,* 55, 133-141.

[119] Yuan, Y. Shimizu, I. Shen, M. Aoyagi, E. Takenaka, H. Itagaki, T. Urata, M. Sannomiya, K. Kohno, N. Tamaki, K. Shono, M. and Takayama, T. (2008). Effects of estradiol and progesterone on the proinflammatory cytokine production by mononuclear cells from patients with chronic hepatitis C. *World J. Gastroenterol.*, 14, 2200-2207.

[120] Schultze, R. L. Gangopadhyay, A. Cay, O. Lazure, D. and Thomas, P. (1999). Tyrosine kinase activation in LPS stimulated rat Kupffer cells. *Cell. Biochem. Biophys.*, 30, 287-301.

[121] Zuckerman, S. H. Bryan-Poole, N. Evans, G. F. Short, L. and Glasebrook, A. L. (1995). In vivo modulation of murine serum tumour necrosis factor and interleukin-6 levels during endotoxemia by oestrogen agonists and antagonists. Immunology, 86, 18-24.

[122] Matsubara, K. and Tokino, T. (1990). Integration of hepatitis B virus DNA and its implications for hepatocarcinogenesis. *Mol. Biol. Med.*, 7, 243-260.

[123] Wang, X. W. Gibson, M. K. Vermeulen, W. Yeh, H. Forrester, K. Sturzbecher, H. W. Hoeijmakers, J. H. and Harris, C. C. (1995). Abrogation of p53-induced apoptosis by the hepatitis B virus X gene. *Cancer Res.*, 55, 6012-6016.

[124] Sasaki, Y. (2006). Does oxidative stress participate in the development of hepatocellular carcinoma? *J. Gastroenterol.*, 41, 1135-1148.

[125] Tanaka, Y. Mukaide, M. Orito, E. Yuen, M. F. Ito, K. Kurbanov, F. Sugauchi, F. Asahina, Y. Izumi, N. Kato, M. Lai, C. L. Ueda, R. and Mizokami, M. (2006). Specific mutations in enhancer II/core promoter of hepatitis B virus subgenotypes C1/C2 increase the risk of hepatocellular carcinoma. *J. Hepatol.*, 45, 646-653.

[126] Shimizu, I. Inoue, H. Yano, M. Shinomiya, H. Wada, S. Tsuji, Y. Tsutsui, A. Okamura, S. Shibata, H. and Ito S (2001). Estrogen receptor levels and lipid peroxidation in hepatocellular carcinoma with hepatitis C virus infection. *Liver*, 21, 342-349.

[127] Villa, E. Camellini, L. Dugani, A. Zucchi, F. Grottola, A. Merighi, A. Buttafoco, P. Losi, L. and Manenti, F. (1995). Variant estrogen receptor messenger RNA species detected in human primary hepatocellular carcinoma. *Cancer Res.*, 55, 498-500.

[128] Villa, E. Dugani, A. Moles, A. Camellini, L. Grottola, A. Buttafoco, P. Merighi, A. Ferretti, I. Esposito, P. Miglioli, L. Bagni, A. Troisi, R. De Hemptinne, B. Praet, M. Callea, F. and Manenti, F. (1998). Variant liver estrogen receptor transcripts already occur at an early stage of chronic liver disease. *Hepatology*, 27, 983-988.

[129] Shimizu, I. Mizobuchi, Y. Ma, Y.-R. Liu, F. Shiba, M. Horie, T. and Ito, S. (1998). Suppressive effect of estradiol on chemical hepatocarcinogenesis in rats. *Gut*, 42, 112-119.

[130] Pinzani, M. Romanelli, R. G. and Magli, S. (2001). Progression of fibrosis in chronic liver diseases: time to tally the score. *J. Hepatol.* 34, 764-767.

[131] Vargas, R. Wroblewska, B. Rego, A. Hatch, J. and Ramwell, P. W. (1993). Oestradiol inhibits smooth muscle cell proliferation of pig coronary artery. *Br. J. Pharmacol.,* 109, 612-617.

[132] Lindner, V. Kim, S. K. Karas, R. H. Kuiper, G. G. Gustafsson, J. A. and Mendelsohn, M. E. (1998). Increased expression of estrogen receptor-β mRNA in male blood vessels after vascular injury. *Circ. Res.*, 83, 224-229.

[133] Bayard, F. Clamens, S. Meggetto, F. Blaes, N. Delsol, G. and Faye, J. C. (1995). Estrogen synthesis, estrogen metabolism, and functional estrogen receptors in rat arterial smooth muscle cells in culture. *Endocrinology*, 136, 1523-1529.

[134] Iafrati, M. D. Karas, R. H. Aronovitz, M. Kim, S. Sullivan-TR, J. Lubahn, D. B. O'Donnell-TF, J. Korach, K. S. and Mendelsohn, M. E. (1997). Estrogen inhibits the vascular injury response in estrogen receptor alpha-deficient mice. *Nat. Med.*, 3, 545-548.

[135] Kwan, G. Neugarten, J. Sherman, M. Ding, Q. Fotadar, U. Lei, J. and Silbiger, S. (1996). Effects of sex hormones on mesangial cell proliferation and collagen synthesis. Kidney Int, 50, 1173-1179.

[136] Colditz, G. A. Hankinson, S. E. Hunter, D. J. Willett, W. C. Manson, J. E. Stampfer, M. J. Hennekens, C. Rosner, B. and Speizer, F. E. (1995). The use of estrogens and progestins and the risk of breast cancer in postmenopausal women. *N. Engl. J. Med.*, 332, 1589-1593.

[137] Collaborative Group on Hormonal Factors in Breast Cancer. (1997). Breast cancer and hormone replacement therapy: collaborative reanalysis of data from 51 epidemiological studies of 52705 women with breast cancer and 108411 women without breast cancer. *Lancet,* 350, 1047-1059.

[138] Alvaro, D. Alpini, G. Onori, P. Perego, L. Svegliata, B. G. Franchitto, A. Baiocchi, L. Glaser, S. S. Le Sage, G. Folli, F. and Gaudio, E. (2000). Estrogens stimulate proliferation of intrahepatic biliary epithelium in rats. *Gastroenterology,* 119, 1681-1691.

In: Estrogens: Production, Functions and Applications
Editor: James R. Bartos, pp. 121-144
ISBN: 978-1-60741-086-7

Chapter IV

The Role of Estrogen-Therapy in Postpartum Psychiatric Disorders: An Update

Salvatore Gentile[2]
Department of Mental Health ASL Salerno, Italy

Abstract

Postpartum period represents one of the most critical phases of a woman's life. A percentage ranging between 10% and 20% of mothers may develop psychiatric disorders after parturition. Postpartum disorders with psychiatric symptoms are represented by three main syndromes: postpartum blues, postpartum depression, and postpartum psychosis.

One of the most exhaustive theories about the etiology of postpartum psychiatric disorders speculates that their onset may be due to the physiological changes in maternal estrogen levels during pregnancy and the first weeks after parturition.

However, in assessing available literature information about the role of estrogen-therapy in preventing and treating puerperal psychiatric diseases, all reviewed studies were found to suffer from severe methodological limitations. For this reason, further, well-designed, and strictly focused multi-center trials are warranted in order to firmly establish the effectiveness of estrogen-therapy in puerperal psychiatric disorders.

Keywords: *estrogen-treatment, postpartum depression, postpartum psychosis.*

---

[2] Dr. Salvatore Gentile, Department of Mental Health ASL Salerno, Head of Mental Health n. 4, Piazza Galdi 84013 Cava de' Tirreni (Salerno) Italy, tel. +39 098 4455439, fax +39 089 4455440, e-mail: salvatore_gentile@aliceposta.it. Each ordinary correspondence should be addressed to: Salvatore Gentile MD, Piazza Galdi 84013 Cava de' Tirreni (Salerno) Italy.

Background

Postpartum period represents one of the most critical phases of a woman's life. A percentage ranging between 10% and 20% of mothers may develop severe psychiatric disorders after parturition, especially affective-type.[1] Furthermore, postpartum mental disorders have been considered as the most frequent forms of maternal morbidity after delivery,[2] and they range in severity from early postpartum blues to puerperal psychosis. Whereas there is no evidence that postpartum (or maternity) blues is associated with detrimental events for the infant, both postpartum major depressive disorder and puerperal psychosis seriously interfere with the infants' later well-being; hence, such children will be at increased risk to suffer from socioemotional, cognitive, and psychiatric difficulties later in life.[3,4.5]

In addition, maternal depression determines significant effects on neonatal physiology: newborns of mothers affected by depressive symptoms during pregnancy and puerperium show elevated cortisol and norepinephrine levels, lower dopamine levels, and greater relative right frontal EEG asymmetry.[6] The repercussions of maternal depression on infant nutritional status and illness should also be stressed.[7]

During the last years, a growing number of studies have evaluated the potential role of different hormones in the etiology and the treatment of psychiatric disorders related to childbearing and, thus, theoretically caused or worsened by the fluctuation of hormonal concentrations. Most of these studies have been conducted on subpopulations of patients with poor response to classic psychotropic medications The majority of such researchers, however, have been specifically focused on investigating the effectiveness of estrogen supplementation as part of the overall management of postpartum mood changes and puerperal psychosis.

Given these premises, the aim of this chapter is to assess and summarize the existing literature data about the efficacy of estrogen-therapy in preventing and treating postpartum psychiatric disorders. A brief analysis of alternative, effective treatments of psychiatric disorders at postpartum onset will be also provided.

Study Selection

An extensive and unrestrictive computerized search (from 1970 to July 2008) on Medline/Pubmed, TOXNET, EMBASE, and Cochrane Databases was conducted, with the following search terms: estradiol, estrogen-treatment, hormonal treatment, treatment, therapy, postpartum depression, postnatal depression, puerperal depression, postpartum blues, postpartum psychosis, lactation, breastfeeding. Searches were mostly limited to randomized controlled trials. Since few studies were available on the topic, open-label trials and significant clinical observations were also reviewed. Secondary searches were performed using the bibliographies of reviewed articles. An extensive manual review of pertinent journals and textbooks was finally performed.

Psychiatric Disorders at Postpartum Onset Epidemiological Background

Maternity Blues

Maternity blues is considered a relatively mild, self-limiting state of emotional reactivity; its incidence ranges from 50% to 80% of new mothers.[8,9,10] Main symptoms are represented by emotional lability, increased anxiety, irritability, tearfulness, crying, sadness, confusion, and sleep disturbance. In the vast majority of cases, the clinical features occur abruptly 3-5 days after delivery and remit within 7-14 days.[1] Although maternity blues is considered by most as a physiological sequelae of childbirth, it must be considered as a strong predictor of postpartum depression: in fact, a percentage ranging from 13 to 20% of women who experience maternity blues will go on to develop major depressive episode in the first postpartum year.[11,12,13] Recently, a significant association has been also demonstrated between maternity blues and the occurrence of anxiety disorders during early postpartum period.[14] Hence, women with maternity blues should be carefully monitored in the first weeks after delivery with the aim of diagnosing those at risk of developing postpartum depression and/or anxiety disorders and providing specific interventions at an early stage of the disorder.[14]Conversely, the likelihood of developing postpartum blues is not related to a previous psychiatric history.[15]

Postpartum Nonpsychotic Depression

In accordance with DSM IV criteria, postpartum nonpsychotic depression has been defined as a major depressive episode occurring within the first 4 weeks after delivery. However, epidemiological studies suggest that the period of elevated risk for recurrence of major depressive episode spreads as far as the 3rd month after parturition.[16] Postpartum nonpsychotic depression represents the most frequent severe mood disorder in childbearing age as it affects a percentage ranging from 10% to 15% of women; as such, postpartum nonpsychotic depression represents a noteworthy health problem.[17,18,19,20] In addition, women with a personal history of depression appear to be more vulnerable to recurrent episodes during periods of relevant reproductive endocrine changes.[9] However, other non-psychotic psychiatric disorders may complicate the course of puerperium: of note, 2% of postpartum women may meet criteria for more than one disorder;[20] notably, antenatal depression, especially if complicated by comorbid anxiety disorders, and a previous history of premenstrual syndrome seem to represent keys risk factor for further episodes of postpartum depression.[21,22]Clinical features that may suggest the diagnosis of postpartum major depressive episode include anhedonia, feeling of guilt and hopelessness, dysphoria, insomnia, tearfulness, somatic symptoms, and suicidal thoughts, despite the overall incidence of suicidality is lower than that shown by non-postpartum depressed women.[23,24] Certain features seem to be useful for distinguishing postpartum nonpsychotic depression from a major depressive disorder occurring at other times in women's live.[25] A study that compared women with postpartum depression and women with major depressive disorder unrelated to childbearing reported that postpartum women tended to experience more severe depressive episodes than the non-postpartum women do; moreover, although both groups of women were equally likely to recover, the women with postpartum depression took significantly longer to respond to antidepressant treatment.[26] Other factors characterizing specifically postpartum non-psychotic depression also include illness onset at younger age, obsessional symptoms, and worse social adaptation after delivery.[27,28,29]

Puerperal Psychosis

Puerperal psychosis does not represent a specific nosological entity, but rather a variety of common functional psychosis puerperally triggered;[30,31] they usually begin between day 1 and week 6 postpartum (however, in 73% of cases the onset of puerperal psychosis is recordable by day 3 after delivery[32]) and occur in 0.1% to 0.2% of all pregnancies.[16,30,31]

Follow-up studies have demonstrated that the vast majority of puerperal psychosis are represented by bipolar disorder and unipolar major depression with psychotic features.[33] Manic episode is usually considered the most frequent acute psychotic event at postpartum onset, as it affects up to 35% of women with a history of bipolar disorder;[30] however, a number of epidemiological studies conversely suggest that postpartum episodes are almost exclusively depressive.[34]. However, until now there is no agreement in literature in individuating what is the most frequent clinical expression of postpartum psychosis: in fact, a recent retrospective study has suggested that hypomanic symptoms (such as feeling excited, reduced need of sleep, feeling active) rather that manic or depressive symptoms characterize particularly the early onset and development of postpartum psychosis.[30] In any case, postpartum psychosis has been associated with high risk of harming the infants.[35,36] It must be also highlighted that episodes of hospitalization for psychiatric morbidity before delivery are a specific predictor of postpartum psychosis: in fact, almost 10% of women with a history of hospitalization due to psychiatric disorders during pregnancy could develop postpartum psychosis:[37] this underscores the need for obstetricians to assess history of psychiatric symptoms and, with pediatrics and psychiatrists, to optimize the treatment of mothers diagnosed with psychiatric disorder through childbirth.[37]

Other Postpartum Psychiatric Disorders

Postpartum psychiatric disorders also include post-traumatic stress disorder, obsessive-compulsive disorder, and a wide spectrum of anxiety disorders;[38] however, there are no reports suggesting the efficacy of estrogen-treatment in such mental diseases.

Neurophysiological Background

Maternity Blues

Recently, maternity blues has been associated with a decreased serotoninergic activity during the first five days after delivery. Noradrenergic activity seems to be also impaired, as methoxy-4-hydroxyphenylglycol (MHPG) serum levels are significantly in mothers with maternity blues than in healthy controls. These findings seem to suggest that women with blues may show a higher stress sensitivity or a decreased stress coping and that these specificities may contribute to the onset of blues.[39]

Postpartum Nonpsychotic Depression

A number of studies have explored whether specific biological characteristics my underlie an increased puerperal psychiatric vulnerability: the literature on hormonal factors (including thyroid hormones, cortisol, prolactin, and melatonin) that have been postulated as etiologic in postpartum depression is wide.[40,41,42,43] However, the most extensively explored theory about the role of hormonal changes in determining postpartum psychiatric disorders has stressed the physiological oscillations of maternal estrogen levels during pregnancy and the first weeks after delivery. As a consequence, it is possible that subpopulations of younger women may have a specific biological vulnerability to psychiatric disorders that could be catalyzed by physiological fluctuations of gonadal steroids.[1]'[44,45,46] At the end of the term of pregnancy serum estradiol levels are very high;[47] this estradiol is of placental origin. After parturition, however, estradiol levels abruptly decline.[48] This well-known physiological event has been defined "estrogen-withdrawal syndrome".[**33**] Ovarian production of sexual hormones may recover slowly: therefore, postpartum estradiol deficiency could be severe, prolonged, and more likely to induce a wide spectrum of repercussions on maternal mood, behavior, and new memory acquisition.[49,50,51,52] Despite the postulated relationship between periods of hormonal changes and affective weakness, however, no abnormalities in maternal estradiol levels have been identified to explain reproductive endocrine-related psychiatric disorders. In fact, more than a few trials have reported the absence of anomalous hormonal levels in women with postpartum depression. Two studies on total estradiol levels in postpartum period obtained between day 1 and week 8 following delivery have found no differences in women with or without postpartum depression.[42,53] In addition, a study performed on a relatively large size (182 women with childbearing potential) have found no significant difference in the magnitude of total or free estradiol changes from late pregnancy to the puerperium among depressed and non depressed women.[54] These findings seem to confirm the possibility of differential behavioral sensitivity to gonadal steroids.[55] However, a recent research has demonstrated that, with respect to total levels of estrogen, at day 3 after parturition estrogen levels were surprisingly higher in women with current major depressive disorder (MDD) than in those with previous history of MDD or healthy controls.[56] This finding seems to minimize the role of "estrogen withdrawal" in contributing to the onset of postpartum depression.

Nonetheless, the mechanism by which estrogens could modulate different neuronal systems is increasingly investigated. Estrogens exert a wide range of action on different neuronal systems and neurons (including serotoninergic, noradrenergic, dopaminergic, cholinergic, and GABAergic pathways and receptors) predominantly through two intracellular estrogen receptors, the α-estrogen receptor (ERα) and the β-estrogen receptor (ERβ).[57,58,59,60,61,62] ERβ are especially abundant in midbrain serotonin system within the dorsal raphe nuclei, where they are believed to influence 5-HT-mediated behaviors such mood, eating, sleep, temperature regulation, libido and cognition.[63] This influence may be due to the estrogen-mediated increase in the density of 5-HT_{2A} binding sites in these neural structures.[64] Furthermore, such hormones enhance serotoninergic activity *via* increased synthesis and reduced breakdown of serotonin,[63] also increasing tryptophan-hydroxylase protein by interacting with ERβ specifically localized in dorsal raphe nuclei.[65] Moreover, decrease in motivation and anhedonia – key MDD-symptoms – may be induced by dysregulation of dopamine neurotransmission; in fact, estrogens provoke up-regulation of dopamine D_{1A} receptors, a direct increase in the number of D_2 receptors, stimulation of synthesis and release of dopamine in the striatum.[66,67,68] In addition, the identification of estrogen receptors in the limbic system supports the assumption that estrogen not only modulates endocrine functions, but also has neuromodulating functions.[69] Finally, estrogen mediates a wide range of intracellular effects:[70] these effects include the transcription of genes that encode enzymes which regulate several pathways involved in the synthesis and metabolism of neurotransmitters, neuropeptides, nerve growth factors, signal transduction proteins, and hypothalamic releasing hormones such as Corticotropin-Releasing Hormone.[60, 71,72,73,74] In particular, estrogen may modulate response to stress through interactions with the hypothalamic-pituitary-adrenal (HPA) axis and noradrenergic systems.[75]

Puerperal Psychosis

The extraordinarily high risk of postpartum mania for women with bipolar disorder has been hypothesized to result from the sharp decline in estrogens and, especially, estradiol, which occur immediately after parturition, along with sleep disruptions that occur before and after the birth.[76] The fall of estrogens serum levels consequently results in a decreased antidopaminergic effects, with the consequential over-exposure of supersensitive dopamine receptors.[77,78] The possible influence of sex steroid-related genes on interindividual differences with respect to susceptibility to psychiatric disorders have been recently reviewed by Westberg and Eriksson.[79] The correlation between changes in estrogens levels and the onset of postpartum psychosis may be mediated by selective polymorphisms[80] in the gene codifying the human estrogen receptor α (*ESR1*, located on chromosome 6q25.1).[81] Nevertheless, the correlation between low maternal estradiol serum levels and increased risk of puerperal psychosis is still controversial.[82]

Psychosocial Background of Postpartum Psychiatric Disorders Maternity Blues

Postpartum Non Psychotic Depression

No specific contributing factors have been associated with increased rates of maternity blues. Conversely, well-known psychosocial factors may contribute to the development of postpartum depression: lower socio-economic status, poor partner relationship, unplanned pregnancy, single motherhood, shorter inter-pregnancy intervals (less than 24 months), and younger maternal age are some features associated with higher risk of postpartum mood disorders.[83,84,85,86] Emerging risk factors are conversely represented by recent immigration, feeling unready for hospital discharge, dissatisfaction with their infant breastfeeding method, pregnancy-induced hypertension, previous history of premenstrual syndrome, and family caregiver role (defined as women who have to take care of disabled or ill relatives).[22,87] Another important risk factor associated with postpartum non-psychotic depression is a decrease in social support, which may result from a lack of traditional cultural rituals. Postnatal rituals (like those existing in selected countries with ancient culture of traditional ceremonies, such as China, Turkey, and Spain) in which women receive attention after birth may protect against postpartum depression.[88,89] Despite it has been hypothesized that the absence of these rituals may be a relevant contributing factor to the occurrence of postpartum depression in Western countries,[90] this finding remains controversial.[91]

Puerperal Psychosis

Some of above mentioned psychosocial factors have also been associated with increased rates of puerperal psychosis.[92]

Findings

Studies Evaluating the Prophylactic Effectiveness of Estrogen in the Recurrence of Postpartum Psychiatric Episodes

Sichel and co-workers evaluated 11 pregnant women with a history of at least one episode of postpartum affective disorders who took no psychotropic medications during pregnancy.[93] Oral estrogens were daily administered immediately following delivery; two patients, however, had also received intravenous estrogens to ensure compliance during the first 2 days of treatment. All but one woman remained symptom-free during the early phase of puerperium and the first postpartum year, despite an expected relapse-risk ranging from 35% to 60%. Table 1 shows some details about the study, as well as its limitations.

A recent trial evaluated 29 pregnant women who had a history of hypomania, mania, or schizoaffective disorder – as defined by Research Diagnostic Criteria – for testing the hypothesis that estrogen administration after childbirth could prevent postpartum disease-relapses (Table 1).[94] Estradiol treatment was started on the first day after delivery or - at latest - within 48 hours. The study showed no evidence that estrogen administration during the early puerperium phase was associated with a reduced recurrence-rate of affective psychosis after childbirth.

Studies Evaluating the Efficacy of Estrogens in the Treatment of Postpartum Psychiatric Episodes.

A double-blind, placebo-controlled study enrolled 61 women with major depression that had begun within 3 months of childbirth and persisted for up 18 months postnatally.[95] Eighty percent of patients treated with estrogen-supplementation improved rapidly, and to a significantly greater extent than controls at Edinburgh Postnatal Depression Scale.[96] None of a range of other factors (age, psychiatric, obstetrical and gynecological history, severity and duration of current episode of depression, and concurrent antidepressant medication) influenced the response to estrogen-treatment. After a 3 month-period of hormonal-supplementation, patients in the active group received 10 mg/day of dydrogesterone for 12 days per month in order to reduce the risk of endometrial hyperplasia. Overall frequency of adverse events did not differ between the active and the placebo group. Nonetheless, the study evidences relevant limitations that partially prejudice the results' validity.[97]

Three very small open-label studies (in total, 6 patients) also suggested the efficacy of 17β-estradiol in the treatment of both depressive and psychotic symptoms at postpartum onset in patients with low serum estradiol levels at baseline.[98,99,100] In the third of these studies women became psychotic within week 4 after parturition.[100] During hormonal treatment, psychiatric symptoms rapidly ameliorated in accordance with the Brief Psychiatric Rating Scale (BPRS).[101] After 3 months of estradiol treatment, dydrogesterone was started (10 mg twice a day, for 10 days every fifth week) in order to minimize the risk of endometrial hyperplasia. Treatment discontinuation, however, resulted in a rebound of florid psychotic features: subsequently, estrogen treatment was effectively resumed in one of these women. Some results of this last study were also described in a successive brief report.[102]

In a further trial, 23 women who met ICD-10 diagnostic criteria for psychosis with postpartum onset were consecutively recruited from a psychiatry duty unit.[61] At baseline, all patients exhibited severe psychiatric symptoms at BPRS. Sixty percent of women underwent psychiatric treatment with psychotherapy or neuroleptic agents without adequate efficacy. After parturition, maternal serum estradiol levels were even lower than the threshold value of gonadal failure, and ranged between 13 and 90 pmol/L. Thus, estrogen-treatment was started in order to reach maternal estradiol levels of 400 pmol/L. After week 1 of hormonal supplementation, the total scores of symptoms significantly decreased and all women substantially became symptom-free at week 2 of treatment.

Ahokas and co-workers subsequently recruited a number of depressed mothers having documented physiological postpartum estradiol deficiency.[103] The mean serum estradiol level after parturition was 79.8 pmol/L. Main inclusion criteria were represented by ICD-10 criteria for major depression, onset of depression within 6 months after delivery, time since parturition of less than 12 months, and serum estradiol concentrations ≤ 200 pmol/L. Estradiol daily dosage was established for reaching a serum hormonal concentration of 400 pmol/L. A 50% of reduction of the baseline depression score at Montgomery-Asberg Depression Rating Scale (MADRS)[104] was defined as *"treatment response"*, whereas *"recovery"* was defined as a total MADRS score of 7 or less. This preliminary study showed the following results: at week 1 of treatment, in 21/23 patients symptomatologic-amelioration exceeded the responder criteria; 9/23 patients also showed a MADRS total score ≤ 7. At week 8 all patients had a MADRS total score ≤ 7. No unwanted reactions were observed both in the mothers and in the breastfed infants. Tables 1 and 2 show some relevant characteristics and limitations of reviewed studies.[61,95,98-100,102,103]

Treatment of Postpartum Psychiatric Disorders

Estrogen Therapy

Estrogen trials are especially interesting because they verify a treatment that may have specific etiological relevance to postpartum psychiatric disorders.[97] Furthermore, most of reviewed studies suggest that estradiol-treatment could be useful in treating women affected by depressive and psychotic disorders both at early and late postpartum onset, and especially in those with documented estradiol-deficiency. Unfortunately, however, all reviewed studies appear anecdotal, fragmentary, poorly systematized, and suffering from other relevant limitations. Efficacy of estrogen-treatment has been evaluated in women affected by either a broad range of affective disorders (such as postpartum monopolar depression, bipolar depression, mania, hypomania, schizoaffective disorders),[105] or severe postpartum psychiatric diseases with uncertain affective components. Reviewed studies have also been dispersed in analyzing the efficacy of estradiol as a) prophylactic treatment for preventing the recurrences of psychiatric episodes; b) acute phase-treatment for extinguishing each single episode.[106] Moreover, most reviewed studies have been performed on small sample sizes. For these reasons, the findings should be considered with great caution until they are better-replicated.[107] In addition, diagnostic and inclusion criteria, estradiol dosage, dose-response relationship,[108] treatment's duration, and time of disease-onset after delivery were widely variable in all reviewed studies.

On the other hand, the routine utilization of estrogen supplementation in treating puerperal mood disorders was limited by several complications:[109] Estrogens are suspected of causing vaginal epithelial changes, endometrial hyperplasia, thromboembolic events, and decreased milk production in lactating women especially when utilized at high doses, as reviewed elsewhere.[110] The free hormonal passage into breast milk was also associated with increased risks of neonatal jaundice and poor weight gain.[93,95, 111,112,113] Furthermore, chronic exposure to estradiol has been associated with increased risk of major depressive disorder (MDD), probably because a direct and/or indirect hormonal effects on brain regions regulating mood.[114,115] The relationship of estradiol to MDD appears to be dose-dependent.[116]

Given these reasons, at present definitive conclusions cannot be reached about the effectiveness of estrogen-treatment in puerperal psychiatric disorders,[117,118] despite the case of a female patient developing psychosis associated with significant hypoestrogenemia independent from menstrual cycle, puerperium, or other conditions related to possible changes in estrogens serum levels described recently by Rettembacher et al.[119] In this woman, oral hormonal treatment (estradiol valerat, 2 mg/day for 11 days, followed by 10 days-treatment with estradiol valerat, 2 mg/day plus norgestrel, 0.5 mg/day) dramatically reduced psychotic symptoms within one week, and with no need of antipsychotic medication.

Given the ethical problems in treating this population of patients, the difficulty in enrolling a significant number of mothers affected by psychiatric disorders with postpartum onset, and the inconclusive findings of reviewed studies, the necessity exists of further, well-designed, and strictly focused studies before making conclusions about the safety and the efficacy of estrogen-therapy in puerperal psychiatric disorders. For this aim, a pilot trial in being conducted in Canada to evaluate the effect of transdermal estradiol patch in combination with sertraline among women with postpartum depression.[120] So far, however, double blind, placebo-controlled studies comparing the efficacy of psychotropic medications alone *vs* estrogens alone *vs* combination therapy are lacking. Preliminarily, however, a careful clinical evaluation of patients with psychiatric disorder at postpartum onset remains an indispensable tool, in order to reduce the risk of both sub-optimal treatment and misdiagnosis of subtle forms of bipolar disorder.[121,122] Hence, large multi-center trials could represent one of the best research-option for obtaining conclusive information about the role of estrogens in psychiatric disorders at postpartum onset. Such studies may be focused on one specific psychiatric disorder (e.g., unipolar recurrent depressive episodes) and then on one definite field of efficacy (e.g., efficacy in the treatment of each single episode **or** efficacy in the prophylaxis of episodes' recurrences)

Classic Psychotropic Medications

More than a few reports have suggested the efficacy of several psychotropic drugs in puerperal mental diseases:[123] among SSRIs, both sertraline and fluvoxamine have been proposed as safe and effective medications for postpartum depression;[124,125,126] two randomized controlled trial have also suggested the usefulness of paroxetine and fluoxetine, and preliminary data on venlafaxine and bupropion are quite reassuring.[127,128,129,130] These findings are not surprising: in fact, Newport et al individuated the role of unique alterations of serotoninergic functions that are puerperium-specific and strongly involved in the pathogenesis of postpartum major depression. Such alterations are mainly represented by selective anomalies in platelet serotonin transporter (SERT) binding.[131,132] However, an important consideration in the treatment of postpartum non psychotic depression is the safety of antidepressants when used by breastfeeding mothers.[133] SSRIs may be certainly preferable for all severe depressive episodes; these compounds appear associated with relatively low risk for detrimental events in breastfed infants.[134,135,136,137] Recent articles concluded that sertraline and paroxetine should be considered as first-line medications in women who need to start antidepressant-treatment during puerperium and wish to continue breastfeeding. The utilization of fluoxetine and citalopram seems conversely to be associated with a relatively higher risk of unwanted events (of low degree of severity, however).[138,139,140,141,142,143] For the other newer and old antidepressant drugs, data are still of no conclusive value to the patient or physician in deciding on the safety of their use in lactation. These considerations, however, are a guide particularly for commencing new antidepressant treatment. It does not imply that established antidepressant treatment should be changed with each childbearing phase. In fact, when a pregnancy occurs in patients already treated with antidepressant medications, it is important to review whether the drug has been effective and is still indicated and the most appropriate clinical decision in these cases may well be to continue ongoing treatment. Finally, it must be stressed that there is no evidence of the effectiveness of antidepressants given immediately postpartum in preventing postnatal depression.

No definitive conclusions can be drawn about the risk/benefit profile of the majority of antipsychotic medications in breastfeeding. Hence, when clinicians are forced to start antipsychotic treatment in drug-naïve patients, until now the choice of the safest option should be based on the general effectiveness profile of each agent, with two possible exceptions: clozapine (the drug should be considered contraindicated during breastfeeding because its liability of inducing potential life-threatening events in the infant), and olanzapine (the drug seems to be associated with an increased risk of inducing extrapyramidal reactions in the breastfed babies). Conversely, in patients who need to continue antipsychotic therapy during breastfeeding, it is suitable to maintain the previous pharmacological regimen, if known as effective.[144] Probably, however, monotherapy with conventional antipsychotic agents may be still preferred for breastfeeding mothers with psychotic features.[145,146,147]

Regarding mood stabilizers, the American Academy of Pediatrics (AAP) has stated that "lithium has been associated with significant effects on some nursing infant and should be given to nursing mothers with caution".[148] The management of mothers who need lithium-treatment continuation in the puerperium and wish for continuing breast-feeding, as well as the monitoring-needs of the infants, have been comprehensively summarized by Yonkers et al.[149] As regards valproate, if a decision is made to breastfeed, vigilance against unwanted hematological events in infants is required.[150] However, 6 infants born to bipolar mothers, for whom exposure to the compound occurred exclusively during breastfeeding, showed low valproate serum levels (0.7-1.5 mcg/mL), thus presenting a relatively low risk compared to the risk of maternal disease relapse.[151] Valproate is considered compatible with breastfeeding by the AAP.[147] Caution is also advisable when mothers take carbamazepine and breastfeed their babies, since there is little information on carbamazepine-related toxicity for suckling infants. However, maternal CBZ intake is considered compatible with breastfeeding by the AAP.[147] Nonetheless, for all these medications it is recommended that for safe breastfeeding the ratio of infant dose exposure to maternal dose not be greater than 10%[152,153].

Psychotherapeutic Interventions

Cognitive-behavioral therapy (CBT), interpersonal psychotherapy (IPT), and couple interventions, all supported by social intervention for reducing social isolation and improving role adjustment after delivery, could be useful in approaching depressive episodes of light-moderate severity.[128],[154,155,156,157] Recently, however, Dennis found that the trials evaluating the effectiveness of CBT related to postpartum depression suffered from significant methodological limitations.[158] Moreover, supportive therapy by paraprofessional health care workers has been found to reduce depressive symptoms in women with postpartum non psychotic depression.[159] A relatively recent study also found that women in the early postpartum who received a number of home visits by a midwife during the first month after parturition experienced a significant improvement in mental health and a lowered risk of depression compared with mothers who did not receive such a support.[160] Conversely, no relevant information is available about the possible role of psychological approaches in ameliorating mental health in women with postpartum psychosis. For this reason, expert opinion would not rely on psychotherapy alone in this specific clinical situation.[161]

Table 1. Summary of existing studies evaluating the efficacy of estrogen treatment in puerperal psychosis

Study and sample size	*Psychiatric diagnosis and drug regimen*	*Main study's limitations*	*Study-population's characteristics*	*Effectiveness*
Sichel, 1995.[93] (N=11)	Recurrent affective disorders Up to 10 mg/day of estrogen-replacement therapy (Premarin ®), in decreasing dosages over 4 weeks.	Open-label clinical trial No control group was used Hormonal daily dose was about 15 times the usual dose for estrogen-deficiency symptoms The patients required heparin-treatment to prevent thromboembolic events No data is available on maternal estradiol-levels at baseline	Patients with previous episodes of either nonpsychotic depression or manic postpartum psychosis All patients were symptom-free and sought consultation because of concerns regarding the current pregnancy	Estrogen was effective in preventing postpartum disease relapse No adverse events were recorded
Kumar, 2003.[94] (N=29)	Recurrent affective psychosis Transdermal 17β-estradiol, at 200, 400, or 800 μg/day, for 12 days Hormonal treatment was started within 48 hours after delivery	Open-label clinical trial No control group was used During estradiol treatment breastfeeding was not permitted No available data on maternal estradiol levels at baseline	Patients who had a history of hypomania, mania, or schizoaffective disorders	Estradiol did not reduce the rate of recurrence of psychosis No available data on possible adverse events associated with hormonal treatment
Ahokas, 1999.[100] (N=2)	Puerperal psychosis Micronized 17β-estradiol, 1 mg sublingually, 4 to 6 times daily for 2-30 weeks Hormonal treatment was started within month 2 and 4 after delivery, respectively	Very small case series Before starting hormonal treatment, one patient also took chlorpromazine up to 200 mg/day for 2 weeks	Time of disease onset after delivery: from 1 to 4 weeks. Estrogen maternal levels at baseline: 79 and 54 pmol/L, respectively	Estradiol was effective in treating postnatal psychosis. No data is available on possible adverse events associated with hormonal -treatment

Study and sample size	*Psychiatric diagnosis and drug regimen*	*Main study's limitations*	*Study-population's characteristics*	*Effectiveness*
Ahokas, 2000.[102] (N=2)	Puerperal psychosis Micronized 17β-estradiol, 1 mg sublingually, 4 to 6 times daily, for 2-5 weeks and more (unspecified) Hormonal treatment was started within month 5 and 2 after delivery, respectively	Very small case series In one case, ineffective haloperidol treatment was suspended only during the first week of hormonal treatment	Time of disease onset after delivery: from 1 to 2 weeks. Estrogen maternal levels at baseline: 69 and 28 pmol/L, respectively	Estradiol was effective in treating postnatal psychosis. No available data on possible adverse events associated with hormonal -treatment
Ahokas, 2000.[60] (N=10)	Puerperal psychosis Micronized 17β-estradiol, 1 mg sublingually, 3 to 6 times daily (mean daily dose: from 3.8 to 4.7 mg), for 6 weeks. Hormonal treatment was started within 2-170 days after delivery. Respectively	Small sample size No control group was used Open-label clinical trial Four patients also received psychotropic medication discontinued during the first week of estradiol treatment	Time from delivery to onset of psychosis: 12.3 ± 8.3 days Mean baseline levels of serum estradiol: 49.5 ± 30.8 pmol/L	Estradiol was effective in treating postnatal psychosis. No available data on possible adverse events associated with hormonal -treatment

Reproduced from: Gentile S. The role of estrogen-therapy in postpartum psychiatric disorders: an update. CNS Spectrums 2005; 10 (12): 944-952.With permission.

Table 2. Summary of existing studies evaluating the efficacy of estrogen-treatment in postpartum depression

Study and sample size	Psychiatric diagnosis and drug regimen	Main study's limitations	Study-population's characteristics	Effectiveness
Gregoire, 1996.[95] (N=61)	Severe postnatal depression Transdermal 17β-estradiol, 200μg/day, for 3 months	Patients also on psychotropic drugs were excluded only if there had been a change of medication in the previous 6 weeks No data is available on maternal estrogen levels at baseline	Women with major depression which began within 3 months of childbirth and persisted for up 18 months postnatally	Estradiol was effective in treating postnatal depression

Table 2. (Continued)

Gregoire, 1996.[95] (N=61)	Hormonal treatment was started about 4 weeks after the first contact			Endometrial curettage at the end of treatment showed endometrial changes in 3 women which resolved on follow-up
Ahokas, 1998.[98] (N=2)	Postnatal depression 17β-estradiol, 1 mg sublingually, 3-4 times daily for 2 weeks Hormonal treatment was started within 4 months after delivery	Very small case series	Time of disease onset after delivery: from 2 to 8 weeks. Estrogen maternal levels at baseline: 140 and 23 pmol/L, respectively	Estradiol was effective in treating postnatal depression No available data on possible adverse events associated with hormonal - treatment
Ahokas, 1999.[99] (N=2)	Postpartum depression Micronized 17β-estradiol, 1 mg sublingually, 4 times daily for 2 weeks Hormonal treatment was started within 2 and 5 months after delivery, respectively	Very small case series Before starting hormonal treatment, one patient also took antidepressants, but the study does not specify psychotropic treatment duration	Time of disease onset after delivery: from 5 to 7 days Estrogen maternal levels at baseline: 23 and 31 pmol/L, respectively	Estradiol was effective in treating postnatal depression No data are available on possible adverse events associated with hormonal treatment
Ahokas, 2001.[103] (N=23)	Severe postpartum depression Micronized 17β-estradiol, 1 mg sublingually, 3 to 8 times daily (mean daily dose: from 3.9 to 4.8 mg), for 8 weeks Mean duration of symptoms before starting hormonal treatment: 74 ± 61 days	Small sample size No control group was used Open-label clinical trial The patients took antidepressants before starting hormonal treatment	Time from delivery to onset of psychosis: 33.7.3 ± 31.7 days Mean baseline levels of serum estradiol: 79.8 ± 41.7 pmol/L	Estradiol was effective in treating postnatal depression No adverse events were recorded in the mothers and breastfed infants

Reproduced from: Gentile S. The role of estrogen-therapy in postpartum psychiatric disorders: an update. CNS Spectrums 2005; 10 (12): 944-952.With permission.

References

[1] Rapkin AJ, Mikacich JA, Moatakef-Imani B. Reproductive mood disorders. *Prim. Psychiatry* 2003;10:31-40.

[2] Stocky A, Lynch J. Acute psychiatric disturbance in pregnancy and the puerperium. *Baillieres Best Pract .Res. Clin. Obstet. Gynaecol.* 2000;14:73-87.

[3] Weimberg MK, Tronick EZ. The impact of maternal psychiatric illness on infant development. *J. Clin. Psychiatry* 1998;59 (suppl. 2):53-61.

[4] Niemi TL, Suvisaari JM, Haukka JK, Wrede G, Lonnqvist JK. Cumulative incidence of mental disorders among offspring of mothers with psychotic disorder. *Br. J. Psychiatry* 2004;185:11-17.

[5] Murray L, Cooper PJ. Postpartum depression and child development. London, England: Guilford Press, 1997.

[6] Diego MA, Field T, Hernandez-Reif M, Cullen C, Schanberg S, Kuhn C. Prepartum, postpartum, and chronic depression effects on newborns. *Psychiatry* 2004;67:63-80.

[7] Rahman A, Iqbal Z, Bunn J, Lovel H, Harrington R. Impact of maternal depression on infant nutritional status and illness: a cohort study. *Arch. Gen. Psychiatry* 2004;61:946-952.

[8] Jones HW, Venis A. Identification and classification of postpartum psychiatric disorders. *J. Psychol. Nurs* 2001;39:23-29.

[9] Llewellyn AM, Stowe ZN, Nemeroff CB. Depression during pregnancy and the puerperium. *J. Clin. Psychiatry* 1997;58 (suppl. 15):26-32.

[10] Seyfred LS, Marcus SM. Postpartum mood disorders. *Int. Rev. Psychiatry* 2003;15:231-242.

[11] O'Hara MW, Schlechte JA, Lewis DA, Wright EJ. Prospective study of postpartum blues: biologic and psychosocial factors. *Arch. Gen. Psychiatry* 1991;48:801-806.

[12] Campbell SB, Cohn JF, Flanaghan C. Course and correlates of postpartum depression during the transition to parenthood. Development and Psychopathology 1992;4:29-47.

[13] Reck C, Stehle E, Reinig K, Mundt C. Maternity blues as predictor of DSM-IV depression and anxiety disorders in the first three months postpartum *J. Affect. Disord.* 2008 [Epub ahead of print].

[14] Watanabe M, Wada K, sakata Y, et al. Maternity blues as predictor of postpartum depression: a prospective cohort study among Japanese women. *J. Psychosom. Obstet.* Gynecol 2008 [Epub ahead of print].

[15] Hapgaod CC, Elkind GS, Wright JJ. Maternity blues: phenomena and relationship to later postpartum depression. *Aust. N .Z. J. Psychiatry* 1988;22:299-306.

[16] Kendell RE, Chalmers JC, Platz C. Epidemiology of puerperal psychosis. *Br. J. Psychiatry* 1987;150:662-673.

[17] Watson JP, Elliott SA, Rugg AJ, Brough DI. Psychiatric disorder in pregnancy and the first postnatal year. *Br. J. Psychiatry* 1984;144:453-462.

[18] Georgiopoulos AM, Bryan TL, Yawn BP, Houston MS, Rummans TA, Therneau TM. Population-based screening for postpartum depression. *Obstet. Gynecol.* 1999;93:653-657.

[19] Robertson E, Grace S, Wallington T, Stewart DE. Antenatal risk factors for postpartum depression: a synthesis of recent literature. *Gen. Hosp. Psychiatry* 2004;26:289-295.

[20] Navarro P, Garcia-Esteve L, Ascaso C, Aguado J, Jelabert E, Martin-Santos R. Non-psychotiv psychiatric dirders afer childbirth: prevalence and comorbidity in a community sample. *J. Affect. Disord.* 2008;109:171-176.

[21] Milgrom J, Gemmill AW, Bilszta JL, et al. Antenatal risl factors for postnatal depression: a large prospective study. *J. Affect Disord.* 2008;108:147-157.

[22] Garcia-Esteve L, Navarro P, Ascaso C, et al. Family caregiver role and premenstrual syndrome as associated factors of postnatal depression. *Arch. Womens Mental Health* 2008;11:193-200.

[23] Cohen LS, Nonacs R, Viguera AC, Reminick A. Diagnosis and treatment of depression during pregnancy. *CNS Spectr*. 2004;9:209-216.

[24] Dennis CLE, Stewart DE. Treatment of postpartum depression, Part 1: a critical review of biological interventions. *J. Clin. Psychiatry.* 2004;65:1242-1251

[25] Flores DL, Hendrick VC. Etiology and treatment of postpartum depression. *Curr. Psychiatr. Rep.* 2002;4:461-466.

[26] Miller L. Linking evidence and experience: postpartum depression. *JAMA* 2002; 287:762-765.

[27] American Psychiatric Association. Diagnostic and statistic manual of mental disorders, text revision, edn 4, Washington DC: American Psychiatric Association 2000;561-562.

[28] Hendrick V, Altshuler L, Strause T, Grosser S. Postpartum and non-postpartum depression: differences in presentation and response to pharmacological treatment. Depress Anxiety 2000;11:66-72.

[29] Pill B. "Atypical" depression following childbirth. *Br. J. Psychiatry* 1968;114:1325-1335.

[30] Pfuhlmann B, Stoeber G, Beckmann H. Postpartum psychosis: prognosis, risk factors, and treatment. *Curr. Psychiatry Rep.* 2002:4:185-190

[31] Freeman MP, Smith KW, Freeman SA, McElroy SL, Kmetz GE, Wright R et al. The impact of reproductive events on the course of bipolar disorder in women. *J. Clin. Psychiatry.* 2002;63:284-287.

[32] Heron J, McGuiness M, Blackmore ER, Craddock N, Jones I. Early postpartum symptoms in puerperal psychosis. *BJOG* 2008;115:348-353.

[33] Stowe ZN, Nemeroff CB. Women at risk of postpartum-onset major depression. *Am. J. Obstet. Gynecol.* 1995;173:639-645.

[34] Rohde A, Marneros A. Postpartum psychosis: onset and long term course. *Psychopathology* 1993;26:203-209.

[35] Attia E, Downey J, Oberman M. Postpartum psychosis. In: Miller LJ, ed. Postpartum mood disorder. Washington DC: *American Psychiatric Press.* 1999:99-117

[36] Parry BL. Postpartum psychiatric syndromes. In: Kaplan HI, Sadock B, eds. Comprehensive Textbook of Psychiatry. Vol. 1, 6th ed. Philadelphia, Pa: William and Wilkins; 1995:1059-1066.

[37] Harlow BL, Vitonis A, Sparen P, Cnattingius S, Joffe H, Hultman CM. Incidence of hospitalization for postpartum psychotic and bipolar episodes in women with and

without prior prepregnancy or prenatal psychiatric hospitalizations. *Arch. Gen. Psychiatry* 2007;64:42-48.

[38] Brockington I. Postpartum psychiatric disorders. *Lancet* 2004;363:303-310.

[39] Doornbos B, Fekkes D, Tanke MA, de Jonge P, Korf J. Sequential serotonin and noradrenalin associated processes involved in postpartum blues. Prog. *Neuropsychopharmacol. Biol. Psychiatry* 2008;32:1320-1325.

[40] Bokhari R, Bhatara VS, Bandettini F, McMillin JM. Postpartum psychosis and postpartum thyroiditis. *Psychoneuroendocrinol.* 1998;23:643-650.

[41] Harris B, Lovett L, Smith J, Read G, Walker R, Newcombe R. Cardiff puerperal mood and hormone study. III. Postnatal depression at 5 to 6 weeks postpartum, and its hormonal correlates across the postpartum period. *Br. J. Psychiatry* 1996;168:739-744.

[42] Harris B, Johns S, Fung H, Thomas R, Walker R, Read G, et al. The hormonal environment of post-natal depression. *Br. J. Psychiatry* 1989;154:660-667.

[43] Suzuki S, Dennerstein L, Greenwood KM, Armstrong SM, Sano T, Satohisa E. Melatonin and hormonal changes in disturbed sleep during late pregnancy. *J. Pineal. Res.*1993;15:191-198

[44] Parry BL, Sorenson DL, Meliska CJ, Basavaraj N, Zirpoli GG, Gamst A et al. Hormonal basis of mood and postpartum disorders. *Curr. Women's Health Rep.* 2003;3:230-235.

[45] Bloch M, Schimdt PJ, Danaceau M, Murphy J, Nieman L, Rubinow DR. Effects of gonadal steroids in women with history of postpartum depression. *Am. J. Psychiatry* 2000;157:924-930.

[46] Born L, Zinga D. Challenges in identifying and diagnosing postpartum disorders. *Prim. Psychiatry* 2004;11:29-36.

[47] Willcox DL, Yovich Jl, Mc Colm SC, Phillips JM. Progesterone, cortisol and estradiol-17 beta in the initiation of human parturition: partitioning between free and bound hormone in plasma. *Br. J. Obstet. Gynaecol.* 1985;92:65-71.

[48] Hendrick V, Altshuler LL, Suri R. Hormonal changes in the postpartum and implications for postpartum depression. *Psychosomatics* 1998;39:93-101.

[49] Shors TJ, Leuner B. Estrogen-mediated effects on depression and memory formations in females. *J. Affect. Disord.* 2003;74:85-96.

[50] Backstrom T, Cartensen H, Sodegard R. Concentration of estradiol, testosterone and progesterone in cerebrospinal fluid compared to unbound and total concentrations. *J. Steroid Biochem.* 1976:7:469-472.

[51] Schwartz S, Pohl P. Steroid hormones and steroid hormone binding globulins in cerebrospinal fluid studied in individuals with intact and with disturbed blood-cerebrospinal fluid barrier. *Neuroendocrinology* 1992;55:174-182.

[52] Rapkin AJ, Mikacich JA, Moatakef-Imani B, Ragson N. The clinical nature and formal diagnosis of premenstrual, postpartum, and perimenopausal affective disorders. *Curr. Psychiatry Rep.* 2002;4:419-428.

[53] Nott PN, Franklin M, Armitage C, Gelder MG. Hormonal changes in mood and puerperium. *Br. J. Psychiatry* 1976;128:379-383.

[54] O'Hara MW, Schlechte JA, Lewis DA, Wright EJ. Controlled prospective study of postpartum mood disorders: psychological, environmental, and hormonal variables. *J. Abnorm. Psychol.* 1991;100:63-73.
[55] Schimdt PJ, Neiman LK, Danaeau MA, Adams LF, Rubinow DR. Differenytial behavioral effects on gonadal steroids in women with and those without premenstrual syndrome. *Sem. Reprod. Endocrionol.* 1998;15:91-100.
[56] Klier CM, Muzik M, Dervic K, et al. The role of estrogen and progesterone in depression after birth. *J. Psychiatr. Res.* 2007;41:273-9.
[57] Rubinow DR, Schmidt PJ, Roca CA. Estrogen-serotonin interactions: implication for affective regulation. *Biol. Psychiatry* 1998;44:839-850.
[58] McEwen BS, Alves SE. Estrogen actions in the central nervous system. *Endocrin. Rev.* 1999;20:279-307.
[59] Rupprecht R, Holsboer F. Neuroactive steroids: mechanism of action and neuropsychopharmacological perspectives. *Trend Neurosci.* 1999;22:410-416.
[60] Payne JL. The role of estrogen in mood disorders in women. *Int. Rev. Psychiatry* 2003;15:280-90.
[61] Ahokas A, Marjatta, A, Rimón R. Positive treatment effect of estradiol in postpartum psychosis: a pilot study. *J. Clin. Psychiatry* 2000;61:166-169.
[62] Fink G, Sumner BE, Rosie R, Grace O, Quinn JP. Estrogen control of central neurotransmission: effect on mood, mental state, and memory. *Cell Mol. Neurobiol.* 1996;16:325-344.
[63] Nomura M, Akama KT, Alves S, et al. Differential distribution of estrogen receptor (ER)-alpha and ER-beta in the midbrain raphe nuclei and periacqueductal gray in male mouse: predominant role of ER-beta in midbrain serotoninergic systems. *Neuriscience* 2005;130:445-456.
[64] Luine VN, Khylchevskaya RI, McEven B. Effects of gonadal steroids on activities of monoamine oxidase and choline acetylase in rat brain. *Brain Res.* 1975; 86:293-306
[65] Lu NZ, Shlaes TA, Gundhal T, et al. Ovarian steroid action on tryptofan hydroxylase protein and serotonin compared to localization of ovarian steroid receptors in midbrain of guinea pigs. *Endocrine* 1999;11:257-267.
[66] Becker JB. Gender differences in dopaminergic function in striatum and nucleus accumbens. *Pharmacol. Biochem. Behavior* 1999;64:803-812.
[67] Lee SH, Mouradian MM. Up-regulation of D1A dopamine receptor gene transcription by estrogen. *Mol. Cell Endocrinol.* 1999;156:151-157.
[68] Le Saux M, Di Paolo T. Influence of oestrogenic compounds on monoamine transporters in rat striatum. *J. Neuroendocrinol.* 2006;18:25-32.
[69] Riecher-Rössler A. Association between oestradiol and puerperal psychosis[Invited comment]. *Acta Psychiatr. Scand.* 2000; 101: 169-170.
[70] McEwen BS. Nongenomic and genomic effects of steroids on neural activity. *Trend Pharmacol. Sci.* 1991;12:141-147.
[71] O' Malley BW, Means AR. Female steroid hormones and target cell nuclei. *Science* 1974;183:610-620.
[72] Magiakou MA, Mastorakos G, Rabin D, Dubbert B, Gold PW, Chrousos GP. Hypothalamic corticotropin-releasing hormone suppression during the post-partum

period: implications for the increase of psychiatric manifestations in this period. *J. Clin. Endocrinol. Metab.* 1996;81:1912-1917.

[73] Cizza G, Chrousos GP. High-dose transdermal estrogen, corticotrophin-releasing hormone, and postnatal depression [letter]. *J. Clin. Endocrinol. Metab.* 1997;82:704.

[74] Warner R, Appleby L, Whitton A, Faragher B. Demographic and obstetric risk factors for postnatal psychiatric morbidity. *Br. J. Psychiatry* 1996;168:139-144.

[75] Maharjan S, Serova L, Sabban EL. Transcriptional regulation of tyrosine hydroxylase by estrogen: opposite effects with estrogens receptors α and β and interactions with cyclic AMP. *J. Neurochem.* 2005;93:1502-1514.

[76] Sharma A, Mazmanian D. Sleep loss and postpartum psychosis. *Bipolar. Disord.* 2003;5:98-105.

[77] Cookson JC. The neuroendocrinology of mania. *J. Affect Disord.* 1985; 8: 233-241.

[78] Wieck A, Kumar R, Hirst AD, Marks MN, Campbell IC, Checkley SA. Increased sensitivity of dopamine receptors and recurrence of affective psychosis after childbirth. *Br. Med. J.* 1991; 303: 613-616.

[79] Westberg L, Eriksson E. Sex steroid-related candidate genes in psychiatric disorders. *J. Psychiatry Neurosci.* 2008;33:319-330.

[80] Feng J, Yan J, Michaud S, et al. Scanning of estrogen receptor alpha (ERalpha) and thyroid hormone receptor alpha (TRalpha) genes in patients with psychiatric diseases: four missense mutations identified in ER alpha gene. *Am. J. Med. Genet.* 2001;105:369-374.

[81] Pomglikitmongkol M, Green S, Chambon P. Genomic organization of the human oestrogen gene. *EMBO J.* 1988;7:3385-3388.

[82] Karrupaswamy J, Vlies R. The benefit of oestrogens and progestogens in postnatal depression. *J. Obstet. Gynaecol.* 2003;23:341-346.

[83] Joffe H, Cohen LS. Estrogen, Serotonin, and mood disturbance: where is the therapeutic bridge? *Biol. Psychiatry* 1998;44:798-811.

[84] Gotlib JH, Whiffen VE, Mount JH, Milne K, Cordy NI. Prevalence and demographic characteristics associated with depression in pregnancy and the postpartum. *J. Consult Clin. Psychol.* 1989;57:269-274.

[85] O'Hara MW. Postpartum depression: causes and consequences. New York, Springer-Verlag. 1995.

[86] Guzel S, Garel II. The evaluation of determinants of early postpartum low mood: the importance of parity and interpregnancy interval. *Hum. J. Obstet. Gynecol. Repr. Biol.* 2000;91:21-24.

[87] Dennis CLE, Janssen PA, Singer J. Identifying women at-risk for postpartum depression in the immediate postpartum period. *Acta Psychiatr. Scand.* 2004;110:338-346.

[88] Niska K, Snyder M, Lia-Hoagberg B. Family ritual facilitates adaptation to parenthood. *Public Health Nurs* 1998;15:329-337.

[89] Danaci AE, Dinc G, Dececi A et al. Postnatal depression in Turkey: epidemiological and cultural aspects.

[90] Stern G, Krackman L. Multidisciplinary perspectives on postpartum depression: an anthropological critique. *Soc. Sci. Med.* 1983;17:1027-1041.

[91] Huang Y, Mathers N. Postnatal depression: biological or cultural? A comparative study of postnatal women in the UK and Taiwan. *J. Adv. Nurs.* 2001;33:279-287.
[92] Benabarre A, Vieta E, Colom F, Martinez-Aran A, Reinares M, Gasto C. Bipolar disorder, schizoaffective disorder and schizophrenia: epidemiological, clinical and prognostic differences. *Eur. Psychiatry* 2001;16:167-72.
[93] Sichel DA, Cohen LS, Robertson LM, Ruttemberg A, Rosenbaum JF. Prophylactic estrogen in recurrent postpartum affective disorders. Biol Psychiatry 1995;38:814-818
[94] Kumar C, McIvor RJ, Davies T, Brown N, Papadopulos A, Wieck A, et al. Estrogen administration does not reduce the rate of recurrence of affective psychosis after childbirth. *J. Clin. Psychiatry* 2003;64:112-118.
[95] Gregoire AJP, Kuman R, Everitt B, Henderson AF, Studd JWW. Transdermal oestrogen for treatment of severe postnatal depression. *Lancet* 1996;347:930-933.
[96] Cox JL, Holden JM, Sagovsky R. Detection of postnatal depression: development of the 10 item Edinburgh Postnatal Depression Scale. Br J Psychiatry 1897:150:782-786
[97] Murray D. Oestrogen and postnatal depression [Commentary]. *Lancet* 1996;347:918-919.
[98] Ahokas A, Turtainen S, Aito M. Sublingual oestrogen treatment of postnatal depression [letter]. *Lancet.* 1998;351:109.
[99] Ahokas A, Kaukoranta J, Aito M. Effect of oestradiol on postpartum depression. Psychopharmacology (Berl) 1999;146:108-110.
[100] Ahokas A, Aito M. Role of estradiol in puerperal psychosis. *Psychopharmacology* (Berl) 1999:147:108-110.
[101] Overall JE, Gorham DR. The Brief Psychiatric Rating Scale. *Psychol. Rep.* 1962;10:799-812.
[102] Ahokas A, Aito M, Turianen S. Association between estradiol and puerperal psychosis. *Acta Psychiatr. Scand.* 2000;101:167-169.
[103] Ahokas A, Kaukoranta J, Wahlbeck K, Aito M. Estrogen deficiency in severe postpartum depression: successful treatment with sublingual physiologic 17β-estradiol. A preliminary study. *J. Clin. Psychiatry* 2001;62:332-336.
[104] Montgomery SA, Asberg MC. A new depression scale designed to be sensitive to change. *Br. J. Psychiatry* 1979;134:382-389.
[105] Grigoriadis S, Kennedy SH. Role of estrogen in treatment of depression. *Am. J. Ther.* 2002;9:503-509.
[106] Gentile S., 2005. *"The role of estrogen-therapy in postpartum psychiatric disorders: an update"*. CNS Spectrums, 10 (12): 944-952.
[107] Soares NC, Joffe H, Cohen LS, Almeida OP. Efficacy of 17β-Estradiol on depression: is estrogen deficiency really necessary? [letter] *J. Clin. Psychiatry.* 2002;63:451
[108] Cattel DL, King EA. Estrogen for postnatal depression. J Fam Pract 1966;43:22-23.
[109] Flores DL, Hendrick VC. Etiology and treatment of postpartum depression. *Curr. Psychiatry Rep.* 2002;4:461-466.
[110] Rössler-Riecher A, de Geyter C. The forthcoming role of treatment with oestrogens in mental health. *Swiss Med Wkly.* 2007;137:565-572.
[111] Parry BL. Treatment of postpartum depression. *Prim. Psychiatry.* 2004;11:48-51.

[112] Ball DE, Morrison P. Oestrogen transdermal patches for postpartum depression in lactating women-a case report. *Cent. Afr. J. Med.* 1999;45:68-70.

[113] Gjerdingen D. The effectiveness of various postpartum treatments and the impact of antidepressant drugs on nursing infant. *J. Am. Board Fam. Pract.* 2003;16:387-392.

[114] Frye CA. An overview of oral contraceptives: mechanism of action and clinical use. *Neurology* 2006;66:S29-S36.

[115] Slap GB. Oral contraceptives and depression: impact, prevalence, and cause. *J. Adolesc. Health Care* 1981;2:53-64.

[116] Lasiuk GC, Hegadoren KM. The effects of estradiol on central serotoninergic systems and its relationship to mood in women. Biol Res Nurs 2007. Available on: http://brn.sagepub.com.

[117] Huber TJ, Rollnik J, Wilhelms J, von zur MÜlhen A, Emrich HM, Schneider U. Estradiol levels in psychotics disorders. *Psychoneuroendocrinology* 2001;26:27-35.

[118] Lawrie TA, Herxheimer A, Dalton K. Oestrogens and progestogens for preventing and treating postnatal depression (Cochrane Review). In: The Cochrane Library, Issue 3, 2004. Chichester, UK: John Wiley and Sons, Ltd.

[119] Rettembacher MA, Mechtcheriakov S, Bergant A, Brugger A, Fleischhacker WW. Improvement of psychosis during treatment with estrogen and progesterone in a patient with hypoestrogenemia. *J. Clin. Psychiatry* 2004;65:275-277.

[120] Dennis CL, Ross LE, Herxheimer A. Oestrogens and progestins for preventing and treating postpartum depression. The Cochrane Library 2008;2:1-18.

[121] Marcus SM, Flynn HA, Blow F, Barry K. A screening study of antidepressant treatment rates and mood symptoms in pregnancy. Arch Womens Ment Health 2005;8:25-27

[122] Sharma V. Pharmacotherapy of postpartum depression. *Expert Opin. Pharmacother.* 2002;3:1421-1431

[123] MacQueen G, Chokka P. Special issue in the management of depression in women. *Can. J. Psychiatry.* 2004;49(3 Suppl 1):27S-40S.

[124] Wisner KL, Perel JM, Peindl KS, Hanusa BH, Piontek CM, Findling RL. Prevention of postpartum depression: a pilot randomized clinical trial. *Am. J. Psychiatry* 2004;161:1290-1292.

[125] Sunder KR, Wisner KL, Hanusa BH, Perel JM. Postpartum depression recurrence versus discontinuation syndrome observations from a randomized controlled trials. *J. Clin. Psychiatry* 2004;65:1266-1268

[126] Suri R, Burt VK, Altshuler LL, Zuckerbrow-Miller J, Fairbanks L. Fluvoxamine for postpartum depression. *Am. J. Psychiatry.* 2001;158:1739-1740.

[127] Misri S, Reebye P, Corral M, Milis L. The use of paroxetine and cognitive-behavioral therapy in postpartum depression and anxiety: a randomized controlled trial. *J. Clin. Psychiatry* 2004;1236-1241.

[128] Appleby L, Warner R, Whitton A, Faragher B. A controlled study of fluoxetine and cognitive-behavioural counselling in the treatment of postnatal depression. *BMJ.* 1997;314:932-936.

[129] Cohen LS, Viguera AC, Bouffard SM, Nonacs RM, Morabito C, Collins MH. Venlafaxine in the treatment of postpartum depression. *J. Clin. Psychiatry* 2001;62:592-596.

[130] Nonacs RM, Soares CN, Viguera AC, Pearson K, Poitras JR, Cohen LS. Bupropion SR for the treatment of postpartum depression: a pilot study. *Int. J. Neuropsychopharmacol* 2005 8:445-449.

[131] Newport DJ, Owens MJ, Knight DL, Ragan DL, Morgan N, Nemeroff CB, Stowe ZN. Alterations in platelet serotonin transporter binding in women with postpartum onset major depression. *J. Psychiatry Res.* 2004;38:467-473.

[132] Howard L, Hoffbrand S, Henshaw C, Boath L, Bradley E. Antidepressant prevention of postnatal depression. *Cochrane Database Syst .Rev.* 2005;18:CD004363.

[133] Gentile S. The safety of newer antidepressants in pregnancy and lactation. *Drug Saf.* 2005; 28:137-152.

[134] Gentile S. SSRIs in pregnancy and lactation with emphasis on neurodevelopmental outcome. *CNS Drugs* 2005;19:623-633.

[135] Hendrick V, Fukuchi A, Altshuler L, Widawski M, Wertheimer A, Brunhuber MV. Use of sertraline, paroxetine and fluvoxamine by nursing infants. *Br. J. Psychiatry* 2001;179:163-166.

[136] Kristensen JH, Hackett LP, Kohan R, Paech M, Ilett KF. The amount of fluvoxamine in milk is unlikely to be a cause of adverse effects in breastfed infants. *Hum. Lact.* 2002;18:139-143.

[137] Piontek CM, Wisner KL, Perel JM, Peindl KS. Serum fluvoxamine levels in breastfed infants. *J. Clin. Psychiatry* 2001;62:111-113.

[138] Gentile S. Psychotropic drugs in pregnancy and during breastfeeding. Clinical aspects. *Eur. Psychiatry* 2008;23 (suppl.2): S373.

[139] Gentile S.SSRIs and mood stabilizers in pregnancy and during breastfeeding. Clinical aspects. *Eur .Neuropsychopharmacol.* 2007;17 (suppl.4): S224

[140] Gentile S. Use of contemporary antidepressants during breastfeeding. A proposal for a specific safety index. *Drug. Saf.*2007;30:107-21.

[141] Gentile S. Escitalopram use late in pregnancy and during breastfeeding. *Ann. Pharmacother.* 2006;40:1696-1697.

[142] Gentile S. Quetiapine-fluvoxamine combination during pregnancy and while breastfeeding. *Arch Womens Ment. Health* 2006;9:158-159.

[143] Gentile S, Rossi A, Bellantuono C. SSRIs during breastfeeding: spotlight on milk-to-plasma ratio. A*rch. Womens Ment. Health* 2007;10:39-51

[144] Gentile S. Infant safety with antipsychotic therapy in breast-feeding. A systematic review. *J. Clin. Psychiatry* 2008;69:666-671.

[145] Gentile S. Atypical antipsychotics in pregnancy and lactation. *Ann. Pharmacother.* 2004;38:1265-1271.

[146] Yoshida K, Smith B, Cragg M, Kumar R. Neuroleptic drugs in breast-milk: a study of pharmacokinetics and possible adverse effects in breast-fed infants. *Psychol. Med.* 1998; 28:81-91.

[147] Whalleu LJ, Blain PG, Prime K. Haloperidol secreted in breast milk. *Br. Med. J.* (Clin Res Ed) 1981; 282:1746-1747

[148] American Academy of Pediatrics Committee on Drugs. The transfer of drugs and other chemical agents into human milk. *Pediatrics* 2001;108:776-789.

[149] Yonkers KA, Wisner KL, Stowe Z, Leibenluft E, Cohen L, Miller L, et al. Management of bipolar disorder during pregnancy and postpartum period. *Am. J. Psychiatry* 2005;161: 608-620.

[150] Dodds S, Berk M. The pharmacology of bipolar disorder during pregnancy and breastfeeding. *Expert Opin. Drug Saf*.2004:3:221-9.

[151] Piontek CM, Baab S, Peindl KS, Wisner KL. Serum valproate levels in 6 breastfeeding mother-infant pairs. *J. Clin. Psychiatry* 2000;61 (3): 79-90.

[152] Bennet PN. Use of the monograph in drugs. In: Bennet PN, ed. Drugs and human lactation: a comprehensive guide to the content and consequences of drugs, micronutrients, radiopharmaceuticals, and environmental and occupational chemicals in human milk. 2nd ed. Amsterdam: *Elsevier,* 1996:67-74.

[153] Gentile S. Prophylactic Treatment of Bipolar Disorder in Pregnancy and Breastfeeding: Focus on Emerging Mood Stabilizers. *Bipolar. Disord.* 2006;8:207-20.

[154] Chabrol H, Teissedre F, Saint-Jean M, Teisseyre N, Roge B, Mullet E. Prevention and treatment of post-partum depression: a controlled randomized study on women at risk. *Psychol. Med.* 2002;32:1039-1047.

[155] Steinberg SI, Bellavance F. Characteristics and treatment of women with antenatal and postpartum depression. *Int. J. Psychiatry Med.* 1999;29:209-233.

[156] O' Hara MW, Hoffman JG, Phillips LIIC, Wright EJ. Adjustment in childbearing women: the postpartum adjustment questionnaire. *Psychol. Assess* 1992;4:160-169.

[157] Misri S, Kosstaras X, Fox D, et al. The impact of partner support in the treatment of postpartum depression. *Can. J. Psychiatry* 2000;45:554-558.

[158] Dennis CLE. Treatment of postpartum depression, Part 2: a critical review of nonbiological interventions. *J. Clin. Psychiatry* 2004;65:1252-1265.

[159] Holden JM, Sagovsky R, Cox II. Counseling in a general practice setting: a controlled study of health visitor intervention in the treatment of postnatal depression. *BMJ* 1989;298:223-226.

[160] McArthur C, Winter HR, Bick DE, et al. Effects of redesigned community postnatal care on women's health four months after birth: a cluster randomized controlled trial. *Lancet* 2002;359:378-385.

[161] Kahn DA, Moline ML, Ross RW, Cohen LS, Altshuler LL. Expert Consensus Guideline Series. Major depression during conception and pregnancy; a guide for patients and families. *Postgrad Med Spec. Rep.* 2001;3:110-111.

In: Estrogens: Production, Functions and Applications
Editor: James R. Bartos, pp. 145-168
ISBN: 978-1-60741-086-7

Chapter V

The Relationship between Estrogen and Schizophrenia

A. M. Mortimer[3]
Department of Psychiatry, Hertford Building,
The University of Hull, United Kingdom

Abstract

There is a wealth of historical and circumstantial evidence to suggest that women patients with schizophrenia may suffer from a deficit in estrogenic function. The prolactin inducing properties of the majority of antipsychotic drugs, and subsequent negative feedback on estrogen levels, is in keeping with this. The functions of estrogen, its complex receptor organization and its numerous actions are the focus of ongoing research activity. Of particular interest are its neuroprotective properties, particularly with regard to cognitive impairment, and its involvement with neurotransmitter systems which are the substrate for psychotropic drugs. Estrogen has now been used as an adjunct to standard antipsychotic medication in quite a few studies of women schizophrenia patients. Most of these are, however, not double blind randomized controlled trials. Only three relatively small double blind RCTs returned positive results: one long term study which selected for hypoestrogenism reported negative findings. Furthermore, recent evidence of the risks of long term hormone replacement therapy is of concern. The advent of specific estrogen receptor modulators, which may avoid excess risks of cancer and cardiovascular events, will have little to add to schizophrenia treatment if estrogen is, essentially, devoid of any specific antipsychotic or adjuvant mechanism of action relevant to the pathophysiology of this disorder.

Keywords: *estrogen, schizophrenia, estrogen receptor, prolactin, antipsychotic*

---

3 Correspondence: A. M. Mortimer, Department of Psychiatry, Hertford Building, The University of Hull, Cottingham Road,HULL HU6 7RX, United Kingdom, Tel. 01482 464565, Fax. 01482 464569 Email a.m.mortimer@hull.ac.uk

Key Issues

- The pathophysiology of schizophrenia remains a matter of debate
- Natural substances with a multiplicity of actions cannot be assumed to possess specific therapeutic properties
- Hypoestrogenism in women schizophrenia patients may not have the implications for aetiology, treatment and prognosis which have been assumed
- 'Gold standard' evidence for the use of estrogen in women with schizophrenia has overall failed to materialize
- Specific estrogen receptor modulators may avoid the unwanted side effects of estrogen, but this will not confer efficacy advantages if estrogen is not efficacious as an adjunct in schizophrenia to begin with

The Relationship between Estrogen and Schizophrenia

Introduction: The Neurophysiology of Estrogen

The term estrogen includes 30 hormones, of which the most widely known are 17β-estradiol (E2) and estrone (E3) [1]. E2 is the most potent form of estrogen, and this is the form to which the term estrogen will refer in this review.

The actions of estrogen are mediated by two receptors, ERα and ERβ. These are ligand induced intracellular transcription factors belonging to the nuclear receptor superfamily. ERα and ERβ differ in two amino acid residues at the ligand binding site [2]. Further estrogen receptors have been isolated as membrane bound receptors, coupled to second messenger systems involving G proteins and cAMP pathways: this affords estrogen the potential to act as a mediator of common intracellular signalling pathways in multiple cell types, including neurons. [3]. For instance, in rats, G protein coupled receptor 30 (GPR30) is found in hippocampal pyramidal neurons, where in response to estrogen it translocates to the cytoplasm and increases calcium levels [4]. A further receptor in guinea pig hypothalamus invokes a signalling pathway consequential to energy homeostasis [5].

In animal brain, ERα is found in the hypothalamus and amygdala, which are involved in neuroendocrine, autonomic and emotive functions [6] while ERβ is found in the hippocampus and cerebral cortex, areas subserving learning and memory (7). ERβ in addition is necessary for neuronal migration and apoptosis during late embryonic development. In human brain, estrogen receptor transcripts similarly prefer limbic sites [8] ERα is again found in the hypothalamus and amygdala. ERβ is expressed in the hippocampal formation, entorhinal cortex and thalamus, suggesting roles in cognition, non-emotional memory and motor functions. The functionality of estrogen receptors is further diversified and enhanced by the expression of alternatively spliced variants from different promoter sites, and the ability of different subtypes to form heterodimers [9].

Estrogen has been demonstrated in animals and in vitro to act as a neuroprotective agent against glutamatergic excitotoxicity, anoxia, oxidative injury and other toxins [10]. Some of estrogen's neuroprotective effects, particularly its antioxidant activities, are not receptor dependent [11]. Estrogens promote the survival and differentiation of cultured neurons: they are active in animal models of Parkinson's disease, Alzheimer's disease and cerebral ischemia, which is corroborated by clinical reports in human patients [12]. For instance, nuclear ERα receptor levels in post-mortem brain of Alzheimer patients correlate with degree of cognitive impairment prior to death [13]. There are associations with risk of dementia and estrogen receptor polymorphisms, although the effects seem small [14]. Furthermore, women with Down syndrome experience early onset of both menopause and Alzheimer's disease: it has been demonstrated that those with low levels of estrogen are much more likely to develop dementia, several years earlier than women with adequate estrogen levels [15]. The earlier the menopause, the greater the risk of and the earlier onset of dementia in these women [16]. Furthermore, there is an association between risk for Parkinson's disease and markers of lower estrogen levels, such as a shorter child-bearing period: estrogen replacement therapy in postmenopausal women may decrease the risk [17]. Finally, surgical menopause is associated with cognitive decline, which varies with the level of reduction of estrogen [18].

Most data suggest that estrogen can benefit the ischaemic brain and reduce cell death [19]. Estrogen is a regulator of apoptosis during maturation [20]. It is likely that these actions are mediated through modulation of genes which affect neuronal survival and the expression of neurotrophins. Estrogen modulates and interacts with a variety of both cell death regulators and growth factors: furthermore estrogen reduces levels of inflammatory factors in the brain [12]. It also reduces homocysteine, elevated levels which are implicated in the risk of dementia [21].

However, estrogen relies on calcium signalling to activate some mechanisms required for morphological plasticity and neuronal survival: it has been pointed out [22] that this implies that the actions of estrogen are dependent on neuronal integrity, whereby healthy neurons which can maintain calcium homeostasis are protected from insult, but degenerating neurons which cannot are more susceptible to insult in the presence of estrogen. Both in vitro and in vivo work converges on this issue: women who receive estrogen therapy at the menopause have a threefold lower risk of developing Alzheimer's disease compared to women not so treated [23]. On the other hand, women who commence estrogen therapy 15-20 years after the menopause, when neuronal integrity may be compromised, have a twofold higher risk of developing Alzheimers [24]. Cognitive test performance in healthy women who began therapy early or late in relation to their menopause is consistent with this [25]. Overall, therefore, neuroprotective effects of estrogen may be preventative, and by contrast there may be deleterious effects of using estrogen as treatment in established neurodegenerative disorder.

Further neuroprotective phenomena include the in vitro prevention of neuronal death from amyloid beta peptide, a toxin which accumulates in brain prior to the formation of plaques and tangles in Alzheimer's disease. The mechanism responsible is thought to consist of increased expression of estrogen receptors, which in turn induce a heat shock protein [26]. Similarly, in a mouse model, agonism of estrogen receptors in the choroid plexus may induce transthyretin, which scavenges and sequesters amyloid beta peptides [27]. A third mechanism against this particular neuropathology is the upregulation by estrogen of seladin-1, itself a neuroprotective agent in respect of beta amyloid toxicity and oxidative stress, which furthermore inhibits the apoptosis mediator caspase-3 [28]. Nongenomic actions of estrogen in the brain include maintaining nitric oxide levels to prevent overactivation of glial cells, with resultant scarring and prevention of axonal repair.

Estrogen is a neuroactive steroid: it may alter neuronal excitability through neurotransmitter receptors located on the cell surface. There is evidence that estrogen modulates monaminergic (dopamine, noradrenergic), indoleaminergic (serotonin) glutamatergic and cholinergic systems, and possibly noradrenergic function [29], [30], [31], [32] [33]. All, especially the dopamine system, have been implicated in the pathophysiology of schizophrenia, the mechanisms of action of antipsychotic treatment, or both. Estrogen enhances the effects of dopamine antagonists in animal models [34]: there may be a direct, rapid effect on presyaptic D2 receptors [35], [36]. The ERα receptor is implicated in dopaminergic neuroprotection, agonists modulating NMDA and AMPA receptor function [37]. Furthermore, estrogen opposes the inhibitory actions of dopamine in the anterior pituitary. It may inhibit tuberoinfundibular dopamine synthesis [38] and downregulate D2 receptors on lactotroph cells which secrete prolactin (10). Furthermore it binds to intracellular lactotroph receptors, enhancing prolactin gene synthesis and transcription, DNA synthesis and mitosis [39]. Prolactin itself feeds back to reduce estrogen via inhibition of the hypothalamic-pituitary-gonadal axis at several levels, thus attenuating estrogen's antidopaminergic activities.

Regarding serotonergic effects, hormone replacement therapy substantially upgrades 5HT2A receptors in the brain [40] : estrogen upgrades the 5HT1A receptor as well [41]. In animal models of depression, specific regional alterations in 5-HT2A receptors are reversed by estrogen (42) an action which may be mediated by induction of the serotonin transporter [43].

These actions overlap, potentially, with the actions of a variety of psychotropic drugs as well as the antipsychotic variety: therefore, estrogen could be implicated in mood and cognition as well as reality testing. Indeed it is generally accepted that gonadal hormones such as estrogen are implicated in mood states: in otherwise healthy women, depression may arise at times when estrogen levels decrease, ie the premenstruum, the postnatal period, the perimenopause [44] and post menopause [45] [46] including after surgical menopause [47]. There is an association of depression with polycystic ovary syndrome (PCOS), a condition in which estrogens are antagonized by hyperandrogenism (Setji ref 13) although the infertility, hirsutism, acne and obesity would no doubt impact independently on mood. Supplementary estrogens may prevent or treat postnatal and postmenopausal depression [48], [49], [50]: estrogen supplementation attenuates glucocorticoid and catecholamine responses to mental stress in perimenopausal women [51].

By contrast, it has been pointed out that women are much more susceptible to major depression and other stress related disorders than men, the majority of the risk occurring during childbearing years: animal work suggests that estrogen enhances stress-induced prefrontal cortex dysfunction [52].

Other actions of estrogen are numerous and varied. These include increasing cerebral blood flow, augmentation of cerebral glucose utilisation, and blunting of hypothalamic-pituitary-adrenal axis reactivity [53].

Estrogen and schizophrenia: evidence for an association?

In women with schizophrenia, there is indirect evidence that estrogen may raise the vulnerability threshold for the onset and manifestations of the disorder [54]. It is generally accepted that the age of onset in women is about four years later than for men [55], [56], [57], [58],[59]. This sex difference in age of onset is reduced in the presence, in women, of additional risk factors, such as a family history of psychosis and birth complications [60], [61]. However, subsequent work has demonstrated that the earlier the age of onset, the less the gender difference: the difference may only hold true for the paranoid subtype of schizophrenia, which has a greater age of onset in any case [42]. It has been suggested that the neuroprotective effect of estrogen delays onset at older ages: this effect is more marked in women, with their greater estrogen levels.

Overall, however, the data do not directly support the notion that estrogen acts, contemporaneously, as an endogenous antipsychotic drug during a period of vulnerability to schizophrenia onset in women. One alternative is that greater synaptic pruning in males, in childhood and adolescence, may lead to earlier onset and severity of schizophrenia: an etiology to which the contribution made by differential levels of estrogen is not clear [62]. Even so, pregnant women with schizophrenia, whose estrogen levels are comparatively very high, may improve symptomatically and require less medication [63].

The menopause is a further state for which there are conflicting views on the effect of estrogen, or lack of it. There is an additional peak in the incidence of schizophrenia in women between ages 45-54, when estrogen levels are in decline [55], [56], [54]. Twice as many women as men encounter an onset of schizophrenia over the age of forty years: their symptoms and natural history are disproportionately severe [64], [65]. Furthermore, there tends to be post-menopausal deterioration in women with schizophrenia of earlier onset [54], [66]. It has been claimed that premenopausal women may require smaller doses of antipsychotic treatment than male patients: after the menopause, this effect is lost [67]. Even so, later work from a large sample does not support this contention ([68]). Another study of post-menopausal women with schizophrenia taking hormone replacement therapy observed that they took half the chlopromazine equivalents and manifested less negative symptoms than similar patients not so treated[69]. However, scrutiny of the numerical differences in negative symptoms suggests that although statistically significant these are too small to be clinically significant. Furthermore, it is possible that women requiring very minor doses of antipsychotic treatment were perceived as only mildly ill and therefore their menopausal symptoms more worthy of treatment. Moreover, in healthy postmenopausal women, hormone replacement therapy modestly increased dopamine transporter availability although some of this was attributed to the progesterone component [70]. This suggests a potential psychotomimetic effect of dopamine agonism, not an antipsychotic effect: indeed, studies in patients with Parkinson's disease suggest that estrogen has an agonist effect on dopaminergic activity. By contrast in women with schizophrenia, hyperkinetic movement disorder was reduced in women during stages of their cycle when estrogen and progesterone were highest, more consistent with dopamine antagonism [71]. Suppression of gonadal secretion of estrogen, for instance in the course of infertility treatment, can result in exacerbation of schizophrenic psychosis[72]

There have been strong recommendations to pay more attention, urgently, to the gonadal axis and estrogen status in women with schizophrenia, both in research and in practice [73] Nonetheless, whether estrogen upgrades or downgrades dopaminergic function in women with schizophrenia, or acts as a partial agonist, and whether there are differential effects across individual dopaminergic systems, remains undetermined.

Some authors consider that women with schizophrenia have a better course and prognosis [74],[75] [64], [53]. Symptoms appear to wax and wane with women's cyclical levels of estrogen [76], [77], [78], [65], and during and after pregnancy and after the menopause (54), (79). However, correlations between symptomatology and estrogen levels are mostly absent or negative from this work (eg [80], [81]. One study demonstrated a weak but significant inverse correlation between estrogen levels and positive symptoms [82]. It has been pointed out [83] that most of the early work on symptom variability across the menstrual cycle in a number of psychiatric disorders included few patients, lacked prospective daily symptoms rating and hormonal evaluations and was confounded by the use of ongoing medication. Furthermore, definitions of the premenstrual phase were inconsistent. Even so a recent well designed study confirmed previous findings [81]

A study of estrogen administration after childbirth found that the relapse rate of affective psychosis was not reduced [84]. Similar work in pregnant women with schizophrenia remains to be carried out [85]. However, some animal work suggests that dopamine function in the forebrain is upgraded by gestation itself [86]. If this can be extrapolated to pregnant women, it would render them more vulnerable to psychosis during pregnancy, and afterwards given the added stress of giving birth. While it is accepted that the pueriperium is a time of great risk of relapse for women with pre-existing schizophrenic illness, the evidence in pregnancy tends to the opposite [54] unless, of course, antipsychotic medication is stopped by the patient or her psychiatrist.

Later menarche, perhaps indicating a relative deficit in estrogen or its actions, was thought to be associated with an earlier age of onset in women who go on to develop schizophrenia [87],[88] although a recent study found no association [89]. Even so, there was a relationship between later menarche, negative symptoms and functional impairment. Indeed, women who go on to develop schizophrenia demonstrate, as a group, a later age at menarche than healthy women [65]. There is more evidence that women with schizophrenia are lacking in estrogen functionality: although much of this may be inextricably confounded by antipsychotic induced hyperprolactinaemia, there is one study [90] of unmedicated patients which demonstrated lower prolactin levels than healthy women. This implies, possibly, lower estrogen levels since estrogen promotes prolactin secretion. Furthermore, before the neuroleptic era a high incidence of amenorrhea was reported in women with schizophrenia (see below).

Post-mortem transcriptomal studies of ERα are difficult to interpret. In the dentate gyrus of women with schizophrenia there was less receptor expression than in control brain, which would be expected subsequent to adequate estrogen levels (ie no upgrading of the receptor in response to estrogen deficit). Furthermore there were no between group differences in the dorsolateral prefrontal cortex, amygdala or basomedial nucleus [91]. There were correlations between receptor expression and age of onset of schizophrenia in opposite directions, depending on whether expression was evaluated in the dentate gyrus or dorsolateral prefrontal cortex. In vivo, there appear to be no differences in estrogen receptor polymorphisms between women with schizophrenia and healthy subjects, and no effect of allele type on clinical or outcome variability in patients [92].

Another piece of circumstantial evidence against an estrogen deficit, at least in prenatal life, is that women with schizophrenia have a more 'feminine' digit pattern (longer index comparative to ring fingers) than healthy women [93]

Circumstantial evidence for an association between lack of estrogen and psychotic states in general, is the precipitation of such states when estrogen levels fall substantially. Apart from the pueperium, these may follow abortion, cessation of oral contraceptives, premenstrual status, removal of hydatidiform mole and treatment with drugs which reduce or antagonize estrogen [94]. Such acute psychotic states tend to be brief, with very mixed symptomatology, may recur in similar circumstances and are associated with a history of puerperal psychosis. It is notable that an excess of premenstrual symptoms, exacerbations and admissions has been observed in several disorders, not just in schizophrenia: this lack of specificity may reflect estrogen's overall diversity of function.

There is reasonable evidence that estrogen levels are related to cognitive function, particularly verbal memory. For instance in healthy elderly men, estrogen enhances brain activation using an fMRI paradigm during a memory task: nevertheless, effects on attention, working memory and behavior are likely to be small [95]. The relevance of this for schizophrenia is that cognitive function is usually impaired in schizophrenia. Memory deficits are ubiquitous in schizophrenia [96] and are felt to be relevant to personal and social function. Even so, it is possible to construe such cognitive deficits as a risk factor for schizophrenia, rather than an integral constituent of its pathophysiology [97]. Furthermore, whether hormone replacement therapy protects against cognitive decline from any cause, or dementing illness in postmenopausal women, has not yet been firmly established [98] Recently it was demonstrated that unopposed estrogen in healthy women over 70 years had no benefits for cognition, mood or quality of life [99].

Even so, in rats, disruption of latent inhibition (a cognitive paradigm for antipsychotic treatment efficacy) is restored by estrogen in ovariectomized rats [100]. Whether this has implications for women patients is perhaps tenuous, given the lack of evidence that estrogen enhances cognition in women patients with schizophrenia, or anybody else for that matter. Even so, one study [101] was able to demonstrate cycle specific variations in cognition in severely ill, early onset women inpatients with schizophrenia, although there was no effect on symptoms: a later study found cyclical estrogen effects on positive symptoms, but not on cognition [82]. Another study demonstrated an unexpected adverse effect on motor performance in women with schizophrenia at a high estrogen phase of their cycle, and no benefit for healthy control women at this time. The authors suspected a Parkinsonian explanation of the deficit owing to the postulated antidopaminergic effects of estrogen, but clearly this could not be implicated in the performance of healthy controls. Furthermore, the women with schizophrenia failed to demonstrate any cyclical variation in symptoms as expected [102].

The Great Confounder: Antipsychotic Medication in Schizophrenia, Hyperprolactinaemia and Hypoestrogenism

All antipsychotic drugs used to treat schizophrenia are D2 receptor antagonists, and this property gives rise to numerous side effects. Hyperprolactinaemia is induced by antipsychotic drugs which reduce the inhibitory effects of dopamine on the lactomorph cells of the anterior pituitary by antagonizing D2 receptors: while antipsychotic drugs and estrogen may both increase prolactin levels, it is not clear that the mechanisms are identical or of similar magnitude. Antipsychotic induced hyperprolactinaemia may reduce estrogen to post-menopausal levels [103]). However, consistent with the hyperdopaminergic hypothesis of schizophrenia, there is some evidence that drug free female schizophrenia patients do have lower prolactin levels than healthy females, as if these levels were reduced by excess dopamine [104]. Conflicting with this is that women with schizophrenia may manifest intrinsic hypoestrogenism, as if there was too much negative feedback from excess prolactin, rather than a removal of this prolactin 'brake' on estrogen levels by hyperdopaminergia, through reducing prolactin and subsequent escalation of estrogen levels. Indeed, the term 'amenorrheal insanity' appeared early in the 20th century [105]. One study from the pre-neuroleptic era demonstrated a greater incidence (73%) of missed periods over five years in schizophrenia inpatients, than those with other diagnoses (12-59%) [106] although it has been pointed that schizophrenia patients may have stayed in hospital for longer, thus increasing the chances of making the observation[107]. Furthermore, women treated with antipsychotic drugs which do not induce hyperprolactinaemia still demonstrate low estrogen levels [108], [109] It has recently been demonstrated that most of 75 women with schizophrenia fulfilled a strict definition of hypoestrogenism: their differing prolactin levels did not account for this [105].

Overall the evidence suggests a more general failure of normal homeostatic mechanisms between prolactin and estrogen, with estrogen levels depressed even in the absence of negative feedback from prolactin, and especially so in untreated or exacerbated psychotic states. Supporting evidence for this can be found in a recent study of 50 acutely psychotic women and 23 healthy controls [11]: the psychotic women were much more likely to be admitted premenstrually, and their estrogen levels were markedly reduced across the cycle: prolactin levels were unrelated to estrogen levels.

The effects of antipsychotic treatment on the whole serve to lower estrogen levels, possibly by direct actions on the hypothalamus as well as on prolactin [111]: even so, antipsychotic drugs are efficacious. The most likely explanation for this apparent paradox is that the antidopaminergic effect of the antipsychotic treatment overrides any escape of dopaminergic activity from the control of much reduced levels of estrogen [112].

Estrogen – A Potential Antipsychotic Drug?

As will be clear from the research evidence discussed, direct evidence that estrogen acts as an antipsychotic drug by antagonizing D2 receptors (still the *sine qua non* of antipsychotic action) across dopaminergic systems, rather than specifically in the tuberoinfundibular pathway, is lacking. The tuberoinfundibular pathway has never been thought relevant to therapeutic effects, only to the side effect of hyperprolactinaemia. This premise is supported by one small study (29) which failed to demonstrate the expected cyclical variation in D2 occupancy in both healthy women, and treated women with schizophrenia, elsewhere in the brain.

It is perhaps the circumstantial evidence of an association between female sex and later age of onset or postmenopausal age of onset, compounded by the tantalizing variety of potentially beneficial actions of estrogen (at least in theory), which has perhaps generated hope that estrogen will prove to have therapeutic actions of clinical relevance in schizophrenia. For instance estrogen's neuroprotective action mediated by nitric oxide may have some relevance to schizophrenia, particularly regarding toxic mechanisms leading to negative symptoms [113] and subtle permanent brain damage [114], [113]: estrogen's effects on liver metabolism may enhance the effects of antipsychotic drugs [35].

Estrogen in Schizophrenia Treatment: The Evidence

Case Reports/Open Studies

Felthous [115] described a patient whose psychosis fluctuated in close association with her menstrual cycle. The prescription of an oral contraceptive abolished the psychosis.

Villeneuve [116] treated 20 male "chronic psychiatric patients" age 29-63, who had tardive dyskinesia, with estrogen for six weeks. 16 patients experienced a decrease in intensity or disappearance of dyskinesia. However the authors admitted that the improvement was often slight and the disappearing dyskinesias mild. The authors considered that estrogen may have a direct antidopaminergic action, and were therefore surprised that Parkinsonism did not supervene. There were no symptom changes.

Koller [117] added estrogen to the treatment of a mixed group of 21 patients with Huntingdon's chorea, tardive dyskinesia or dystonia. Less than a third of patients made any response despite estrogen's supposed antidopaminergic effect.

O'Connor [118] used progesterone in three violent treatment resistant schizophrenic patients, two of whom responded with a decrease in violence.

Korhonen [119] treated a 48 year old schizophrenia patient whose relapses were confined to the premenstrual stage with daily estradiol. 1 month into treatment the patient discontinued her antipsychotic drug, and remained well at the time of the report, after 12 months treatment. She maintained a regular menstrual cycle.

Kulkarni [106] added estrogen to the treatment as usual of 11 acutely psychotic women, and compared them to 7 women on usual treatment only, for 8 weeks. The treated group demonstrated more rapid resolution of their symptoms but by the end of the trial there were no differences.

Lindamer [120] described a postmenopausal schizophrenia patient prescribed estrogen replacement for 4 months alongside antipsychotic treatment: her PANSS positive score fell from 15 to 9 although her negative and general psychopathology scores were very slightly higher. Six weeks after stopping the estrogen, and having needed an increase in the dose of her antipsychotic drug, the positive PANSS total was 22, the negative score slightly better but the general score again slightly worse. This course is reminiscent of that described by Liao below ie worsening on discontinuation of estrogen treatment.

Ahokas [121] treated ten women with severe postpartum psychosis with estradiol alone for two weeks, at which point the symptoms had virtually disappeared. These women had baseline estradiol levels in the gonadal failure range, and there was an association between the attenuation of their symptoms and increasing estradiol levels on treatment. This is a very interesting study, despite it applying to postpartum psychosis rather than schizophrenia *per se*. Unusually the women were admitted 10 weeks post-partum rather than requiring admission within the first 4 weeks as is routinely the case with this disorder: the authors stated that the women had suffered mild but progressive symptoms from a week or two after the birth. This is even more unusual given the tendency of post-partum psychosis to develop suddenly and quite floridly.

Liao [122] prescribed estrogen supplements to 4 chronic female inpatients noted to suffer from premenstrual exacerbation of symptoms for 3 months. Only 2 patients benefited: 3 became worse when the treatment was stopped.

Tunde-Ayinmode [123] treated a paranoid schizophrenia patient, who was severely functionally impaired and poorly compliant with antipsychotic treatment, with an oral contraceptive pill. The patient improved on her additional treatment.

Studies with blinding, randomization or both

Glazer (124) studied tardive dyskinesia for 3 weeks in 10 postmenopausal patients randomized to estrogen or placebo in a double blind design. Although the estrogen and placebo groups' dyskinesia decreased by 38% and 9% respectively, this did not reach statistical significance. There were no diffcrences in psychopathology or Parkinsonian symptoms.

Kulkarni [125] conducted a double-blind RCT of two doses of estradiol versus placebo added to 'treatment as usual' (mainly risperidone) in 36 women (ie 12 per group) in acute relapse of schizophrenia, for 28 days. Total PANSS decreased by 14, 8 and 3 points in the higher estradiol, lower estradiol and placebo groups respectively: the difference between high estradiol and placebo was statistically significant, but a difference of 14 PANSS points would not fulfill criteria for response in most commercial antipsychotic drug trials, which stipulate >20% improvement in symptoms rating scale scores. The patients randomized to higher dose estradiol were 8 PANSS points worse than the other two groups at baseline, although this was not statistically significant. The mean PANSS improvement on placebo, of less than 3 points in 28 days, is remarkably small considering that these patients were prescribed effective antipsychotic treatment. Furthermore, there were no between group differences in estrogen levels across the study.

Akhondzadeh [126] reported a double-blind RCT of estrogen versus placebo added to haloperidol, variable dose, in 32 women with highly symptomatic chronic schizophrenia (mean PANSS score ~110) for 8 weeks. Psychopathology improved substantially in both groups, with a mean drop in PANSS total score of 58 points for estrogen and 38 for placebo. The between groups difference was statistically significant. The PANSS improvement on active treatment is impressive and of undoubted clinical significance, but that so much of it appears to constitute a placebo effect makes the finding very difficult to interpret. These women were an unusually severely ill group, with substantial room for improvement. The author's original analysis output files demonstrated that about two thirds of the overall improvement was in general psychopathology scores, with about one third from positive symptoms and hardly any from negative symptoms, in both groups. It may be that previous antipsychotic treatment was inadequate, that variable dose haloperidol by contrast did afford adequate treatment (alongside the general beneficial effects of being in a trial), and that the extra estrogen supplementation acted on mood and wellbeing primarily rather than specifically on schizophrenia psychopathology.

Gattaz [78] reported a double-blind RCT of conjugated estrogens versus placebo added to haloperidol 5mg daily in 40 women patients admitted with acute schizophrenia for 28 days. There were no benefits in efficacy or side effects.

Louza (10) reported a study of 44 acutely psychotic women randomized to a double blind trial of estrogen or placebo added to haloperidol 5mg for 28 days. Both groups improved but there were no between group differences.

Bergemann [127] reported a double-blind cross-over study of combined 17 βestradiol and norethisterone acetate, versus placebo, in 46 hypoestrogenic women with schizophrenia taking their 'treatment as usual' antipsychotic drug, over 8 months. Plasma assays confirmed fluctuating estrogen levels as expected, but there were no effects of active treatment on psychopathology, side effects or relapse events.

Kulkarni [128] compared 100mcg estradiol transdermal patches with placebo in 102 women on antipsychotic treatment, for 28 days. Total PANSS scores fell from approximately 78 to approximately 68 (results are reported as figures not tables) with statistically significant diminution in positive and general symptoms but not negative symptoms. Hormone assays indicated significant suppression of luteinising hormone in the active treatment group but no other differences. Again, a fall in symptom scores of 13% would not be considered a response in commercial clinical trials. This study is really too short to derive any firm conclusions.

The Cochrane Review (129)

This review considered all eligible randomized controlled trials: of 19 trials identified, only five fulfilled methodological criteria, including 122 patients. The remaining 14 were excluded owing to lack of randomization, lack of patients, lack of useable data etc. Many excluded studies were only available as conference abstracts, lacking later substantive publication. The studies included were Glazer 1985, Good 1999 [130], which is a conference abstract, Kulkarni 1996 and 2001, and Louza 2004. With the exception of Good 1999, all studies are described above. However the results of the review were based on Kulkarni 2001 as this was the only study reporting useable non-skewed data. Kulkarni's RCT of 2008 described above post-dated the publication of the review. Regarding Good 1999, this was a study with useable data from 10 women randomized to estrogen plus progesterone or placebo, alongside antipsychotic treatment for 6 months. There were no significant differences except for negative symptoms, with a mean PANSS subscale advantage of 9 points favoring the hormone treated patients. The PANSS negative syndrome score ranges from 7 to 49 points, so this mean difference would not constitute evidence of response in ordinary efficacy studies, and its clinical significance is probably low.

The authors of the review concluded that there is no evidence of any benefit of adjunctive estrogen over placebo. Even though the studies available were small and their methodology far from ideal, the authors pointed out that giving estrogen treatment to women (particularly unopposed by progesterone) was not without risk.

Discussion

The preclinical evidence for neuroprotective and neuroactive effects of estrogen suggests the possibility of therapeutic potential in schizophrenia. This, linked with the evidence for hypoestrogenism in this disorder, and differential age of onset, has led to an understandable interest in estrogen as a factor modifying risk and more recently as a treatment option. However, the evidence that endogenous estrogen acts through similar mechanisms on the same dopaminergic substrates, and at a similar magnitude, to standard antipsychotic drugs, is almost completely lacking. Indeed, there remains the paradox that antipsychotic treatment is associated with a reduction in estrogen levels yet is usually efficacious. It seems plausible, therefore, that any significant or worthwhile therapeutic activity afforded by estrogen must rest on some of its other actions: it is at least possible that estrogen may be of value in women who are particularly hypoestrogenic, rather than when it is used as a blanket approach. Unfortunately the only trial to examine this group [127] did not return any positive finding. With the exception of the trials of Kulkarni and Akhondazeh, there are hardly any positive findings in any study.

It is recognized that antipsychotic monotherapy is not effective in a significant minority of patients with schizophrenia: adjunctive treatment is widely used despite a limited evidence base [131]. By contrast in medical conditions, polypharmacy is well accepted, although overall this probably comprises true combination treatment rather than mainstay treatment plus adjuncts. It is more likely that because the effectiveness of schizophrenia treatment remains far from ideal, over the years psychotropic drugs of most other classes have been added to antipsychotic drugs in an attempt to augment antipsychotic efficacy: lithium, benzodiazepines, anticonvulsants and antidepressants have all been tried. However, adjuvant drugs may have little effect on unresolved symptoms even when used appropriately [132]. The latest reviews of antipsychotic polypharmacy and psychotropic adjunctive treatment came to opposite conclusions [133];[134].

Estrogen is not primarily a psychotropic drug, but at least the scientific rationale behind its experimental use as adjunctive treatment has some merit, albeit from, to some extent, circumstantial origins. However, an issue not addressed by acute relapse trials is that the role of adjunctive medication in schizophrenia becomes relevant in the context of a partial response: when the acute episode is over, but the patient has failed to make acceptable improvements in general or in specific regards. It is at this point, not in acute psychotic relapse, that trials of adjunctive medication are contemplated. Therefore there seems limited value in adding adjuncts in the acute stage, at least until their value has been proven in partial response. In this regard, rational adjunctive treatment must raise the issue of for what sorts of symptoms the treatment is added: in what way is the patient failing to get better? Most adjuncts should be directed at specific problems: benzodiazepines for anxiety and agitation, antidepressants for depression, extra antipsychotic for resistant positive symptoms, mood stabilizers for elation and grandiosity, etc. There is no such obvious indication for estrogen, with the possible exception of depression, which again has never been tested.

One is left with the rather non-specific notion that absolute or relative estrogen deficiency may contribute to poor response in schizophrenia, and thus supplementation may enhance response to antipsychotic treatment. Therefore, for a patient to benefit from estrogen supplementation it must be determined that the patient manifests such deficiency. This has implications for clinical practice: as a general rule it may be better to prescribe prolactin sparing atypical antipsychotic drugs to women, and to enquire routinely regarding menstrual irregularity in the premenopausal group, referring on women who may be hypoestrogenic for gynecological and endocrinological opinion. Women manifesting postmenopausal worsening of symptoms or an increased requirement for medication at this time may benefit from hormone replacement therapy. Those in whom premenstrual (or other phase) symptom exacerbation occurs may require dosage adjustments, although the delayed action believed to attach to the antipsychotic effects of antipsychotic drugs (as opposed to the side effects) may render such strategies impractical.

That the adjunctive estrogen trials reported to date may be substantially flawed cannot be denied. Even so it is disappointing that nearly all of the evidence points in the same direction, which is that estrogen added to antipsychotic treatment has no value. Even those results reported in a positive light are frankly unconvincing in terms of the clinical usefulness of routine estrogen treatment. It is difficult, therefore, to make a case for any further study in this area, unless women were selected for treatment on the grounds of, for instance, premenopausal hypoestrogenism in the presence of a partial response to a prolactin neutral antipsychotic drug. Such trials would need to be much longer than most short existing trials, and include large numbers of patients whom because of the entry criteria would be difficult to recruit. However it remains possible that estrogen deficient women with incompletely treated schizophrenia may demonstrate benefits in cognition, residual symptoms and function in these circumstances. The study of Akhondzadeh would tend to support this, given the incompleteness of the subjects' treatment and the magnitude of the response, even allowing for placebo effects and the undetermined nature of pretrial estrogen status.

Even so, there are important risks associated with giving women estrogen, the most ominous being breast and uterine cancer. Indeed, the Women's Health Initiative RCT [135] was stopped after 5 years' follow up, when the incidence of invasive breast cancer exceeded the predetermined criterion in the active treatment arm, and the absolute excess risk of adverse events was 19 per 10,000 person years. The authors stated that the risk-benefit profile found in the trial was not consistent with the requirements for a viable intervention for primary prevention of chronic diseases.

Because estrogen is not a patentable entity, it is not likely that schizophrenia trial resources will or have been forthcoming from the pharmaceutical industry: indeed, this may be one of the reasons for the limited and far from ideal nature of the studies published to date. However, selective estrogen receptor modulators (SERMS) have now been developed, with differential affinity properties across tissues. For instance raloxifene is an estrogen agonist in bone, but an antagonist in the breast and uterus. A drug which acted as an agonist in the brain but which was otherwise similar to raloxifene may have adjunctive benefits in the treatment of estrogen deficient women with schizophrenia. Raloxifene itself is an estrogen antagonist in brain: it abolishes estrogen mediated upgrading of serotonergic transmission in rats [33]. Given that serotonergic action can decrease arousal, this is consistent with a report that raloxifene can increase brain activation, and prevent attenuated performance on a facial recognition task in healthy elderly males over time compared to placebo [136]. On the other hand, estrogen can abolish prepulse inhibition deficits induced by buspirone in healthy volunteers (137). The relevance of this to schizophrenia is that schizophrenia patients reliably demonstrate deficits in prepulse inhibition intrinsic to the disorder.

The neuroprotective potential of estrogen and SERMS is more apparent in studies of stroke and cerebrovascular disease [19] [138]and in attempts to design treatments for the prevention of Alzheimer's disease [139] than in schizophrenia. It should be emphasized that such potential is currently conceptualized in terms of prevention, not active treatment. Indeed, a randomized placebo controlled trial of raloxifene [140] indicated that a higher dose of raloxifene did reduce the incidence of cognitive impairment and Alzheimer's disease.

It has been pointed out that while estrogen antagonism in the uterus and breast has anti-cancer effects, estrogen antagonism in the bone and brain may be deleterious [141]. On potential solution would be to combine a SERM with dihydroxyepiandosterone (DHEA), the precursor of both estrogen and androgen, to keep these tissues supplied with optimal levels of estrogen postmenopausally. Another is the use of enabling excipients to target estrogen or its derivatives to brain tissues [142].

There is much interest in the development an efficacious 'NeuroSERM' [22] to treat menopausal symptoms of cerebral origin, and to prevent age-associated neurodegenerative disorders: several ERβ selective phytoestrogens have been identified, which may enhance neuroprotection and cognition in men, while reducing the risk of prostate cancer [2]. Then again, whether such NeuroSERMs, with or without DHEA, would have anything to offer to schizophrenia patients of either sex is a matter for conjecture. The fundamental question is, why should estrogen be of benefit at all? Its actions are extremely complex, numerous and disparate: while some may have potential relevance to schizophrenia pathophysiology (which is itself mostly conjectural) there is no proven hypothesis which would support the notion that estrogen is efficacious. Furthermore, the suggestion that estrogen can be used as prevention, but harm may ensue if it is used as a cure [22], should lead to very serious caveats. Essentially, the question of specific mechanisms which should render estrogen effective in schizophrenia appears to have been obscured by a morass of circumstantial evidence, to which has been adduced a not insubstantial degree of optimistic speculation.

Conclusions

It is likely that the disappointing results of trials to date will discourage further research endeavor in this field. Only the publication of a large double blind RCT with clinically significant positive findings may serve to reawaken enthusiasm for estrogen as an adjunct to antipsychotic treatment in schizophrenia. That such an endeavor should be attempted now seems unlikely. Although selective estrogen modulators may be worth looking at in partially responding subacute hypoestrogenic patients, it seems unlikely that specific development of these will become a priority of pharmaceutical company strategy because of the minority status, perceived or otherwise, of this group.

Eventually, one would expect SERMS of proven efficacy in prevention (or even treatment) of dementing illness to be tried out in patients with schizophrenia, alongside antipsychotic treatment: this has already happened with antidementia drugs, without substantial benefit [143].

Accepted wisdom regarding atypical antipsychotic drugs has become that, overall, they do not differ in efficacy (with the exception of clozapine): therefore, treatment decisions are increasingly predicated on tolerability. There is a growing awareness of the importance of adverse effects: what amounts to iatrogenic disease, such as severe weight gain and metabolic disorder, is unlikely to be tolerated by health care funders, doctors, patients and relatives in the current climate of increasing managerialism, consumerism and defensive medicine. Treatments such as estrogen, whose actions are not well understood by psychiatrists and which afford potentially very serious side effects, are unlikely to be attractive to any stakeholder. Currently other avenues of intervention, such as early psychosis services and new drugs with claimed tolerability advantages, appear to hold more promise than theoretically attractive, but practically problematic, adjunctive treatments of dubious efficacy.

Acknowledgments

Adapted from Expert Rev. Neurotherapeutics. 7(1), 45-55 (2007) with permission of Expert Reviews Ltd

The author is grateful for Dr Akhondzadeh, who was kind enough to supply original analytic printouts of his data at the author's request.

Reference List

[1] Cho J, Lannucci F, Fraile M, et al. The role of the estrogen in neuroprotection: implications for neurodegenerative diseases. *Neuroendocrinology Letters* 2003; 24(3/4):141-147.

[2] Zhao L, Brinton R. Estrogen receptor beta as a therapeutic target for prooting neurogenesis and preventing neurodegeneration. *Drug Development Research* 2005; 66(2):103-117.

[3] Mhyre A, Dorsa D. Estrogen activates rapid signaling in the brain: role of estrogen receptor a and estrogen receptor beta in neurons and glia. *Neuroscience* 2006; 138(3):851-858.

[4] Funakoshi T, Yanai A, Shinoda K, et al. G protein-coupled receptor 30 is an estrogen receptor in the plasma membrane. *Biochemical and Biophysical Research Communications* 2006; 346(3):904-910.

[5] Qiu J, Bosch M, Tobias S, et al. A G-protein-coupled estrogen receptor is involved in hypothalamic control of energy homeostasis. *Journal of Neeuroscience* 2006; 26(21):5649-5655.

[6] Doncarlos L, Greene G, Morrell J. Distribution of estrogen receptor-immunoreactive cells in the forebrain of the female guinea pig. *Journal of Comp Neurol* 1991; 305:591-612.

[7] Kuppers E, Beyer C. Expression of estrogen receptor alpha and beat mRNA in the developing and adult mouse stratium. *Neurosci Letters* 1999; 276:95-98.

[8] Ostlund H, Keller E, Nordstrom A-L. Estrogen receptor gene expression in relation to neuropsychiatric disorders. *Annals New York Academy of Sciences* 2003; 1007:54-63.

[9] Cowley S, Hoare S, Mosselman S, et al. Estrogen receptor alpha and beta form heterodimers on DNA. *Journal of Biological Chemistry* 1997; 272:18862-19858.

[10] Kukstas L, Domec C, Bascles L, et al. Different expression of the two dopaminergic D2 receptors, D2415 and D2444, in two types of lactotroph each characterised by their response to dopamine, and modification of expression by sex steroids. *Endocrinology* 1991; 129:1101-1103.

[11] Manthey D, Behl C. From structural biochemistry to expression profiling: neuroprotective activities of estrogen. *Neuroscience* 2006; 138(3):845-850.

[12] Amantea D, Russo R, Bagetta G, et al. From clinical evidence to molecular mechanisms underlying neuroprotection afforded by estrogens. *Pharmacological Research* 2005; 52(2):119-132.

[13] Kelly J, Bienias J, Shah A, et al. Levels of estrogen receptors alpha and beta in frontal cortex of patients with Alzheimer's disease: Relationship to mini-mental state examination scores. *Current Alzheimer Research* 2008; 5(1):45-51.

[14] Yaffe K, Lui L-Y, Grady D, Stone K, Morin P. Estrogen receptor 1 polymorphisms and risk of cognitive impairment in older women. *Biological Psychiatry* 2002; 51(8):677-682.

[15] Schupf N, Winsten S, Patel B, et al. Bioavailable estradiol and age at onset of Alzheimer's disease in postmenopausal women with Down syndrome. *Neuroscience Letters* 2006; 406(3):298-302.

[16] Schupf N, Pang D, Patel B, et al. Onset of dementia is associated with age at menopause in women with Down's syndrome. *Annals of Neurology* 2003; 54(4):433-438.

[17] Chen L, Zhang B-S, Chen R-J, Zhang M-Y. Influence of fertility characteristics on Parkinson's disease in Chinese women. *Chinese Journal of Contemporary Neurology and Neurosurgery* 2006; 6(2):119-123.

[18] Farrag A-K, Khedr E, Abdel-Aleem H, Rageh T. Effect of surgical menopause on cognitive functions. *Dementia and Geriatric Cognitive Disorders* 2002; 13(3):193-198.

[19] Murphy S, McCullough L, Littleton-Kearney M, et al. Estrogen and selective estrogen receptor modulators: neuroprotection in the women's health initiative era. *Endocrine* 2003; 21(1):17-26.

[20] Duenas M, Luquin S, Chowen J, et al. Gonadal hormone regulation of insulin growth factor-I-like immunoreactivity in hypotalamic astroglia of developing and adult rat. *Neuroendocrinology* 1994; 59:528-538.

[21] Whitmer R, Haan M, Miller J, Yaffe K. Hormone replacement therapy and cognitive performance: The role of homocysteine. Journals of Gerontology - Series A Biological *Sciences and Medical Sciences* 2003; 58(4):324-330.

[22] Zhao L, O'Neill K, Brinton R. Selective estrogen receptor modulators (SERMs) for the brain: current status and remaining challenges for developing neuroSERMs. *Brain Research Reviews* 2005; 49(3):472-493.

[23] Zandi P, Carlso B, Plassman K, et al. Hormone replacement therapy and incidence of Alzheimer disease in older women: the Cache County Study. *Journal of the American Medical Associatio*n 2002; 288:2123-2129.

[24] Shumaker S, Legault C, Rapp S, et al. Estrogen plus progestin and the incidence of dementia and mild cognitive impairment in postmenopausal women: The Women's Health Initiative Memory Study: a randomized controlled trial. *Journal of the American Medical Association* 2003; 289:2651-2662.

[25] MacLennan A, Henderson V, Paine B, et al. Hormone therapy, timing of initiation, and cognition in women aged older than 60 years: *The REMEMBER pilot study. Menopause* 2006; 13(1):28-36.

[26] Zhang Y, Champagne N, Beitel L. Estrogen and androgen protection of human neurons against intracellular amyloid beta 1-42 toxicity through heat shock protein 70. *Journal of Neuroscience* 2004; 24(23):5315-5321.

[27] Tang Y, Haslam S, Conrad S, et al. Estrogen increases brain expression of the mRNA encoding transthyretin, an amyloid beta scanenger protein. *Journal of Alzheimer's Disease* 2004; 6(4):414-420.

[28] Peri A, Danza G, Serio M. Seladin-1 as a target of estrogen receptor activation in the brain: a new gene for a rather old story? *Journal of Endocrinological Investigation* 2005; 28(3):285-293.

[29] Nordstrom A-L, Olsson H, Halldin C. A PET study of D2 dopamine receptor density at different phases of the menstrual cycle. *Psychiatry Research* 1998; 83:1-6.

[30] Cyr M, Calon F, Morissette M, et al. Estrogenic modulation of brain activity: implications for schizophrenia and Parkinson's disease. *Journal of Psychiatry and Neuroscience* 2002; 27:12-27.

[31] Oesterlund M. The role of estrogens in neuropsychiatric disorder. *Current Opinion in Psychiatry* 2002; 15:307-312.

[32] Di Paolo T. Modulation of brain dopamine transmission by sex steroids. *Reviews in the Neurosciences* 1994; 5:27-41.

[33] Sumner B, Grant K, Rosie R, Hegele-Hartung Ch, Fritzemeier K-H, Fink G. Raloxifene blocks estradiol induction of the serotonin transporter and 5-hydroxytryptamine_{2A} receptor in female rat brain. *Neuroscience Letters* 2007; 417(1):95-99.

[34] Gruzelier J. Syndromes of schizophrenia and schizotypy, hemispheric imbalance and sex differences: implications for developmental psychopathology. *International Journal of Psychophysiology* 1994; 18:167-178.

[35] Yonkers K, Kando J, Cole J. Gender differences in pharmacokinetics and pharmacodynamics of psychotropic medication. *American Journal of Psychiatry* 1992; 149:587-595.

[36] Di Paolo T, Poyet P, Labrie F. Effect of prolactin and estradiol on rat striatal dopamine receptors. *Life Science* 1982; 31:2921-2929.

[37] Morissette M, La Saux M, D'Astous M, et al. Contribution of estrogen receptors alpha and beta to the effects of estradiol in the brain. *Journal of Steroid Biochemistry and Molecular Biology* 2008; 108(3-5):327-338.

[38] Arita J, Kimura F. Director inhibitory effect of long term estradiol treatment on dopamine synthesis in tuberoinfundibular dopaminergic neurons: studies using hypothalamic slices. *Endocrinology* 1987; 121:692-698.

[39] Molitch M. The pituitary. Prolactin. Cambridge (MA): Blackwell Science, 1995: 136-186.

[40] Moses E, Drevets W, Smith G, et al. Effects of estradiol and progesterone administration on human serotonin 2A receptor binding: a PET study. *Biological Psychiatry* 2000; 48:854-860.

[41] Wissink S, Van der Burg B, Katzenellenbogen B, Van der Saag P. Synergistic activation of the serotonin-1A receptor by nuclear factor-kappaB and estrogen. *Molecular Endocrinology* 2001; 15(4):543-552.

[42] Salokangas R, Honkonen T, Saarinen S. Women have later onset than men in schizophrenia - but only in its paranoid form. Results of the DSP project. *European Psychiatry* 2003; 18:274-281.

[43] Fink G, Sumner B, Rosie R, Wilson H, McQueen J. Androgen actions on central serotonin neurotransmission: Relevance for mood, mental state and memory.S. *Behavioural Brain Research* 1999; 105(1):53-68.

[44] Rasgon N, Shelton S, Halbreich U. Perimenopausal mental disorders: Epidemiology and phenomenology. *Source CNS Spectrums* 2005; 10(6):471-478.

[45] Pearlstein T, Rosen K, Stone A. Mood disorders and menopause. *Endocrinol Metab Clin N Am* 1997; 26:279-294.

[46] Almeida O, Lautenschlager N, Vasikaram S, Leedman P, Flicker L. Association between physiological serum concentration of estrogen and the mental health of community-dwelling postmenopausal women age 70 years and over. *American Journal of Geriatric Psychiatry* 2005; 13(2):142-149.

[47] Shifren J, Avis N. Surgical menopause: Effects on psychological well-being and sexuality. *Menopause* 2007; 14(3):586-591.

[48] Sichel D, Cohen L, Robertson L, et al. Prophylactic estrogen in recurrent postpartum affective disorder. *Biological Psychiatry* 1995; 38:814-818.

[49] Gregoire A, Kumar R, Everitt B, et al. Transdermal oestrogen for treatment of severe postnatal depression. *Lancet* 1996; 347:930-933.

[50] Best N, Rees M, Barlow D, et al. Effect of estradiol implant on noradrenergic function and mood in menopausal subjects. *Psychoneuroendocrinology* 1992; 17:87-93.

[51] Komesaroff P, Esler M, Sudhir K. Estrogen supplementation attenuates glucocorticoid and catecholamine responses to mental stress in perimenopausal women. *Journal of Clinical Endocrinology and Metabolism* 1999; 84(2):606-610.

[52] Shansky R, Arnsten A. Estrogen enhances stress-induced prefrontal cortex dysfunction: Relevance to Major Depressive Disorder in women. Dialogues in Clinical *Neuroscience* 2006; 8(4):478-481.

[53] Grigoriadis S, Seeman M. The role of estrogen in schizophrenia: implications for schizophrenia practice guidelines for women. *The Canadian Journal of Psychiatry* 2002; 47(5):437-442.
[54] Riecher-Rossler A, Hafner H. Schizophrenia and oestrogens - is there an association? *European Arch Psychiatry Clinical Neuroscience* 1993; 242:323-328.
[55] Hafner H, Riecher-Rossler A, Maurer K, et al. First onset and early symptomatology of schizophrenia. *European Arch Psychiatry Clinical Neuroscience* 1992; 242:109-118.
[56] Hambrecht M, Maurer K, Hafner H. Evidence for a gender bias in epidemiological studies of schizophrenia. *Schizophrenia Research* 1992; 8:223-231.
[57] Galdos P, Van Os J, Murray R. Puberty and the onset of psychosis. *Schizophrenia Research* 1993; 10:7-14.
[58] Faraone S, Chen W, Goldstein J, et al. Gender differences in age at onset of schizophrenia. *British Journal of Psychiatry* 1994; 164(625):629.
[59] Szymanski S, Lieberman J, Alvir J, et al. Gender differences in onset of illness, treatment response, course and biological indexes in first-episode schizophrenic patient. *American Journal of Psychiatry* 1995; 152:698-703.
[60] Konneke R, Hafner H, Maurer K, et al. Main risk factors for schizophrenia: increased familial loading and pre- and peri-natal complications antagonize the protective effect of oestrogen in women. *Schizophrenia Research* 2000; 44:81-93.
[61] Hafner H. Gender differences in schizophrenia. In: Bergemann N, Riecher-Rossler A, editors. Estrogen effects in psychiatric disorders. Wien, New York: Springer, 2003.
[62] De Bellis M, Keshavan M, Beers S, et al. Sex differences in brain maturation during childhood and adolescence. *Cereb Cortex* 2001; 11:552-557.
[63] Chang S, Renshaw D. Psychosis and pregnancy. *Compr Therapy* 1986; 12:36-41.
[64] Riecher-Rossler A, Loffler W, Munk-Jorgenssen P. What do we really know about late-onset schizophrenia? *European Arch Psychiatry Clinical Neuroscience* 1997; 247:195-208.
[65] Riecher-Rossler A. Estrogen effects in schizophrenia and their potential therapeutic implications: review. *Archives of Women's Mental Health* 2002; 5:111-118.
[66] Riecher-Rossler A, Rossler W. The course of schizophrenic psychoses: what do we really know? A selective review from an epidemiological perspective. *European Arch Psychiatry Clinical Neuroscience* 1998; 248:189-202.
[67] Seeman M. Interaction of sex, age and antipsychotic dose. *Comprehensive Psychiatry* 1983; 24:125-128.
[68] Salokangas R. Gender and the use of neuroleptics in schizophrenia. *Schizophrenia Research* 2004; 66:41-49.
[69] Lindamer L, Buse D, Lohr J, et al. Hormone replacement therapy in postmenopausal women with schizophrenia: positive effect on negative symptoms? *Biological Psychiatry* 2001; 49(1):47-51.
[70] Gardiner S, Morrison M, Mozley P, et al. Pilot study on the effect of estrogen replacement therapy on brain dopamine transporter availability in healthy, postmenopausal women. *American Journal of Geriatric Psychiatry* 2004; 12(6):621-630.

[71] Thompson K, Sergejew A, Kulkarni J. Estrogen affects cognition in women with psychosis. *Psychiatry Research* 2000; 94:201-209.

[72] Abu-Tair F, Strowitzki T, Bergemann N. Exacerbation of a schizoaffective psychosis after in vitro fertilization with leuproreline acetate. *Nervenarzt* 2007; 78(6):691-695.

[73] Riecher-Rossler A. Estrogens and the gonadal axis - Implications for the therapy of women with schizophrenia. *Nervenarzt* 2003; 74(5):398-405.

[74] Seeman M. Current outcome in schizophrenia: women vs men. *Acta Psychiatrica Scandinavica* 1986; 73:609-617.

[75] Hafner H, Riecher-Rossler A, an der Heiden W, et al. Generating and testing a causal explanation of gender difference in age at first onset of schizophrenia. *Psychological Medicine* 1993; 23:925-940.

[76] Riecher-Rossler A, Hafner H, Maurer K, et al. Schizophrenic symptomatology varies with serum estradiol levels during menstrual cycle. *Schizophrenia Research* 1992; 6:114-115.

[77] Hallonquist J, Seeman M, Lang M, et al. Variation in symptoms severity over the menstrual cycle of schizophrenics. *Biological Psychiatry* 1993; 33:207-209.

[78] Gattaz W, Vogel P, Riecher-Rossler A, et al. Influence of the menstrual cycle phase on the therapeutic response in schizophrenia. *Biological Psychiatry* 1994; 36:137-139.

[79] Seeman M. The role of estrogen in schizophrenia. *Journal of Psychiatry and Neuroscience* 1996; 21:123-127.

[80] Choi S, Kang S, Joe S. Changes in premenstrual symptoms in women with schizophrenia: a prospective study. *Psychosom Medicine* 2001; 6:822-829.

[81] Akhondzadeh S, Mokhberi K, Amini H, et al. Is there a relationship between estrogen serum level and symptom severity throughout the menstrual cycle of patients with schizophrenia? *Therapy* 2005; 2(5):745-751.

[82] Halari R, Kumari V, Mehrotra R, et al. The relationship of sex hormones and cortisol with cognitive functioning in schizophrenia. *Journal of Psychopharmacology* 2004; 18(3):366-374.

[83] Hendrick V, Altshuler L, Burt V. Course of psychiatric disorders across the menstrual cycle. *Harvard Review of Psychiatry* 1996; 4(4):200-207.

[84] Kumar C, McIvor R, Davies T, et al. Estrogen administration does not reduce the rate of recurrence of affective psychosis after childbirth. *Journal of Clinical Psychiatry* 2003; 64:112-118.

[85] A.Bosanac P, Buist A, Burrows G. Motherhood and schizophrenic illnesses: a review of the literature. *Australia and New Zealand Journal of Psychiatry* 2003; 37:24-30.

[86] Byrnes E, Byrnes J, Bridges R. Increased sensitivity of dopamine systems following reproductive experiences in rats. *Pharmacol Biochem Behav* 2001; 68:481-489.

[87] Cohen R, Seeman M, Gotowiec A, et al. Earlier puberty as a predictor of later onset of schizophrenia in women. *American Journal of Psychiatry* 1999; 156:1059-1064.

[88] Cohen R, Seeman M. Puberty and schizophrenia onset. In: Bergemann N, Riecher-Rossler A, editors. Estrogen effects in psychiatric disorders. Wien, New York: *Springer,* 2003.

[89] Hochman K, Lewine R. Ages of menarche and schizophrenia onset in women. *Schizophrenia Research* 2004; 69:183-188.

[90] Warner M, Walker A, d'Souza D, et al. Lower prolactin bioactivity in unmedicated schizophrenic patients. *Psychiatry Research* 2001; 102:249-254.

[91] Perlman W, Tomaskovic-Crook E, Montague D, et al. Alteration in estrogen receptor mRNA levels in frontal cortex and hippocampus of patients with major mental illness. *Biological Psychiatry* 2005; 58:812-824.

[92] Ouyang W-C, Wang Y-C, Hong C-J, Tsai S-J. Estrogen receptor alpha gene polymorphism in schizophrenia: Frequency, age at onset, symptomatology and prognosis. *Psychiatric Genetics* 2001; 11(2):95-98.

[93] Arato M, Frecska E, Beck C, et al. Digit length pattern in schizophrenia suggests disturbed prenatal hemispheric lateralization. *Progress in Neuro-Psychopharmacology and Biological Psychiatry* 2004; 28:191-194.

[94] Mahe V, Dumaine A. Oestrogen withdrawal associated psychoses. *Acta Psychiatrica Scandinavica* 2001; 104:323-331.

[95] Goekoop R, Duschek E, Knol D, et al. Raloxifene exposure enhances brain activation during memory performance in healthy elderly males; its possible relevance to behavior. *Neuroimage* 2005; 25(1):63-75.

[96] McKenna PCLMMBA. Memory in schizophrenia: what is impaired and what is preserved. *Neuropsychologia* 1993; 31:1225-1241.

[97] Mortimer A. The neuropsychology of schizophrenia. *Psychiatry* 2005; 4(10):26-29.

[98] Craig M, Cutter W, Norbury R, et al. Ostrogens, brain function and neuropsychiatric disorders. *Current Opinion in Psychiatry* 2004; 17:209-214.

[99] Almeida O, Lautenschlager N, Vasikaram S, Leedman P, Gelavis A, Flicker L. A 20-week randomized controlled trial of estradiol replacement therapy for women aged 70 years and older: Effect on mood, cognition and quality of life. *Neurobiology of Aging* 2006; 27(1):141-149.

[100] Arad M, Weiner I. Loss of latent inhibition in ovariectomized female rats: possible link to the estrogen hypothesis of schizophrenia. *European Neuropsychopharmacology* 2006; 16(suppl.4):S396.

[101] Hoff A, Kremen W, Wieneke M, et al. Association of estrogen levels with neuropsychological performance in women with schizophrenia. *American Journal of Psychiatry* 2001; 158:1134-1139.

[102] Thompson K, Kulkarni J, Sergejew A. Extrapyradmidal symptoms and oestrogen. *Acta Psychiatrica Scandinavica* 2000; 101(2):130-134.

[103] Kinon B, Gilmore J, Liu H, et al. Prevalence of hyperprolactinemia in schizophrenic patients treated with conventional antipsychotic medications or risperidone. *Psychoneuroendocrinology* 2003; 28(supplement 2):55-68.

[104] Rao M, Gross G, Halaris A, et al. Hyperdopaminergia in schizophreniform psychosis: a chronobiological study. *Psychiatry Research* 1993; 47:187-203.

[105] Bergemann N, Mundt C, Parzer P, et al. Plasma concentrations of estradiol in women suffering from schizophrenia treated with conventional versus atypical antipsychotics. *Schizophrenia Research* 2005; 73:357-366.

[106] Gregory B. The menstrual cycle and its disorders in psychiatric patients: 11. *Journal of Psychosom Research* 1957; 2:199-224.

[107] Haddad P, Wieck A. Antipsychotic-induced hyperprolactinaemia, mechanisms, clinical features and management. *Drugs* 2004; 64(20):2291-2314.
[108] Bergemann N. Hypooestrogenism in schizophrenic women. Archives of Women's Mental Health 2001; 3(supplement 2):S154.
[109] Canuso C, Goldstein J, Wojcik J, et al. Antipsychotic medication, prolactin elevation, and ovarian function in women with schizophrenia and schizoafffective disorder. *Psychiatry Research* 2002; 111:11-20.
[110] Huber T, Borsutzky M, Schneider U, et al. Psychotic disorders and gonadal function: evidence supporting the oestrogen hypothesis. *Acta Psychiatrica Scandinavica* 2004; 109:269-274.
[111] Baptista T, Lacruz A, Angeles F, et al. Endocrine and metabolic profile in the obesity associated to typical antipsychotic drug-administration. *Pharmacopsychiatry* 2001; 34:223-231.
[112] Baptista T, Beaulieu S. The hypothesis of oestrogen withdrawal associated psychoses and the paradox of antipsychotic drug-induced hypoestrogenaemia. *Acta Psychiatrica Scandinavica* 2002; 105(6):473-474.
[113] Rao M, Kolsch H. Effects of estrogen on brain development and neuroprotection - implications for negative symptoms in schizophrenia. *Psychoneuroendocrinology* 2003; 28:83-96.
[114] Hafner H. Gender differences in schizophrenia. *Psychoneuroendocrinology* 2003; 2:17-54.
[115] Felthous A, Robinson D, Conroy R. Prevention of recurrent menstrual psychosis by an oral contraceptive. *American Journal of Psychiatry* 1980; 137(2):245-246.
[116] Villeneuve A, Cazejust T, Cote M. Estrogens in tardive dyskinesia in male psychiatric patients. *Neuropsychobiology* 1980; 6(3):145-151.
[117] Koller W, Barr A, Biary N. Estrogen treatment of dyskinetic disorders. *Neurology* 1982; 32(5):547-549.
[118] O'Connor M, Baker H. Depo-medroxy progesterone acetate as an adjunctive treatment in three aggressive schizophrenic patients. *Acta Psychiatrica Scandinavica* 1983; 67:399-403.
[119] Korhonen S, Saarijarvi S, Aito M. Successful estradiol treatment of psychotic symptoms in the premenstrual phase: a case report. *Acta Psychiatric Scandanavica* 1995; 92:237-238.
[120] Lindamer L, Lohr J, Harris M, Jeste D. Gender, estrogen and schizophrenia. *Psychopharmacology Bulletin* 1997; 33(2):221-228.
[121] Ahokas A, Aito M, Rimon R. Positive treatment effect of estradiol in postpartum psychosis: a pilot study. *Journal of Clinical Psychiatry* 2000; 61:166-169.
[122] Liao D-L, Chen H, Lee S-M, et al. Estrogen supplementation for female schizophrenics treated with atypical antipsychotics. *General Hospital Psychiatry* 2002; 24(5):357-359.
[123] Tunde-Ayinmode M, Singh A, Marsden K. Improved functioning in a woman with schizophrenia on exclusive therapy with oestrogen pills. *Australasian Psychiatry* 2002; 10(4):403-404.
[124] Glazer W, Naftolin F, Morgenstern H. Estrogen replacement and tardive dyskinesia. *Psychoneuroendocrinology* 1985; 10(3):345-350.

[125] Kulkarni J, Riedel A, de Castella A, et al. Estrogen - a potential treatment for schizophrenia. *Schizophrenia Research* 2001; 48:137-144.

[126] Akhondzadeh S, Nejatisafa A, Amini H, et al. Adjunctive estrogen treatment in women with chronic schizophrenia: a double-blind, randomized, and placebo-controlled trial. *Progress in Neuro-Psychopharmacology and Biological Psychiatry* 2003; 27:1007-1012.

[127] Bergemann N, Mundt C, Parzer P, et al. Estrogen as an adjuvant therapy to antipsychotics does not prevent relapse in women suffering from schizophrenia: results of a placebo-controlled double-blind study. *Schizophrenia Research* 2005; 74:125-134.

[128] Kulkarni J, de Castella A, Fitzgerald P, et al. Estrogen in severe mental illness: A potential new treatment approach. *Archives of General Psychiatry* 2008; 65(8):955-960.

[129] Chua W, de Izquierdo Santiago A, Kulkarni J, Mortimer A. Estrogen for schizophrenia (review). *The Cochrane Database of Systematic Reviews* 2005;(4).

[130] Good K, Kopala L, Martzke J, et al. Hormone replacement therapy in postmenopausal women with schizophrenia: preliminary findings. *Schizophrenia Research* 1999; 12(3):131.

[131] Mortimer A. Another triumph of hope over experience?: revisiting... treatment of the patient with long-term schizophrenia. *Advances in Psychiatric Treatment* 2005; 11:227-285.

[132] Buchanan R, Kreyenbuhl J, Zito J, Lehman A. Relationship of the use of adjunctive pharmacological agents to symptoms and level of function in schizophrenia". *American Journal of Psychiatry* 2002; 159(6):1035-1043.

[133] Lerner V, Libov I, Kotler M, Strous R. Combination of atypical antipsychotic medication in the management of treatment resistant schizphrenia and schizoaffective disorder. *Progress in Neuro-Psychopharmacology and Biological Psychiatry* 2004; 28(1):89-98.

[134] Stahl S, Grady M. A critical review of atypical antipsychotic utilization: comparing monotherapy with polypharmacy and augmentation. Current Medicinal Chemistry - *Central Nervous System Agents* 2004; 11(3):313-327.

[135] Rossouw J, Anderson G, Prentice R, et al. Risks and benefits of estogen plus progestin in healthy postmenopausal women: principal results from the women's health initiative randomized controlled trial. *Journal of the American Medical Association* 2002; 288(3):321-333.

[136] Goekoop R, Barkhof F, Duschek E, et al. Raloxifene treatment enhances brain activation during recognition of familiar items: a pharmacological fMRI study in healthy elderly males. *Neuropsychopharmacology* 2006; 31(7):1508-1518.

[137] Gogos A, Nathan P, Guille V, Croft R, Van Den Buuse M. Estrogen prevents 5-HT_{1A} receptor-induced disruptions of prepulse inhibition in healthy women. *Neuropsychopharmacology* 2006; 31(4):885-889.

[138] Viscoli C, Brass L, Kernan W, Sarrel P, Suissa S, Horwitz R. Estrogen therapy and risk of cognitive decline: Results from the Women's Estrogen for Stroke Trial (WEST). *American Journal of Obstetrics and Gynecology* 2005; 192(2):387-393.

[139] Brinton R. Requirements of a brain selective estrogen: advances and remaining challenges for developing a neuroSERM. *Journal of Alzheimer's Disease* 2004; 6(Supplement):S27-S35.

[140] Yaffe K, Krueger K, Cummings S, et al. Effect of raloxifene on prevention of dementia and cognitive impairment in older women: the multiple outcomes of raloxifene evaluation (MORE) randomized trail. *American Journal of Psychiatry* 2006; 162(4):683-690.

[141] Labrie F. Future perspectives of selective estrogen receptor modulators used alone and in combination with DHEA. *Endocrine-Related Cancer* 2006; 13(2):335-355.

[142] Brewster M, Loftsson T, Bodor N. Applications of chemically-modified cyclodextrins: Use of hydroxypropyl-beta-cyclodextrin as an enabling excipient for brain targeting, redox-based derivatives of estradiol: A review of preclinical and clinical findings. *Journal of Drug Delivery Science and Technology* 2004; 14(1):21-34.

[143] Mazeh D, Zemishlani H, Barak Y, et al. Donezepil for negative signs in schizophrenia: an add-on, double -blind, placebo controlled crossover study. *International Psychogeriatrics* 2006; 18(3):429-436.

In: Estrogens: Production, Functions and Applications
Editor: James R. Bartos, pp. 169-181
ISBN: 978-1-60741-086-7

Chapter VI

Estrogen Treatment in Children

Tutku Soyer[1] and Olcay Evliyaoğlu[2]
[1]Assistant Professor of Pediatric Surgery, Kırıkkale University, Medical Faculty, Department of Pediatric Surgery, Kırıkkale, Turkey
[2]Associate Professor of Pediatric Endocrinology, Kırıkkale University, Medical Faculty, Department of Pediatrics, Pediatric Endocrinology Unit, Kırıkkale, Turkey

1. Abstract

Estrogen treatment is rarely indicated during childhood. A limited number of patients requires either topical or systemic estrogens in selected cases. Labial adhesions in which the labia minora fused over the vestibule is the most common indication for topical estrogen treatment in children. Although the most accepted theory of labial adhesions is low estrogen levels, the use of topical estrogen treatment is still controversial.

The systemic application of estrogen is used in girls with hypogonadism. Either in hypo or hypergonadotropic hypogonadism, low doses of estrogen treatment is initiated at pubertal age as a replacement treatment, to mimic normal puberty. In Turner syndrome, which is an example of hypergonadotropic hypogonadism, estrogen treatment should be also initiated at pubertal age in addition to growth hormone replacement. Although in girls, 'constitutional growth and pubertal delay' is not observed as frequently as in boys, very low doses of estrogen therapy for a short duration can be considered to induce normal puberty. Another indication of systemic estrogen treatment is for tall stature in carefully selected cases to fuse epiphysis.

Though topical estrogen treatment in labial adhesions is preferred and used by many practitioners, systemic use of this hormonal therapy is only constituted by pediatric endocrinologists. In this chapter, our aim is to discuss the estrogen treatment in children with special emphasis on indications, treatment doses and results.

2. Introduction

Estrogen is a sex steroid mainly produced by the follicle cells of the ovary utilizing the same initial steps of testosterone production with finally aromatization. At puberty with the surge of LH, theca cells of the ovary are affected and steroid hormone biosynthesis is stimulated. FSH acts on granulosa cells of the ovary and stimulates the aromatization of testosterone to estrogen. In humans the main active estrogen is estradiol which is bound to Sex Hormone Binding Protein in circulation.

Although estrogen's main functions are on uterine and breast development, pregnancy and parturition, it also effects immuno- inflammatory systems, endothelium functions [1], neuroprotection [2], and hepatic fibrosis [3]. Estrogen's effect on the skeletal system is well known — accretion of bone minerals and epiphyseal maturation [4].

In view of this, estrogen has therapeutic effects on a relatively wide range of disorders. In this chapter we will focus on systemic and topical treatment of estrogens in childhood and adolescents.

3. Topical Estrogen Treatment in Children

The topical application of estrogen ointment has been shown to be an effective prophylaxis against ageing of the skin [5]. Conjugated estrogen therapy is a generally accepted method in the treatment of cutaneous degeneration and has been shown to contribute to the connective tissue of the dermis, reflected by increased mucopolysaccharide incorporation, hyaluronic acid turnover and collagen biosynthesis [6]. It has been demonstrated that estradiol may enhance wound reepithelialization by promoting heparin-binding epidermal growth factor-like growth factor production in keratinocytes [7]. Estrogen has an important role in maintenance of tissue integrity, response to inflammation, and healing in the vulvar area [8]. Therefore, topical application of estrogen ointment is commonly used in degenerative epithelial pathologies of the genitourinary region like labial adhesions, vulvovaginitis and phimosis. As an alternative treatment to surgery, topical use of estrogens was reported in the case of urethral prolapse and carincule [9,10].

The most common prescribed formula for topical estrogen contains 0.625 mg conjugated estrogen. It is a mixture of sodium estrone sulfate and sodium equilin sulfate. Conjugated estrogens are soluble in water and are well absorbed through the skin, mucous membranes and the gastrointestinal tract. The distribution of exogenous estrogens is similar to that of endogenous ones and widely distributed in the body, especially in the sex hormone target organs. It is contraindicated in undiagnosed vaginal bleeding, estrogen dependent neoplasia, deep vein thrombosis, pulmonary embolism, liver dysfunction or disease and in known or suspected pregnancy.

Topical estrogen treatment in children is usually limited because of adverse events like vulvar hyperpigmentation, breast enlargement, vaginal bleeding and true precocious puberty [11]. In this chapter, we aim to discuss the most common indications of topical estrogens in these subheadings; labial adhesions in prepubertal girls, vulvuvaginitis and phimosis.

3.1. Labial Adhesions in Prepubertal Girls

The most common use of topical estrogens is labial adhesions in children. Labial adhesion is an acquired pediatric gynecologic problem in which labia minora are fused over the vestibula [12]. Labial adhesions are estimated to occur in 0.6% to 3.0% of prepubertal girls with a peak incidence of 13 to 23 months [13,14]. Its prevalence may be greater since many children with labial adhesions are asymptomatic and remain unreported.

The cause of labial adhesions is not known but is probably associated with low estrogen status and vulvar irritation in prepubertal children [13]. It has been suggested that the skin covering the labia minora may be denuded by local irritation and scratching which results in labial agglutination in the midline [13].

The low estrogen levels are the most accepted theory for which the topical estrogen treatment is the mainstay of the therapy [15]. Labial adhesions are rarely encountered in infants less than 3 months of age and in children older than 5 years of age [16]. Since estrogen levels are much higher in those periods. Furthermore, the role of estrogens in the etiology of labial adhesions is still controversial. It has been found that estrogen levels of infants with labial adhesions were not lower than the level in those without adhesions [16]. Papagainni et al. reported a case of labial adhesion coexisting with an isolated premature telearche and suggested the existence of other factors besides the hypoestrogenism in the etiology [14]. However, topical estrogen application is still the first choice of treatment in labial adhesions. It has been suggested that estrogen treatment enhances the resolution of the labial adhesions by promoting wound healing in the vulva [16].

Although most of the patients are asymptomatic, they can be recognized when the adhesions become inflamed or interfere with voiding [15]. Dysuria and recurrent vulvar or vaginal infections are presenting symptoms [15].

The diagnosis of labial adhesions depends on careful inspection of vulva. The fused labial area may range from a thin, transparent film of tissue to thick, firm adhesions in the midline [12,13].

Since labial adhesions rarely persist after puberty and 80% of cases spontaneously resolve within one year, some pediatric gynecologists suggest only observation of asymptomatic patients [17]. Since many asymptomatic patients are misdiagnosed as absent vagina, parental anxiety is very common among their parents [15]. Therefore, a treatment algorithm including asymptomatic patients is proposed [15] (Figure 1).

Topical treatment with conjugated estrogens is the mainstay of the conservative treatment. Although there is no consensus for the duration of treatment, common accepted treatment protocol consists of two or three times daily administration of conjugated estrogens for two weeks [18]. Warm sitz baths and introital hygiene are also advised [18].

Successful separation with estrogen cream varies from 50% to 88% [16,19]. After successful separation with estrogen creams, 19% of patients experienced recurrence [20]. When patients do not respond to topical estrogens and/or develop recurrences, surgical treatment either by manual separation or surgical lysis should be performed [15]. In the manual separation technique, topical jelly lidocaine can be used to separate mid to moderate adhesions with a success rate of 85% and recurrence rate of 14% [13].

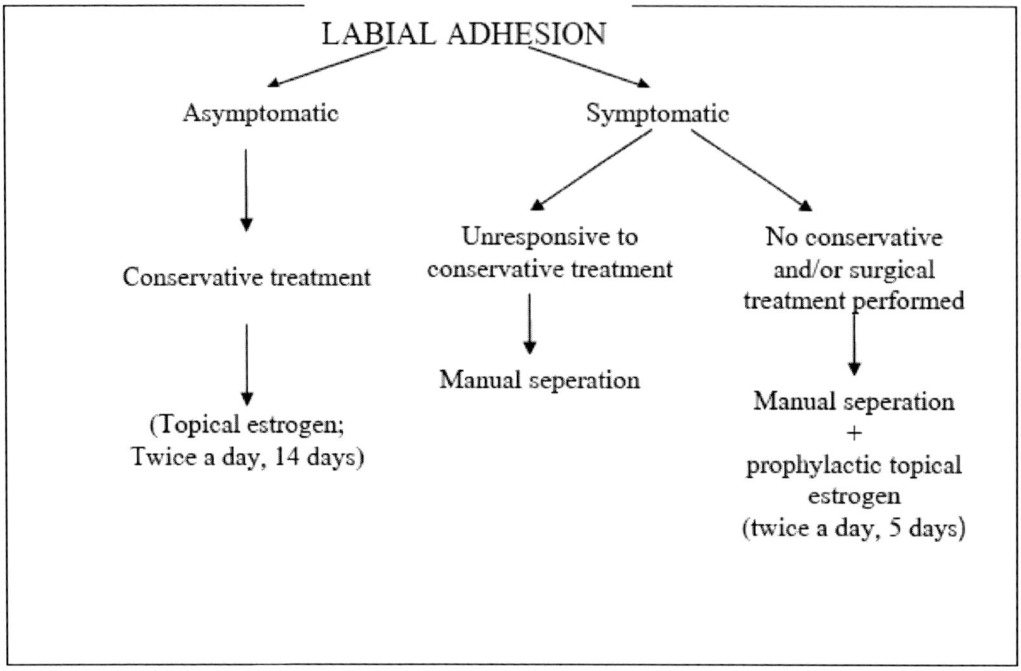

Figure 1. An algorithm of labial adhesions in children.

The prophylactic use of estrogen treatment after manual separation of labial adhesions was suggested by Soyer with a success rate of 100% [15]. In that protocol, conjugated estrogens were recommended to be applied twice a day for the 5 days following manual separation [15].

Because operative procedures are avoided because of general anesthesia, surgical lysis is reserved only for the patients who are unresponsive to conservative treatment and manual separation. Nurzia et al. suggested that thick adhesions should be treated with formal surgical repair under general anesthesia [20].

In conclusion, asymptomatic patients with labial adhesions should also require treatment in which topical estrogens are adequate. Topical estrogens have limited satisfactory results with considerable adverse events. Manual separation should be performed on all symptomatic patients. Topical estrogens prevent recurrences when used as prophylaxis after manual separation in labial adhesions.

2.2. Vulvovaginitis

Vulvovaginitis is the commonest gynecological disorder of prepubertal children [21]. It may be associated with a foreign body or sexual abuse [21]. Between the neonatal period and puberty, the vaginal mucosa is atrophic from estrogen deficiency [21]. The skin is thin, lacks cornification and the pH is alkaline [22]. Therefore it is very prone to infection. Since, the anus is close to the vulva, poor hygiene and a tendency to fecal contamination is claimed as the commonest cause of childhood vulvuvaginitis [21,22].

For specific infections, gonococcus was thought to account for the 80% of all childhood cases [22]. Haemophilis influenza, Staphylacoccus aureus, streptococci, candida and chlamidya are also isolated from vaginal and vulvar swab cultures. Jones R reported that 69% of vulvar swabs showed mixed bacterial growth in prepubertal girls with vulvovaginitis [21]. Treatment with topical estrogens has been suggested for non-specific bacterial infections [21]. The treatment of vulvuvaginitis should be planned according to clinical onset. Acute painful vulvitis with purulent discharge should be treated with oral antibiotics; those with more insidious onset can be treated with estrogens [21,23]. The suggested treatment of topical estrogens in vulvuvaginitis consist application of 0.01% dienoestrol creams twice a day for 14 days [21]. Also, patients should be advised for vulvar hygiene and avoidance of irritants and detergents.

The results of topical estrogen treatment are poor in specific bacterial infections but it has been found successful in cases with non-specific infections or negative swab cultures. It has been shown that topical estrogens resolved vulvuvaginitis in 23 patients among 26 prepubertal girls and oral antibiotics are included in 3 persisted cases [21].

Finally, topical estrogen creams can be used to resolve the vulvuvaginitis in children who had mild symptoms and mixed bacterial swab cultures. In these selected cases, topical estrogens have satisfactory results with limited complications.

2.3. Phimosis

Phimosis is defined as the inability to retract the foreskin [24]. At birth physiologic phimosis is present as adhesions between the prepuce and glans. With spontaneous erections or manipulation over 90% of foreskin becomes retractable by age 3-4 years [25]. The unretractable prepuce predisposes to ballooning of the foreskin on micturation, difficulty to directing the stream of urine, recurrent balanitis and paraphimosis [5].

The predominant treatment of pathologic phimosis is circumcision or dorsal slit [5,24]. Conservative treatment options are introduced to avoid surgical complications and discomfort to the child. However, forceful retraction of the foreskin may produce recurrent adhesions between glans and the prepuce and cause secondary phimosis [5]. Lund L et al. used betamethasone cream (0.05%) two times a day for 1–2 weeks and found that this conservative treatment is successful in 90% of cases [26]. Thereafter, another conservative treatment with topical estrogens was put forward by Yanagisawa et al. [5]. In their protocol, treatment consisted of application of estrogen ointment (0.1% conjugated equine estrogen) once daily on the tip of the foreskin for 2 weeks [5]. If the phimosis persisted, topical estrogen treatment was continued and the patient was examined in every second week. At the end of 8 weeks, patients who have fully retractable foreskins were regarded as cured. They found that topical estrogen ointment was successful in 87% of cases and the recurrence rate was 7% [5]. The average time of treatment was reported as 5 weeks [5]. The results were poor in cases with scarred fibrosis that suggest lichen sclerosus et atrophicus [5]. Prolonged application of estrogen ointments on a poorly responding skin may increase the risk of side effects and surgical treatment should be reserved for that instances.

In conclusion, topical estrogen treatment can be considered as an initial conservative treatment in boys with phimosis. However, topical estrogens obviate the need for surgery; surgical procedures are still the first choice of treatment in symptomatic cases.

3. Systemic Estrogen Therapy in Children

3.1. Hypogonadism

Between childhood and adulthood puberty is the transitional period when physical, sexual, and psychosocial maturation occurs. The onset of puberty is controlled by the gonadotropin-releasing hormone (GnRH) neuron, and is triggered when inhibition of the neuron is lifted [27]. Normally puberty in a girl starts when pulsatile release of GnRH from the hypothalamus begins [28]. Subsequently, GnRH induces secretion of pituitary hormones, follicle-stimulating hormone (FSH), and luteinizing hormone (LH) which in turn stimulate gonads. Concurrently, increases in estrogen levels in both boys and girls stimulate growth hormone (GH), and insulin-like growth factor -1 (IGF-1) secretion, which are responsible for the pubertal growth spurt [27]. Late activation of the pulse generator of hypothalamic GnRH and /or late and/or reduced release of LH and FSH lead to central delay of puberty; hypogonadotropic hypogonadism (Table 1). Whereas primary gonadal disorders lead to peripheral delay in puberty resulting in hypergonadotropic hypogonadism (Table 2) [28]. Delay in puberty is clinically diagnosed in girls in the absence of breast development at the age of 13 and onset of menarche is delayed beyond 15 years [29]. In children with hypogonadism due to either hypothalamic/pituitary defects or gonadal diseases these hormones are not produced and the onset of puberty is precluded.

3.2. Constitutional Delay

Constitutional delay describes a girl with delayed puberty and short stature who is otherwise healthy with relatively normal growth velocity. Referrals for constitutional delay are not much common in females [30]. In these girls, puberty occurs spontaneously and progresses normally at an age later than average. In these patients bone age is also delayed giving more time for growth and resulting in height within genetic potential [29].

Table 1. Etiologic distribution of hypogonadotropic hypogonadism

Constitutional delay	
Congenital	Lack of GnRH synthesis Defective GnRH release or action Isolated LH deficiency Multiple pituitary hormone deficiencies Associated with syndromes Idiopathic

Constitutional delay	
Acquired	Central nervous system tumors Cranial irradiation Chemotherapy Infectious disease Granulomatous disorders Trauma

Table 2. Etiologic distribution of hypergonadotropic hypogonadism

Congenital	Turner syndrome Mutations in gonadotropin and gonadotropin receptor genes Galactosemia Enzyme deficiencies that block estrogen synthesis
Acquired	Autoimmune ovarian failure Irradiation Chemotherapy Infectious disease

3.3. Turner Syndrome

Turner syndrome is the most frequent disorder causing hypergonadotropic hypogonadism in girls with an incidence of 1 out of every 2500 female newborns. Its incidence is much higher in first trimester abortions. In Turner syndrome, the second X chromosome is totally or partially lost. The most common karyotypes are 45, XO, 45, XO/ 46, XX, and isochromosome X in 45–54%, 17%, and 8.5% of cases respectively [31–33].

Short stature, gonadal dysgenesis causing hypergonadotropic hypogonadism, cardiac and renal abnormalities are abnormalities of Turner syndrome. Intelligence is normal in most of the girls with Turner syndrome. Although some patients with Turner syndrome have main phenotypic abnormalities like low posterior hairline, inverted nipples, and cubitus valgus others may have very mild phenotypic characteristics or even have no specific findings [31-33].

Gonadal failure is observed in more than 90% of the patients with Turner syndrome, thus puberty should be initiated by hormonal replacement therapy [31,33]. However, puberty can start spontaneously in up to 15% of the patients [31–33]. Patients with mosaic karyotypes such as 45, X/46, XX or 45, X/ 47, XXX are the most likely to have spontaneous puberty and even fertility [34].

3.4. Estrogen Replacement Therapy

In the treatment of the patients with hypogonadism, deficient gender hormone should be replaced. Although estrogen replacement therapy is the treatment for hypogonadal girls [27], timing for the initiation of therapy and the doses are still controversial even when the underlying disorder is appropriately diagnosed. The aim of the estrogen replacement therapy is to mimic normal puberty by inducing feminization at appropriate time and rate with normal growth velocity and final height.

3.5. Estrogen Preparations

Multiple estrogen preparations are available. The most widely used have been oral estrogens. Oral ethinyl estradiol is a potent synthetic estrogen and is not metabolized by the liver. Oral administered natural estrogens such as micronized estradiol undergo first-pass metabolism in the liver; therefore, they must be given in high doses [35]. Conjugated equine estrogens are extracted from the urine of pregnant mares and contain at least ten different types of estrogen [36]. Choosing the estrogen preparation depends on pediatric endocrinologist. In the workshops held in Europe and United States practices and attitudes of pediatric endocrinologist in choosing estrogen preparations have been questioned. The majority of respondents in the Unites States used conjugated estrogens [37] whereas respondents in Europe mostly used 17 β-estradiol or ethinylestradiol [28].

Timing and Dosing of Estrogen Therapy:

There is no single regimen for the hormone replacement therapy [31, 38]. Main principle of hormone treatment is to initiate estrogen at a low dose and increase the doses gradually. Once the full estrogen dose has been reached cyclic progesterone can be added. Previously delaying treatment until 15 years of age was recommended to optimize height potential [39,40]. This seems unwarranted today unless the diagnosis has been delayed and growth is a priority [41,42]. Recent studies show that estradiol treatment initiated at 12 years of age permit a normal tempo of puberty without interfering with growth and if started positive effect of growth hormone therapy on final height [43-46].

Estrogen can be started orally as 0,3 mg of conjugated estrogens every other day, 5μg of ethinyl estradiol daily or transdermal estrogen (17-β estradiol) preparations (0,025mg) twice weekly. Transdermal estrogen replacement can be preferred in the girls with a history of poor compliance or a family history of thromboembolism [29]. The dose of estrogen is increased every 6 to 12 months aiming to reach full replacement doses after two or three years of therapy. Full replacement doses are 0,625mg/day of conjugated estrogen or 20μg/day ethinyl estradiol. Once full estrogen treatment has been achieved cyclical progesterone 5 to 10 mg of medroxyprogesterone acetate or 200 to 400 mg of micronized progesterone daily for 12 days has to be added every month to induce monthly menstrual bleeding [29].

Patients with constitutional pubertal delay can only be followed without hormone treatment. If estrogen treatment is considered, dose should be low and the duration short. In constitutional delay aim of estrogen therapy is to stimulate hypothalamus-hypophysis-gonadal axis and induce spontaneous puberty. Low dosage patches can be used only at night to induce spontaneous puberty [43].

3.6. Effects of Estrogen Treatment

Effect of estrogen treatment on growth is biphasic; it is stimulatory at low doses and inhibitory at high doses [47]. Estrogens accelerate bone maturation and are the hormones responsible for epiphyseal fusion, therefore they may result in decreased adult height [48–49]. Estrogen therapy induces normal rate of breast development [50–51]. The effects on uterine dimensions are not clear; some studies show beneficial effects [50–52] whereas others report suboptimal uterine development [53–54].

Other benificial effects of estrogen are on bone mineral density, lipid profiles, liver enzymes, physical fitness [55], cardiovascular health [56] and neurocognitive development [57].

3.7. Aromatase Deficiency

Aromatase deficiency is rare in humans. Aromatase is the enzyme that catalyzes conversion of androgens into estrogens. Inactivating mutations in the aromatase gene cause estrogen deficiency with normal or elevated levels of gonadotropins and testosterone in affected individuals of both genders. The aromatase deficient females are born with ambiguous genitalia due to hyperandrogenism and virilization. Later in life they have delay in bone age and puberty with absent breast development, primary amenorrhea, and worsening of virilization. Males with aromatase deficiency do not have obvious clinical phenotype at birth. They are presented later in life with tall stature, delayed epiphyseal closure, osteopenia, osteoporosis, eunuchoid body proportions and impairment of fertility. Estrogen replacement therapy reverses the symptoms both in females and males [58,59].

3.8. Tall Stature

Intrinsic tall stature is defined as a stature greater than 2 SD above mean height for age and gender but within the broadest range of normal including 99.9th centile (+4 SD) [60]. Intrinsic tall stature can be constitutional; a variant of normal or due to a pathological state. Definition of constitutional tall stature depends on the society where the subjects reside. Although previously tall stature was considered as a handicap and was treated with estrogens regarding to its effect on closure of epiphysis, it is no longer considered as a disadvantage [61]. Thus it is rarely treated at present [62]. However two data about estrogen treatment indicate that in girls with a bone age less than 13 years adult height might be foreshortened by approximately 5 cm and 5,2 cm when ethinyl estradiol 0,1mg /day [63] and conjugated estrogens 7,5 to 11,25mg/day [64] is administered until the bone age reaches 15 years (Greulich and Pyle).

4. Conclusion

Estrogen treatment is rarely indicated during childhood. A limited number of patients requires either topical or systemic estrogens in selected cases. Though topical estrogen treatment in labial adhesions is preferred and used by many practitioners, systemic use of this hormonal therapy should be only constituted by pediatric endocrinologists

References

[1] Arnal JF, Scarabin PY, Tremollieres F, Laurell H, Gourdy P. Estrogens in vascular biology and disease: where do we stand today? *Curr Opin Lipidol* 2007;18:554-60.

[2] Prokai L, Simpkins JW. Structure-nongenomic neuroprotection relationship of estrogens and estrogen-derived compounds. *Pharmacol Ther* 2007;114:1-12.

[3] Shimizu I, Omoya T, Kondo Y et al. Estrogen therapy in a male patient with chronic hepatitis C and irradiation-induced testicular dysfunction. *Intern Med* 2001;40:100-4.

[4] Rochira V, Zirilli L, Madeo B et al. Skeletal effects of long-term estrogen and testosterone replacement treatment in a man with congenital aromatase deficiency: evidences of a priming effect of estrogen for sex steroids action on bone. *Bone* 2007;40:1662-8.

[5] Yanagisawa N, Baba Katsuyuki, Yamagoe M, Iwamoto T. Conservative treatment of childhood phimosis with topical conjugated equine estrogen ointment. *Int J Urol* 2000;7: 1-3

[6] Mor Z, Caspi E. Cutenous complications of hormone replacement theraphy. *Clin Dermatol* 1997;15:147-54

[7] Kanda N, Watanabe S. 17beta estradiol enhances heparin-binding epidermal grwoth factor-like growth factor production in human kerotinocytes. *Am J Physiol Cell Physiol* 2005; 288:13-23

[8] Shober J, Dulabon R, Martin-Alguacil N, Kow LM, Pfaff D. Significance of topical estrogens to labial fusion and vaginal introital integrity. *J Pediatr Adolesc Gynecol* 2006; 19:337-9

[9] Wright M. Urethral prolapse in children-alternative management. *S Afr Med J* 1987; 72:551-2

[10] Chen YM, Chen YH, Li PX. Urethral caruncle treated with local applications of stilbestrol. *Zhonghua Wai Ke Za Zhi* 1981; 19:48

[11] Myers JB, Sorensen CM, Wisner BP, Furness PD, Passamaneck M, Koyle MA. Betametasone cream for the treatment of pre-pubertal labial adhesions. *J Pediatr Adolesc Gynecol* 2006; 19:407-11

[12] Omar HA. Management of labial adhesions in prepubertal girls. *J Pediatr Adolesc Gynecol* 2000; 13:183-5

[13] Muram D. Treatment of prepubertal girls with labial adhesions. J Pediatr Adolesc Gynecol 1999; 12:67-70

[14] Papagianni M, Stanhope R. Labial adhesions in a girl with isolated premature thelarche: the importance of estrogenization. *J Pediatr Adolesc Gynecol* 2003; 16:31-2

[15] Soyer T. Topical estrogen theraphy in labial adhesions in children:Therupathic or prophylactic? *J Pediatr Adolesc Gynecol* 2007; 20:241-4

[16] Cağlar KM. Serum estrodiol levels in infants with and without labial adhesions: The role of estrogen in the etiology and treatment. *Pediatr Dermatol* 2007; 24: 373-5

[17] Leung AK, Robson WL, Kao CP, Liu EK, Fong JH. Treatment of labial fusion with topical estrogen theraphy. *Clin Pediatr* 2005; 44: 245-7

[18] Kumetz LM, Quint EH, Fisseha S, Smith YR. Estrogen treatment success in recurrent and persistent labial agglutination. *J Pediatr Adolesc Gynecol* 2006; 19:381-4

[19] Smith C, Smith DP. Office pediatric urologic procedures from a parenteral perspective. *Urology* 2000; 55:272-6

[20] Nurzia MJ, Eickhorst KM, Ankem M, Barone JG. The surgical treatment of labial adhesions in pre-pubertal girls. *J Pediatr Adolesc Gynecol* 2003; 16:21-3

[21] Jones R. Childhood vulvovaginitis and vaginal discharge in general practice. *Fam Pract* 1996;13:369-72

[22] Gray LA, Kotcher E. Vaginitis in childhood. Am J Obstet Gynec 1961; 82:530-539

[23] Smail P. Vulvovaginitis. *Arch Dis Child* 1992; 67:1519-20

[24] Murphy JP, Gatti JM. Abnormalities of the uretha, penis, and scrotum. In Grosfeld JL, O'Neil JA, Fonkalsrud EW, Coran AG. *Pediatric Surgery*, Philedelphia, Mosby Elsevier, Sixth edition, 2006, 1899-1910

[25] Oster J. Further fate of the foreskin: Incidance of preputial adhesions, phimosis, and smegma among Danish schoolboys. *Arch Dis Child* 1968; 43:200-203

[26] Lund L, Wai KH, Mui LM, Yeung CK. Effect of topical steroid on non-retractile prepubertal foreskin by a prospective, randomized, double-blind study. *Scand J Urol Nephrol* 2000; 34: 267-9

[27] MacGillivray MH. Induction of puberty in hypogonadal children. *J Pediatr Endocrinol Metab* 2004;17 Suppl 4:1277-87

[28] Kiess W, Conway G, Ritzen M et al. Induction of puberty in the hypogonadal girl--practices and attitudes of pediatric endocrinologists in Europe. *Horm Res* 2002;57:66-71.

[29] Lee PA HC. Puberty and its disorders. In: F L, ed. *Pediatric Endocrinology*. 2 vol. 5 ed. New York: Informa health care USA, Inc; 2007:272-303.

[30] Rosenfeld R, Cohen, P. Disorders of growth hormone/insulin-like growth factor secretion and action. In: MA S, ed. *Pediatric Endocrinology*. 2 ed. Philadelphia, Pennsylvania: Saunders; 2002:211-288.

[31] Sybert VP, McCauley E. Turner's syndrome. *N Engl J Med* 2004;351:1227-38.

[32] Saenger P. Turner's syndrome. *N Engl J Med* 1996;335:1749-54.

[33] Saenger P, Wikland KA, Conway GS et al. Recommendations for the diagnosis and management of Turner syndrome. *J Clin Endocrinol Metab* 2001;86:3061-9.

[34] Singh RP, Carr DH. The anatomy and histology of XO human embryos and fetuses. *Anat Rec* 1966;155:369-83.

[35] Leung KC, Johannsson G, Leong GM, Ho KK. Estrogen regulation of growth hormone action. *Endocr Rev* 2004;25:693-721.

[36] de Muinck Keizer-Schrama SM. Introduction and management of puberty in girls. *Horm Res* 2007;68 Suppl 5:80-3.

[37] Drobac S, Rubin K, Rogol AD, Rosenfield RL. A workshop on pubertal hormone replacement options in the United States. *J Pediatr Endocrinol Metab* 2006;19:55-64.
[38] Saenger P. Transition in Turner's syndrome. *Growth Horm IGF Res* 2004;14 Suppl A:S72-6.
[39] Brouchet L, Krust A, Dupont S, Chambon P, Bayard F, Arnal JF. Estradiol accelerates reendothelialization in mouse carotid artery through estrogen receptor-alpha but not estrogen receptor-beta. *Circulation* 2001;103:423-8.
[40] Pare G, Krust A, Karas RH et al. Estrogen receptor-alpha mediates the protective effects of estrogen against vascular injury. *Circ Res* 2002;90:1087-92.
[41] Rossouw JE. Hormone replacement therapy and cardiovascular disease. *Curr Opin Lipidol* 1999;10:429-34.
[42] Zhu Y, Bian Z, Lu P et al. Abnormal vascular function and hypertension in mice deficient in estrogen receptor beta. *Science* 2002;295:505-8.
[43] Ankarberg-Lindgren C, Elfving M, Wikland KA, Norjavaara E. Nocturnal application of transdermal estradiol patches produces levels of estradiol that mimic those seen at the onset of spontaneous puberty in girls. *J Clin Endocrinol Metab* 2001;86:3039-44.
[44] Rosenfield RL, Devine N, Hunold JJ, Mauras N, Moshang T, Jr., Root AW. Salutary effects of combining early very low-dose systemic estradiol with growth hormone therapy in girls with Turner syndrome. *J Clin Endocrinol Metab* 2005;90:6424-30.
[45] van Pareren YK, de Muinck Keizer-Schrama SM, Stijnen T et al. Final height in girls with turner syndrome after long-term growth hormone treatment in three dosages and low dose estrogens. *J Clin Endocrinol Metab* 2003;88:1119-25.
[46] Bondy CA. Care of girls and women with Turner syndrome: A guideline of the Turner Syndrome Study Group. *J Clin Endocrinol Metab* 2007;92:10-25.
[47] Ross JL, Cassorla FG, Skerda MC, Valk IM, Loriaux DL, Cutler GB, Jr. A preliminary study of the effect of estrogen dose on growth in Turner's syndrome. *N Engl J Med* 1983;309:1104-6.
[48] Ross JL, Long LM, Skerda M et al. Effect of low doses of estradiol on 6-month growth rates and predicted height in patients with Turner syndrome. *J Pediatr* 1986;109:950-3.
[49] MacGillivray MH, Morishima A, Conte F, Grumbach M, Smith EP. Pediatric endocrinology update: an overview. The essential roles of estrogens in pubertal growth, epiphyseal fusion and bone turnover: lessons from mutations in the genes for aromatase and the estrogen receptor. *Horm Res* 1998;49 Suppl 1:2-8.
[50] Piippo S, Lenko H, Kainulainen P, Sipila I. Use of percutaneous estrogen gel for induction of puberty in girls with Turner syndrome. *J Clin Endocrinol Metab* 2004;89:3241-7.
[51] Chernausek SD, Attie KM, Cara JF, Rosenfeld RG, Frane J. Growth hormone therapy of Turner syndrome: the impact of age of estrogen replacement on final height. Genentech, Inc., Collaborative Study Group. *J Clin Endocrinol Metab* 2000;85:2439-45.
[52] McDonnell CM, Coleman L, Zacharin MR. A 3 year prospective study to assess uterine growth in girls with Turner syndrome by pelvic ultrasound. *Clin Endocrinol* 2003;58:446-450.

[53] Paterson WF HA, Donaldson MD. Poor uterine development in Turner syndrome with oral estrogen therapy. *Clin Endocrinol (Oxf)* 2002;56:359-365.

[54] Bannink EMN LM, de Muinck Keizer-Schrama SMPF. Results of estrogen therapy on uterine dimensions in Turner syndrome (abstract). *Horm Res* 2004;62:456.

[55] Gravholt CH, Naeraa RW, Fisker S, Christiansen JS. Body composition and physical fitness are major determinants of the growth hormone-insulin-like growth factor axis aberrations in adult Turner's syndrome, with important modulations by treatment with 17 beta-estradiol. *J Clin Endocrinol Metab* 1997;82:2570-7.

[56] Gravholt CH, Naeraa RW, Nyholm B et al. Glucose metabolism, lipid metabolism, and cardiovascular risk factors in adult Turner's syndrome. The impact of sex hormone replacement. *Diabetes Care* 1998;21:1062-70.

[57] Ross JL, McCauley E, Roeltgen D et al. Self-concept and behavior in adolescent girls with Turner syndrome: potential estrogen effects. *J Clin Endocrinol Metab* 1996;81:926-31

[58] Zirilli L, Rochira V, Diazzi C, Caffagni G, Carani C. Human models of aromatase deficiency. *J Steroid Biochem Mol Biol* 2008;109:212-8.

[59] Jones ME, Boon WC, McInnes K, Maffei L, Carani C, Simpson ER. Recognizing rare disorders: aromatase deficiency. *Nat Clin Pract Endocrinol Metab* 2007;3:414-21.

[60] Allen DB RS, Reiter EO. Normal growth and growth disorders. In: Kappy MS AD, Geffner ME, ed. *Principles and practice of pediatric endocrinology*. Springfield: Charles C Thomas; 2005:77-216.

[61] Iughetti L, Bergomi A, Bernasconi S. Diagnostic approach and therapy of overgrowth and tall stature in childhood. *Minerva Pediatr* 2003;55:563-82.

[62] Bernard ND SA, Bobela S. The current use of estrogens for growth suppressant therapy in adolescent girls. *J Pediatr Adolesc Gynec* 2002;15:23-26.

[63] Gruters A, Heidemann P, Schluter H, Stubbe P, Weber B, Helge H. Effect of different oestrogen doses on final height reduction in girls with constitutional tall stature. *Eur J Pediatr* 1989;149:11-3.

[64] Weimann E, Bergmann S, Bohles HJ. Oestrogen treatment of constitutional tall stature: a risk-benefit ratio. *Arch Dis Child* 1998;78:148-51.

In: Estrogens: Production, Functions and Applications ISBN: 978-1-60741-086-7
Editor: James R. Bartos, pp. 183-214

Chapter VII

Estrogens and Dentistry

***Ana Lia Anbinder*[1] *and Vanessa Ávila Sarmento Silveira*[2]**
1. Department of Dentistry, University of Taubaté (UNITAU), Taubaté, São Paulo, Brazil
2. University of Pindamonhangaba (FAPI), Pindamonhangaba, São Paulo, Brazil

Abstract

The connection between estrogens and oral health has been a concern and the subject of much research in several areas of dentistry, such as periodontology, implantodontology, endodontology, prosthodontics, orthodontics, maxillofacial surgery, and oral pathology. However, this link still remains controversial. Therefore, the purpose of this chapter is to review and summarize the available literature regarding the role of estrogen in stomatognathic tissues and the consequences of estrogenic variations to this system. Estrogen depletion results in bone loss and may lead to a reduced bone repair capacity, which has been implicated in several clinical complications experienced by postmenopausal women. Among them, a residual alveolar ridge reduction increases the difficulty of dental prosthesis adaptation. Delayed bone repair may modify the wound healing process after intraosseous neoplasm removal or alter the course of endodontic treatment of periradicular lesions, as well as for implant osseointegration. Estrogen deficiency could be an aggravating factor in periodontal diseases and may cause significant rapid orthodontic tooth movement. Estrogenic action has been suggested to be responsible for the high prevalence of autoimmune diseases in women, such as Sjogren's syndrome; the occurrence of burning and dry mouth seems to be generally associated with climacteric symptoms, which are related to estrogen deficiency. Temporomandibular disorders, common clinical conditions involving pain, are more prevalent in women of reproductive-age than in men. Furthermore, women may present different patterns of periodontal disease during pregnancy, the menstrual cycle, or when using contraceptives or hormone replacement therapy. In conclusion, estrogens significantly affect the oral cavity, but further studies are needed to elucidate the extension and molecular mechanisms of those interactions.

Introduction

Hormonal variation experienced by women under physiological conditions, such as puberty, pregnancy, and menopause, as well as under non-physiological conditions, such as hormonal replacement therapy or the use of oral contraceptives, exert significant influence on physiology throughout life [1]. Significant attention to women's health issues has only recently occurred in the medical research within the past few decades, and since then, an increasing body of sex-specific literature has emerged regarding issues related to women [2]. Such studies regarding women have also recently occurred in dentistry, and the connection between estrogen variations, especially deficiency and postmenopausal osteoporosis, and oral health has been a concern in several dental areas, such as periodontology, implantodontology, endodontology, prosthodontics, orthodontics, maxillofacial surgery, and oral pathology. Estrogenicity is a property that has also been studied in dental materials. Although the relationship between estrogens and dentistry has been the focus of much research, it still remains a matter of controversy. For these reasons, the purpose of this chapter is to review and summarize the available literature regarding the role of estrogens in stomatognathic tissues, the consequences of estrogenic variations to this system, and the role of dentist in the diagnosis of related systemic diseases.

1. Estrogen and Oral Neoplasms

The connection between hormones and breast cancer development and growth has been recognized for a long time. Estrogen stimulates the proliferation of breast epithelial cells and estrogenic action at target sites in the body is mediated through related, but distinct, estrogen receptors (ERs) (ERalpha and ERbeta) which result in altered gene expression [3]. However, estrogen signaling in non-reproductive tract tissues is less well characterized [4].

The expression of sex hormone receptors in some tumors suggests a role for these receptors in tumor pathogenesis and therapy. Previous studies on the expression of estrogen and progesterone receptors in salivary gland tumors have reported conflicting results [5].

Of the eight salivary gland tumors exhibiting differential histology (pleomorphic salivary adenoma, adenocarcinoma, mucoepidermoid carcinoma, and carcinoma ex-pleomorphic salivary adenoma), which were investigated by Lamey et al.[6], none demonstrated high affinity receptors for estrogen or progesterone. Salivary tissue from patients with non-neoplastic salivary gland disease has also been studied and did not contain high affinity receptor sites. Pires et al. [7] analyzed the estrogen receptor expression of 136 mucoepidermoid carcinomas and 72 adenoid cystic carcinomas, and all cases were negative. These results do not support a role for estrogens in the lesions studied.

Ozono et al.[8] performed immunohistochemical analyses of estradiol, progesterone, and progesterone receptors in human salivary gland and salivary adenoid cystic carcinoma and found immunoreactivity to estradiol and progesterone in the cytoplasm of cells from the excretory duct system within normal salivary glands. In comparison, the progesterone receptor was restricted to the nuclei of cells for which both sex steroids were positive. This investigation demonstrated the presence of both sex steroids and the progesterone receptor in salivary adenoid cystic carcinomas, suggesting that the human salivary gland is one of the target tissues for estrogen. Nasser et al. [5] evaluated the immunohistochemical expression of androgen, estrogen, and progesterone receptors in 78 salivary gland tumors. The majority [91%] of these salivary gland tumors were negative for both estrogen and progesterone receptors, while androgen receptor expression was found for 54% of 52 malignant salivary gland tumors. The frequency of androgen receptor expression varied from 20% in carcinomas, such as mucoepidermoid, adenoid cystic, and acinic cell, to 100% in carcinoma ex pleomorphic adenoma, salivary duct carcinoma, and basal cell adenocarcinoma. All of the benign salivary gland tumors were negative for the receptors tested. The observed disparity in these reported results could be related to differences in tissue fixation, the sensitivity and specificity of antibodies, methods used by each group, the criteria adopted for determining if a tumor was positive for the marker, or even due to the relatively small number of cases studied [5].

In an investigation of experimentally 9,10-dimethyl-l,2-benzanthracene (DMBA)-induced submandibular epidermoid carcinomas in rats, estrogen receptors were found in the nuclei of tumor cells that occupied the peripheral rim of the tumor cell nests. In contrast, reactivity found in the normal submandibular glands without tumor cells was mostly confined to the nuclei of the duct cells [9]. Based on these results, Ozono et al. proposed that estrogens might be involved in not only duct cell functions, but also in the development or growth of submandibular gland tumors [9].

In cultured oral squamous cell carcinoma cells that over-expressed the estrogen receptor β, an estrogen receptor antagonist (tamoxifen), but not an agonist (estradiol), was able to induce apoptosis through interfering with adhesion and disrupting survival signals. The treatment with tamoxifen resulted in cell structure disorders by destroying F-actin filaments and reducing the invasive ability of squamous cell carcinoma. The authors identified a potentially important role for estrogen antagonists in the treatment of human oral squamous cell carcinoma, which may prevent tumor invasion and metastasis [10].

The evidently lower incidence of squamous oral cancer among women than men suggest endocrine involvement in the development of this disease [11]. According to Suba [11], this gender-specific risk for oral cancer raises two different assumptions: 1) there are noxious factors that selectively affect male patients, and 2) there are common risk factors affecting both sexes, but females have developed defense mechanisms due to specific hormonal and metabolic features. However, there is no available data yet that provides an explanation for the gender-specific incidence rate of oral cancer. In a case-control study [11] that included 2660 inpatients with squamous cell oral carcinoma, almost all female oral cancer patients were postmenopausal, while 25% of control women in the same age group were pre-menopausal. These results raised a new concept concerning oral cancer initiation that a deficiency in estrogen may provoke malignant transformation. An abrupt decrease of estrogen levels after menopause may cause disturbances in gene regulation. As cancer initiation requires many years, the longer the postmenopausal estrogen deficiency period, the higher the possibility of cancer development [11].

There is growing evidence to support the role of steroid hormonal regulation and squamous cell cancer of the upper aerodigestive tract [12]. Yoo et al. [12] measured urinary metabolite levels of 16α-hydroxyestrone (16α-OHE1) and 2-hydroxyestrone(2-OHE1), estrogen metabolites that demonstrated proliferative and anti-proliferative effects, respectively, from 50 head and neck cancer patients compared to 50 age- and sex-matched controls. The most common location of cancer was the larynx (60%), followed by the oropharynx (32%), and the oral cavity (8%). When absolute levels of 16α-OHE1 among cancer patients were compared with controls, there was no statistical difference. However, 30% of head and neck cancer patients exhibited low 2/16α-OHE1 ratios compared with only 4% among the healthy population. This study suggests that low 2-/16 α -OHE1 may constitute a risk factor in the development of cancers of the upper aerodigestive tract; 2-/16 α -OHE1 may also serve as a potential biological marker of individuals with an increased risk for cancer development [12].

2. Estrogens and Non-Neoplastic Soft Tissue Oral Lesions

Estrogens play important roles in the pathogenesis of some oral diseases with a higher prevalence in females, such as pyogenic granulomas and peripheral giant cell granulomas. The pyogenic granuloma (Figure 1) is an exuberant inflammatory response to local irritation or trauma, composed of proliferating capillaries and endothelial cells, typically accompanied by a mixed inflammatory cell infiltrate [13]. The lesion is usually seen on the gingiva, but may also be present on the lips, tongue, or buccal mucosa. When pyogenic granuloma develops in a pregnant woman, the terms "pregnancy tumor" or "granuloma gravidarum" are often used [14]. The lesion will either regress [1] or develop into a smaller mass post-partum if left untreated, so surgical removal is usually performed after parturition. No significant differences in estrogen and progesterone receptor staining were noted among pyogenic granuloma in pregnant women, nonpregnant women, or men; consequently, it appears that the levels of circulating hormones may play a strong role in the development of the pregnancy tumor[13]. Female steroid hormones may not only enhance the expression of angiogenic factors in inflamed tissue, but also decrease apoptosis of granuloma cells to extend angiogenic effects in pregnant woman [15].

Díaz-Guzmán and Castellanos-Suárez [16] examined oral lesions in 7,952 women, and found the greatest prevalence of pyogenic granuloma and benign migratory glossitis during pregnancy. Benign migratory glossitis has not conventionally been included among oral lesions associated with pregnancy, and may constitute only a casual observation in this study [16].

Peripheral giant cell granuloma is also a reactive lesion caused by local irritation, and occurs exclusively on the gingival or edentulous alveolar ridge. The giants cells within the lesion exhibit features of osteoclasts [14]. Günhan et al. [17] studied the presence of estrogen and progesterone receptors in 26 peripheral giant cell granulomas and concluded that cells forming the lesion are potential targets for estrogen, but not progesterone.

Paracoccidioidomycosis (Figure 2), the most important systemic mycosis in Latin America, is much more common in men than in women [18], and often affects oral tissues. Frequently, the dentist is the professional that is responsible for the diagnosis, due to the presence of oral lesions.

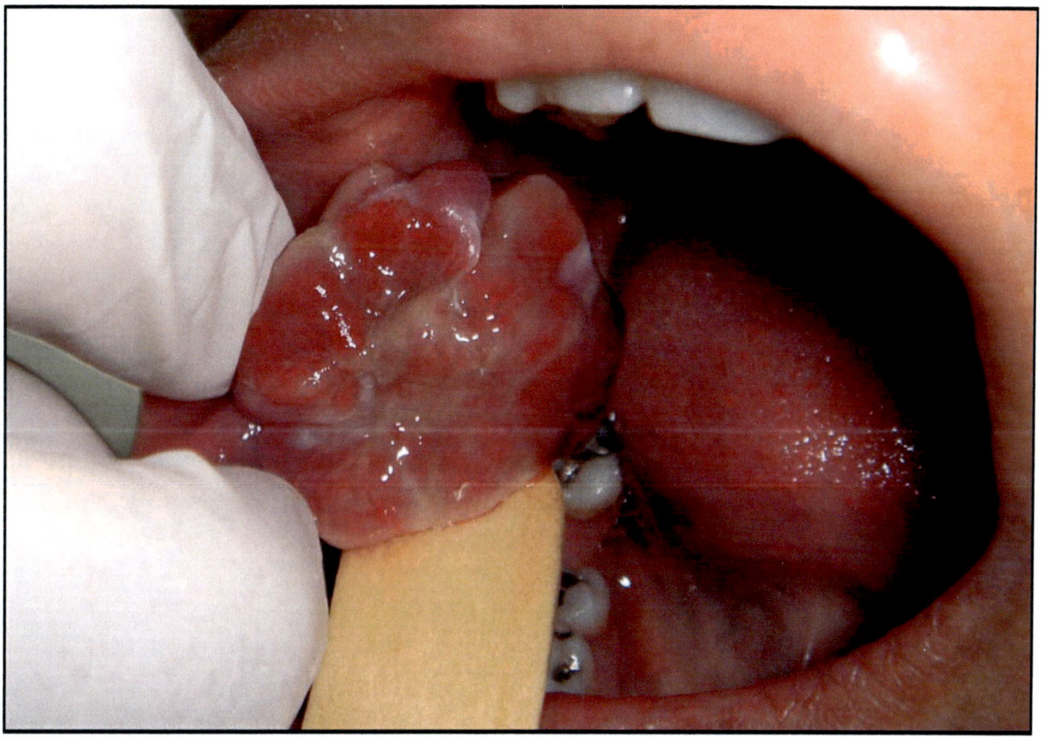

Figure 1. Pregnancy granuloma on buccal mucosa of a post-partum patient.

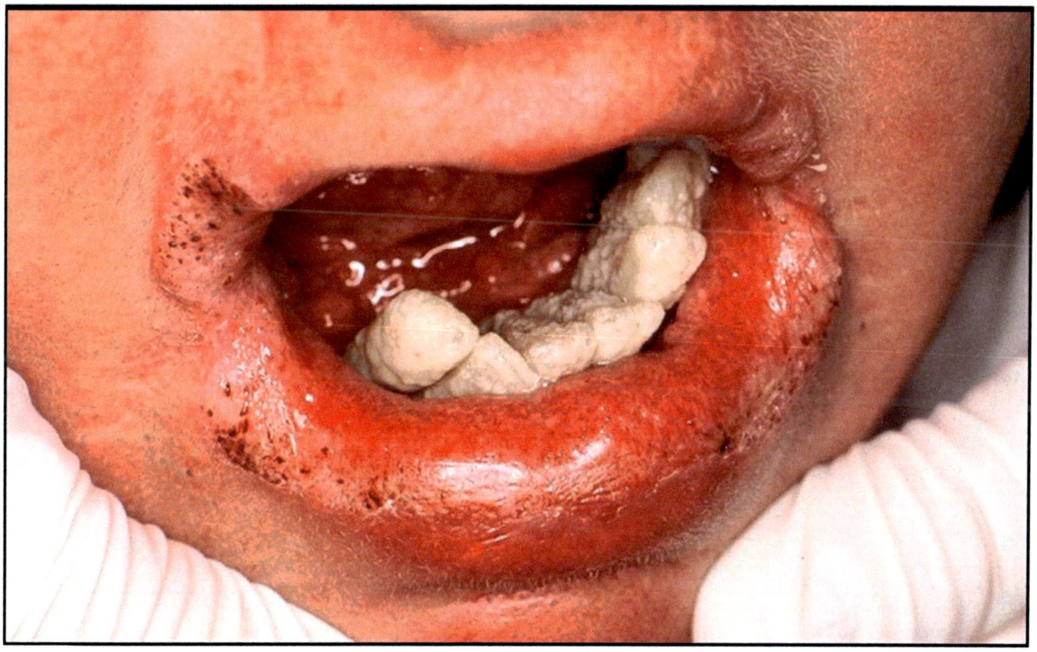

Figure 2. Rare case of paracoccidioidomycosis in woman. Large painful granular ulcers in commissural areas and mouth floor resulted in oral hygiene difficulties.

The etiological agent of this mycosis is the dimorphic fungus *Paracoccidioides brasiliensis*. *In vitro* studies have demonstrated that estrogen inhibits the transition of mycelia or conidia (the saprophytic form of the fungus) to yeasts (the parasitic form) [19, 20]. The same has also been shown *in vivo*, suggesting that female hormones block transition and are responsible for resistance. In male mice that were infected intranasally (mimicking natural infection), the transition from conidia into intermediate forms and yeasts did occur after 96 h, while transition did not occur and the infection cleared in females. Thus, these *in vivo* data are consistent with *in vitro* observations [18].

3. Estrogenicity of Dental Materials

Estrogenicity can be defined as the ability of a chemical, such as bisphenol A (BPA), to bind to the estrogen receptor, which can occur *in vivo* or *in vitro*. These hazardous substances that have predominantly estrogenic activity, are termed endocrine-disrupting chemicals (EDCs) [21] and may cause abnormalities in the reproductive system of wildlife, and probably in humans, although mechanisms of EDCs that affect human health are poorly understood [22, 23]. During the last few years, considerable research reporting biological effects associated with these compounds has been published [24] and the subject has attracted the interest of many investigators as well as legislative bodies [22, 23, 25]

In general, estrogenic action is confined to molecules possessing a double benzoic ring. In dentistry, such polymers include bisphenol A-glycidyl dimethacrylate (Bis-GMA) and polycarbonate products. Potential BPA sources in dental materials are confined to sealants, composites, adhesives, and polycarbonate aesthetic brackets [26].

Olea et al. [27] reported that 90 to 931 μg of BPA was identified in the saliva of patients 1h after treatment with a commercially-available dental sealant, and confirmed the estrogenicity of this resinous material with proliferation tests using human breast cancer cells[27]. These results have generated considerable concern regarding the safety of dental resin materials and incited future research on this topic. Tarumi et al. [28] confirmed estrogenic activity of two commercially available sealants that presented hydrophobic monomer bisphenol A dimethacrylate (BPA-DMA), which is also estrogenic, in an amount greater than the minimum concentration. The authors suggested that these sealants may not cause adverse effects to human health, since the amounts of BPA-DMA would be much less than the maximum acceptable concentration. To Fung et al. [29], the concern regarding the potential estrogenicity of sealants may be unfounded, since they have demonstrated that BPA released orally from a common dental sealant may not be absorbed or may be present in non-detectable quantities in systemic circulation.

Wada et al. [21] observed that the estrogenic activity of 6 commercially available resin composites was associated with the elution of either 2-hydroxy-4-methoxy-benzophenone (HMBP), a photostabilizer, or 2,2- dimethoxy-2-phenyl-acetophenone (DMPA), a photoinitiator.

Plasticizers used in tissue conditioners were also found to have estrogenic activities by Hashimoto et al. [30], who suggest the need for further studies on the accumulation, metabolism, and excretion of these chemicals after oral ingestion.

No trace of BPA released from orthodontic adhesives was found after artificial accelerated aging, implying that the amount of BPA did not exceed the detection limit of the analytical technique used (0.1 ppm or 0.1 μg/L), if BPA was actually present at all [31]. The estrogenic action of orthodontic adhesive resin was investigated by determining the potential effects of these compounds on the proliferation of estrogen-responsive MCF-7 breast cancer cells [26]. Orthodontic adhesive resin did not stimulate proliferation of these cells, indicating the absence of estrogenic activity by orthodontic adhesive eluents [26].

4. Estrogens and Temporomandibular Joint

Temporomandibular joint (TMJ) disorders (TMDs) are defined as a set of clinical conditions characterized by pain and dysfunction of the masticatory muscles, TMJ, and associated hard and soft tissues [32]. Common symptoms are pain, limitation in jaw function, and sounds from the TMJ [33]. A combination of factors, such as occlusion, mental stress, strength, and endurance, has been assumed to be the etiological cause of TMDs [34].

Current literature [33, 35] suggests the TMDs are more prevalent in women than men, and that the severity of symptoms is also related to the age of patients. Pain onset tends to occur after puberty, and peaks during the reproductive years, with the highest prevalence observed in women aged 20–40 [33, 35]. The gender and age distribution of TMD patients suggests a possible link between its pathogenesis and the female reproductive system [34].

Estrogen may influence the development, restitution, and metabolism of the TMJ as well as associated structures, and some studies have shown the presence of high affinity estrogen receptors in the synovial membrane, articular disc and mandibular condyle of humans [33]. The influence of sex hormones on the collagen and protein contents of the TMJ disc in rats was demonstrated by Abubaker et al. [36], as greater contents of both components were found in male than female rats. The effects on the biochemical composition of the disc could theoretically alter the biomechanical properties of the connective tissue. These differences were markedly decreased after gonadectomy.

The effects of estrogen deficiency on the osseous oral structures and the implications for therapy have been extensively studied. Many of these studies are related to periodontology, endodontics or bone repair. Besides the functional significance of the mandibular condyle, the quantitative data regarding the effects of estrogen deficiency in the condyles were far fewer than those on the mandibular body [37] and alveolar bone. Tanaka et al. [38] found no significant differences in bone mineral density (evaluated by dual-energy X-ray absorptiometry- DXA) of the mandibular condyle between ovariectomized and sham group rats, but estrogen deficiency resulted in a significantly larger marrow area. In a later study, the same authors verified that estrogen deficiency induced transient subchondral bone loss and recovery on rat condyle, what suggested that mechanical (occlusal) loading modulates the normal ovariectomized-induced bone loss found in other parts of the skeleton [37]. This group also discovered that estrogen deficiency caused a region-specific net bone loss in the rat mandibular condyle, which may be attributable to the differences in mechanical stress by occlusion [39]. The more pronounced bone loss of the ovariectomized rat condyle in the posterior part compared with the anterior part suggests that mechanical loading of occlusion is important for postmenopausal women to maintain bone mass and physiologic structure of the condyles. Fujita el al. [40] studied the influence of estrogen and androgen on the mandibular condyle of castrated male and female rats and, their results suggested that estrogen could strongly influence normal bone modeling in the mandibular condyle of both men and women, and the hormonal imbalance may predispose the condyle to degenerative changes [40]. Accordingly, estrogens have a protective effect on the structural facets of the TMJ.

Estrogen can regulate the neurotransmission of pain affecting many kinds of neuropeptides in sensory neurons or modulating the pain level [33]. Estrogens may reduce short-term TMJ inflammation, while worsening inflammation over the long term, which is associated with greater tissue damage and pain [41]. Estrogen also participates in the pathogenesis of TMDs by overproduction of pro-inflammatory cytokines, such as IL-1β, IL-6, and IL-8, and may not affect the production of anti-inflammatory cytokines, such as IL-4 and IL-10. That is, TMD may be caused by estrogen through an imbalance among cytokines [32].

Several studies have examined the relation between exogenous hormone use and TMD. LeResche et al. [42] found that the odds of being a TMD case were approximately 30% higher among women receiving estrogen compared to those not exposed, and concluded that the use of oral contraceptives was associated with an approximately 20% increased risk. In contrast, Hatch et al. [43] found that the muscle and joint symptoms of women taking or not taking estrogen were not significantly different. There is substantial evidence to support the hypothesis that estrogen play a role in the incidence of TMD, but this women's health issue demands further exploration and explanation [33].

5. Estrogens and Periodontium

Changes in hormone levels at different life stages, such as puberty, pregnancy, during the menstrual cycle and menopause, as well as those that occur with the use of hormonal supplements, have been associated with the health of the periodontium [2, 44-46]. This influence is recognized by the currently accepted periodontal disease classification [47], which includes the following hormone-related disease categories: puberty-associated gingivitis, menstrual cycle-associated gingivitis, and pregnancy-associated gingivitis.

Human gingiva have receptors for progesterone and estrogen [48]. These receptors indicate that the gingiva is a target tissue for both gestational hormones [49]. Periodontal ligament cells also express estrogen receptors, and these cells exhibited positive modulation on alkaline phosphatase activity and osteocalcin production when exposed to estradiol [50].

Mealey and Moritz [51] reviewed the effects of female sex steroid hormones on the periodontium and described their influences on the gingival vasculature, the local immune system, and cells of the periodontium. The effects on vasculature could explain the increased edema, erythema, gingival crevicular exudates, and hemorrhagic tissues noted by some researches during hormonal oscillations. Both estrogen and progesterone may affect fibroblast proliferation and collagen maturation in gingival connective tissues, in addition to inhibiting tissue repair. Nevertheless, enough information is available to suggest that hormonally-related immunologic changes during pregnancy might increase susceptibility to gingival inflammation.

5.1. Puberty

During puberty, the production of sex hormones reaches a level that remains constant for the entire normal reproductive period [45]. Circumpubertal children demonstrated increased levels of *Prevotella intermedia* relative to prepubertal children. In post-pubertal children, *P. intermedia* populations were replaced by populations of *P. loeschii* and *P. denticola* [52]. These qualitative changes occurred in the presence of approximately equal quantities of supragingival biofilm. Nakagawa et al. [53] confirmed that there is a statistically significant increase in gingival inflammation and the proportion of *P. intermedia* in gingivitis free puberty girls compared to gingivitis free puberty boys. Mombelli et al. [54] and Gusberti et al. [55] annually monitored boys and girls, between the ages of 11 and 14 years old, and found that the bleeding tendency increased significantly with the start of the pubertal phase; moreover, a decrease was noted after the age of 14. However, there was no significant difference in the plaque index [54]. They also verified that the frequency of detection of *Actinomyces odontolyticus* and of *Capnocytophaga sp.* increased with time, while the frequency of detecting *P. intermedia* and *P. melaninogenica* increased at the onset of puberty only in boys [55]. *P. intermedia* is able to replace vitamin K, an essential growth factor, with estradiol and progesterone [56]. Consequently, higher levels of sex hormones can lead to better growth of these bacteria [56, 57]. In summary, hormonal changes during puberty are associated with temporary shifts in the oral microbiota, and an increased tendency for gingival bleeding, which apparently may be controlled over time by a normal, non-compromised host [55].

5.2. Menstrual Cycle

In 1967, Lindhe and Attström [58] studied variations in gingival fluid during the menstrual cycle of a group of women with mild gingivitis. They found significantly greater exudate values on the ovulatory day, when the production of female sex hormones is higher, than during the menstrual phase, when the production of female sex hormones is limited. In contrast, Holm-Pedersen and Löe [59] found that neither menstrual cycle nor pregnancy influenced the flow of fluid from normal gingival. The difference between these results may be credited to differences in methodology and the selection of test persons [58]. While Lindhe and Attström's [58] subjects had mild gingivitis, Holm-Pedersen and Löe's [59] had well-controlled oral hygiene. Therefore, manifestation of hormonal influences in flow of crevicular fluid of susceptible individuals may depend on the simultaneous presence of gingival inflammation [46].

Machtei et al. [60] compared the gingival and periodontal status of pre-menopausal women at different time points during the cycle. They found significantly higher gingival index during the ovulation and pre-menstruation time points than in the menstruation period, regardless of the similarities in plaque index. Several women studied by Machtei et al. [60] reported appreciable oral symptoms just before or during menses, which included erythema, slight burning sensation, bleeding with minor irritation, and general pain and discomfort in the gums. Higher bleeding index during the ovulatory period than the menstrual phase was observed also in a case reported by Koreeda et al.[61]. These results may be due to increased estradiol levels during ovulation and just before menstruation.

5.3. Pregnancy

During pregnancy, some of the most remarkable endocrine alterations occur, and the great increase in plasma hormone levels over several months has a dramatic effect on the periodontium [46]. Periodontal health in pregnancy has been a subject of concern during the last few decades; however, the information available is somewhat controversial [62].

Jensen et al. [63] found increased scores in gingival index and gingival crevicular fluid flow, as well as a 55-fold increase in the recovery of *Bacteroides* species in pregnant women compared with non-pregnant ones. More nutrients for bacteria are provided by a higher sulcus fluid flow rate; in contrast, chemotaxis and phagocytosis were reduced by sexual steroids leading to a better growth of microorganisms [57]. Studies by Kornman and Loesche [64] and Raber- Durlacher et al.[65] also demonstrated an increase in the proportion of *P. intermedia* during pregnancy, which was associated with gingivitis and gingival bleeding. No increase in *P. intermedia* was found during experimental gingivitis post-partum [65], which indicates that oral microbiological aspects altered during pregnancy are reversible. The percentage of sites with periodontal pocket depth (PPD) greater than 4 mm, but with no attachment loss, and salivary estradiol concentrations significantly higher in pregnant than non-pregnant women were also observed by Yokoyama et al. [66]. In addition, the percentage of bleeding at probing sites and the levels of *Campylobacter rectus* in the saliva tended to be higher in pregnant than non-pregnant women. Bleeding upon probing and probing pocket depth increased simultaneously without relation to plaque in the first two trimesters of pregnancy, and then decreased, which was indicative that changes in clinical parameters during pregnancy are also reversible [62], and that pregnancy gingivitis does not predispose or proceed to periodontitis [62, 67]. An immunosuppressive activity of the lymphocyte response was observed during the second trimester of pregnancy and was also resolved after parturition [68]. Raber-Durlacher et al. [69] hypothesized that cytotoxicity directed against B cells and macrophages may result in diminished immuno-responsiveness during pregnancy gingivitis.

In contrast, the results of Jonsson et al.[70] did not indicate that increased hormone levels cause more severe periodontal disease in pregnant women or that high steroid levels result in an increased recovery of *P. intermedia* from subgingival plaque. The authors suggested that the disparity among results may be due to different degrees of disease in the studied population, since Jonsson et al.[70] evaluated areas of definite attachment loss, while others observed no pronounced gingivitis. Díaz-Guzmán and Castellanos-Suárez [16] indicated that pregnancy is not a risk factor for increased gingivitis and early periodontitis. They observed similar prevalence of gingivitis and periodontitis in pregnant and non-pregnant women; nevertheless, severe periodontitis was more frequent among the former.

5.4. Contraceptives

Hormonal contraceptives induce a hormonal condition that stimulates a state of pregnancy to prevent ovulation by the use of gestational hormones [45]. Historic evidence suggests that use of high–dose combined oral contraceptives is related to an increased risk for periodontal diseases [63, 71, 72]. Almost 30 years ago, these drugs contained >50 μg of estrogen and ≥1 mg progestin, but more recently, available formulations contain significantly lower levels of hormones, which can affect experimental results. There is not a consensus between previous and current data, and, similar to periodontal health during pregnancy, the effect of contraceptive use and the periodontium remains controversial.

In 1981, Jensen et al.[63] reported a 16-fold higher percentage of *P. intermedia* occurrence under hormonal contraception. In the same year, it was found that there was a statistically significant increase in gingival inflammation related to duration of oral contraceptive therapy; however, there was no difference in the level of attachment [71].

Seventeen years later, Klinger et al.[57] compared the periodontal influence of two oral contraceptives on a sample of women with healthy periodontal tissues and observed no significant difference in bleeding during probing, pocket depth, or plaque during the 3 weeks of the study. However, groups that received the pill with smaller amounts of estradiol reported a higher prevalence of *P. intermedia* after 20 days from the beginning of the study. The authors found distinct short-term effects of different oral contraceptives, both with lower doses of hormones than earlier studies.

In a cross-sectional study by Tilakaratne et al.[49], the usage of contraceptive preparations resulted in an increased prevalence of gingivitis and a significant higher loss of periodontal attachment with prolonged use. However, the authors did not differentiate between participants using oral contraceptives or injectable progestin-exclusive hormones, which is of potential importance, since although the dose of progestin used was lower than the dosage used in earlier studies, it is much higher than in current oral contraceptive formulations [73].

Using a prospective, splint-mouth, experimental gingivitis model, in pre-menopausal women with no attachment loss that were using or not using low doses of oral contraceptives, Preshaw et al.[73] concluded that low dose oral contraceptive usage was not related to increased plaque, gingival index, or gingival crevicular fluid volume. These results were supported by a large population-based representative sample survey [72], which investigated the association between oral contraceptive use and periodontal diseases among 4,930 National Health and Nutrition Examination Survey (NHANES) I and 5,001 NHANES III pre-menopausal U.S. women, before and after the reduction of hormone levels in oral contraceptives.

Although low-dose contraceptive usage might have no effect on the periodontal health of most pre-menopausal women, Mullally et al. [74] speculate that those drugs could be a risk for pre-menopausal women with a susceptibility to develop aggressive forms of disease. The authors evaluated 50 women with aggressive periodontitis and found deeper mean probing depths, more severe attachment loss, and more sites with bleeding on probing in current pill users.

5.5. Menopause and Post-Menopause

Unlike the rhythmic patterns of the menstrual cycle or pregnancy, when hormone levels are significantly elevated during menopause, ovarian function declines and there is a reduction in the output of sex hormones [46, 51]. During and after menopause, the alterations found in gingiva are somewhat different from others periods of female life [46]. Friedlander [75] described the development of a senile atrophic gingivitis, characterized by an abnormal paleness of the gingival tissues, and menopausal gingivostomatitis, characterized by dry and shiny, easily bleeding, and pale erythematous gingival. Bacterial species in the subgingival plaque of postmenopausal women are among the most important during periodontal disease. In a large community-based sample, it was determined that infections with *Porphyromonas gingivalis*, *Tanarella forsythensis*, *P. intermedia* and *C. rectus* were associated with more severe oral bone loss in postmenopausal women [76]. Estrogen deficiency leads to reduction in the cellular structure and density of collagen fibers on periodontal ligament [77], in addition to inducing osteoclastogenesis in rat periodontium [78] .

Osteoporosis is defined worldwide as a systemic skeletal disease characterized by low bone density and microarchitectural deterioration of bone tissue, which leads to increased bone fragility and risk of fracture [79]. The disease should be considered a public health problem due to its social, physical, and economic impact. The majority of osteoporosis cases occur in post-menopause women, due to estrogen deficiency, and this condition is associated with a rapid increase of bone resorption.

Like periodontitis, osteoporosis could be considered a "silent disease", since severe stages are reached without obvious symptoms in the patients. Since both periodontitis and osteoporosis are characterized by bone loss, these diseases may share common etiologic agents, which may either affect or modulate their processes [80]. Although the etiology of periodontitis is multi-factorial, especially in relation to pathogenic bacterial plaque and susceptible individuals, some risk factors are the same for periodontal disease and osteoporosis, such as the higher prevalence associated with tabagism and increased age, in addition to the influence of some medications, such as steroids [81].

The relationship between osteoporosis and periodontal disease has been suggested in a number of studies. The results of some previous studies have indicated a correlation between osteoporosis and periodontal disease [80, 82-88], while others have not shown any significant relationship [89-91]. Studies discussing this subject are summarized in Table 1.

The use of tooth loss as an indicator of the extent of periodontal disease has numerous limitations because the reason for tooth lose is often unknown and a tooth can be lost due to causes other than direct loss of bone support, such as trauma, endodontic problems, caries, and prosthetic problems. In these analyses, the extent of periodontal disease around the remaining teeth is not taken into account [92, 93]. However, many studies intend to correlate tooth count, alone or in combination with other periodontal measures, and systemic bone loss due to postmenopausal osteoporosis. Several of those studies are summarized in Table 2.

According to Lerner [94], two hypothetical mechanisms may be involved in the association between postmenopausal osteoporosis and the progression of bone loss in periodontal disease: 1) if alveolar jawbones present bone mass reduction as a consequence of systemic osteoporosis, it is possible that super-imposed inflammation and bone resorption due to periodontitis may lead to the enhanced progression of bone loss in comparison to healthy individuals; and 2) the production of the bone resorbing cytokines IL-1, TNF-α, and IL-6 is inhibited by estrogens; consequently, these molecules might be produced in larger amounts during an inflammatory process in an estrogen-deficient woman than in an inflammatory process in an estrogen-sufficient woman.

Due to small sample sizes, non-comparable study populations, varying study methods used to assess periodontitis and osteoporosis, as well as inadequate control of confounding factors, the extent of this relationship remains unclear [2]. Since the data from clinical studies on the degree of periodontal disease in postmenopausal patients with simultaneous periodontitis are inconclusive, well-controlled prospective studies are needed in which the progression of periodontal bone loss is followed in relation to estrogen levels [94]. The clinical consequence of elucidating the relationship between osteoporosis and periodontal diseases would be that physicians should be encouraged to send their osteoporotic patients to dentists for a periodontal examination and dentists should be encouraged to send their patients with severe periodontal disease for a medical examination for osteoporosis [80].

Considering the limitations of cross-sectional studies, since variables are difficult to establish and control, as well as the challenges that disturb prospective studies in humans, experimental animal models are extensively used to study the relationship between osteoporosis/osteopenia and periodontium. The experimental model for osteopenia induced by ovariectomy in female rats is the most commonly used animal model for evaluation of problems related to bone loss in postmenopausal women. As for studies in humans, most of the experimental animal studies have previously supported the association between diminished bone mineral density and periodontal disease [95, 96], although many failed to establish such an association [97, 98].

Table 1. Correlation between skeletal bone and periodontal diseases

Authors, year (ref)/ Type of study	Population	Systemic bone assessment	Oral parameters (studies regarding tooth loss will also be described in Table 2)	Major outcome
Kribbs [89], 1990/ cross-sectional	85 osteoporotic postmenopausal women and 27 normal women (ages 50-84)	Radiographic evidence of vertebral fractures in osteoporotic women	Mandibular bone mass and density, cortical thickness and height of the edentulous ridge (X-ray), PPD, gingival recession, and bleeding after probing	Osteoporotic group had less mandibular bone mass and density as well as a thinner cortex at gonion than normal group. No differences in periodontal measures were found between groups

Table 1. (Continued)

Authors, year (ref)/ Type of study	Population	Systemic bone assessment	Oral parameters (studies regarding tooth loss will also be described in Table 2)	Major outcome
Elders et al.[90], 1992/ cross-sectional	286 women (ages 46-55)	Lumbar BMD (DXA), metacarpal cortical thickness (X-ray)	ABH (X-ray), mean PPD, bleeding after probing	No relationship between systemic bone and oral parameters
Klemetti et al.[99], 1994/ cross-sectional	227 postmenopausal women (ages 48-56)	Femoral neck and lumbar spine BMD (DXA)	Bone support (X-ray), PPD, CPITN	Individuals with higher systemic BMD seem to maintain their teeth with deeper periodontal pockets than osteoporotic ones
Von Wowern et al.[82], 1994/ cross-sectional	12 women with osteoporotic fractures and 14 normal women	Bone mineral content of forearm (DPA)	Plaque index, gingival bleeding, CAL, mandibular bone mineral content	Osteoporosis group presented less mandibular bone mineral content and greater CAL
Wactawski-Wende et al.[100], 1996/ cross-sectional	70 postmenopausal women with periodontitis (ages 51-78)	Lumbar spine and femur BMD (DXA)	CAL and inter-proximal ABH	Osteopenia is related to ABH, but not to CAL
Payne et al.[83], 1999/ longitudinal (2 years)	38 postmenopausal woman with a history of periodontitis	Lumbar spine BMD (DXA)	Alveolar bone density (X-ray-CADIA), ABH (X-ray), supragingival plaque, and bleeding on probing	Osteoporosis/osteopenia group presented a higher frequency of ABH and density loss besides higher bleeding on probing
Tezal et al.[84], 2000/ cross-sectional	70 postmenopausal women with periodontitis (ages 51-78)	Femur and lumbar spine BMD (DXA)	CAL and interproximal alveolar bone loss (X-ray)	Skeletal BMD is related to inter-proximal alveolar bone loss and, to a lesser extent, to CAL
Inagaki et al.[85], 2001/ cross-sectional	190 pre- or postmenopausal women	Metacarpal BMD (X-ray densitometry)	CPITN	Subjects were more likely to have periodontitis as the metacarpal BMD level decreased
Pilgram et al.[91], 2002/ longitudinal (3 years)	135 postmenopausal women	Femur and lumbar spine BMD (DXA)	CAL	No relationship between systemic bone and oral parameters
Mohammad et al.[86], 2003/ cross-sectional	30 postmenopausal women	Calcaneus BMD (DXA)	Plaque index, PPD, and CAL	Decreasing BMD was associated with increased CAL
Yoshihara et al.[80], 2004/ longitudinal (3 years)	179 men and women (age 70)	BMD of the heel (ultrasound bone densitometer)	CAL	Subjects with osteopenia had higher number of sites with attachment loss
Takaishi et al.[87], 2005/ cross-sectional	40 postmenopausal women with minimal or mid-	Vertebral BMD (DXA) and calcaneus speed of sound (SOS)	PPD, CAL, tooth mobility, alveolar BMD (X-ray)	Alveolar BMD is correlated with vertebral BMD, calcaneus SOS, PPD, and mobility of the teeth. SOS

Authors, year (ref)/ Type of study	Population	Systemic bone assessment	Oral parameters (studies regarding tooth loss will also be described in Table 2)	Major outcome
	periodontitis	(quantitative ultrasound)		can to predict CAL
Brennan et al.[88], 2007/ cross-sectional	1329 postmenopausal women	Spine, hip, forearm, and whole body BMD (DXA)	CAL	Strongest association between systemic bone and CAL among women without subgingival calculus

ABH= Alveolar bone height; BMD= Bone mineral density; CAL= Clinical attachment loss; CPITN= Community periodontal index of treatment needs; DPA= Dual photon absorptiometry; DXA= Dual X-ray absorptiometry; PPD= Periodontal pocket deep; SOS= Speed of sound.

Table 2. Correlation between skeletal bone and tooth loss

Authors, year (ref)/ Type of study	Population	Systemic bone assessment	Major outcome
Kribbs[89], 1990/ cross-sectional	85 osteoporotic postmenopausal women and 27 normal women (ages 50 to 84)	Radiographic evidence of vertebral fractures in osteoporotic women	Osteoporotic group had a greater percentage of edentulous subjects and there was a great tooth loss in dentate subjects
Klemetti et al.[99], 1994/ cross-sectional	227 postmenopausal women (ages 48 to 56)	Femoral neck and lumbar spine BMD (DXA)	No relationship between systemic bone and tooth loss
Krall et al.[101], 1996/ longitudinal (7 years)	189 postmenopausal women	Whole body, femoral neck and spine BMD (DXA)	Systemic BMD loss is related to increased tooth loss
Mohammad et al.[102], 1997/ cross-sectional	44 women (ages 50-75)	Spine BMD (DXA)	No relationship between systemic bone and tooth loss
Earnshaw et al.[103], 1998/ cross-sectional	1365 women (ages 45-59)	Lumbar spine and femur BMD (DXA)	No relationship between systemic bone and tooth loss
Taguchi et al.[104], 1999/ cross-sectional	90 women (ages 40-68)	Lumbar spine BMD (DEQCT)	Systemic BMD loss is related to increased tooth loss
Inagaki et al.[85], 2001/ cross-sectional	190 pre- or postmenopausal women	Metacarpal BMD (X-ray densitometry)	Systemic BMD loss is related to tooth loss
Mohammad et al. [86], 2003/ cross-sectional	30 postmenopausal women	Calcaneus BMD (DXA)	Systemic BMD loss is related to tooth loss
Bollen et al.[105], 2004/ cross sectional	154 subjects born before 1936	Osteoporotic fractures	Fractures status do not affect tooth loss
Inagaki et al.[106], 2005/ cross sectional	356 women	Metacarpal BMD (X-ray densitometry	Systemic BMD loss is related to tooth loss
Drozdzowska et al.[107], 2006/ cross sectional	67 postmenopausal women	Hip and lumbar spine BMD (DXA) and hand phalangeal quantitative ultrasound	Hip BMD loss and phalanges amplitude-dependent speed of sound are related to tooth loss

BMD= Bone mineral density; DEQCT= Dual energy computed tomography; DXA= Dual X-ray absorptiometry.

5.6. Hormone Replacement In Postmenopausal Women

Estrogen-hormone replacement therapy (HRT) has a well-known positive effect on the post-cranial skeleton. However, the effects of these drugs on oral bone is still controversial due to a lack of longitudinal studies [108].

Women taking estrogen supplements exhibited lower gingival bleeding than controls aged 50 to 64; however, there was no significant difference in attachment loss or alveolar bone loss [109]. The authors suggested that in this study women on estrogen supplementation most likely exhibited normal rather than elevated levels of sex hormones, which may increase bleeding, similar to that observed during pregnancy. Therefore, the balanced hormone level in the group using estrogen compared to the control group that may present unbalanced levels of sex hormones, probably accounts for the difference observed in gingival bleeding [109]. In contrast, postmenopausal women that reported use of estrogen supplementation presented significantly lower mean clinical attachment loss (CAL) than those who never used estrogen in the study by Ronderos et al. [110]. In addition to the reduced frequency of CAL, Reinhard et al. [111] indicated that estrogen supplementation was associated with reduced gingival inflammation[111]. Beneficial effects of hormone replacement therapy were also reported by Lopez-Marcos et al. [112], who found a protective effect of the therapy in dental pain and the improvement of tooth mobility and PPD.

Paganini-Hill et al. [113] evaluated tooth loss and the need for dentures among 3,921 women, ages of 52 to 109, and found that tooth loss and rates of edentia were significantly lower in estrogen users than in non-users. A reduced risk of tooth loss was also observed among postmenopausal hormone users in a large prospective study in which 42,171 postmenopausal women were followed for two years [114]. In a longitudinal study that took place over the course of three years, there was an increase in femur bone mineral density (BMD) and alveolar bone mass as well as a tendency for the improvement of alveolar bone height (ABH) in postmenopausal women taking estrogen replacement therapy compared to the placebo group [115]. Taguchi et al.[116] observed that the duration of estrogen use was significantly associated with the number of total and posterior teeth remaining, but they did not find relationship between estrogen use and oral bone height or oral bone porosity. Based on these results, estrogen may promote tooth retention by strengthening the periodontal attachment surrounding the teeth.

Two recent longitudinal studies demonstrated no improvement of oral parameters due to estrogen supplementation. Evio et al. [117] compared the effects of HRT, alendronato, and their combination on oral health of elderly postmenopausal women with osteoporosis and found no difference between the initial examination and after two years in the group that received HRT. Tarkkila et al. [118] examined 161 women using or not using HRT and also recorded dental and periodontal status at the initial visit and two years later. Similarly, they found no significant difference in any dental parameters or salivary flow between groups. Nevertheless, women in the HRT group underwent more dental restoration during the period of study, which may indicate a more health conscious attitude in this group. Authors suggest more prospective long-term studies to elucidate whether the use of HRT and oral health are related.

6. Postmenopausal Osteoporosis and Oral and Maxillofacial Radiology

Numerous attempts have been made to identify methods for identifying individuals with osteoporosis at an early stage, because preventive therapy can limit the disease process [119]. BMD can be measured using a variety of techniques, including single photon absorptiometry, dual photon or dual energy X-ray absorptiometry (DPA or DXA), quantitative ultrasound, and quantitative computed tomography (QCT)[119]. BMD testing for the elderly population by DXA, the most reliable way to determine BMD, is considered an immediate action to reduce the incidence of osteoporotic fractures and the subsequent complications[120]. However, it is difficult in clinical practice to refer all postmenopausal women for BMD testing, especially in developing countries, when the cost-effectiveness, limited number of facilities, and amount of trained personnel are considered [116].

Panoramic radiographs constitute an integral part of almost every routine dental evaluation, and many people visit the dentist, at least once per year. As a result, several studies have suggested the use of panoramic radiographs for the early diagnosis of osteoporosis. Different techniques of X-ray image analysis have been described for estimation of changes in oral bones due to osteoporosis[121], such as fractal dimension, microdensitometry, pixel intensity[122], records of linear measures [119-121, 123-127] (morphometric analysis), or classification of mandibular cortical shape [120, 123-125, 128, 129].

Klemetti et al.[130] tried to relate the panoramic mandibular index (PMI), which is the ratio of the cortical thickness to the relatively constant distance between the inferior margin of the mental foramen and the inferior mandibular border [131], to the BMD of the femoral neck, lumbar area and trabecular, and cortical parts of the mandible, measured by DXA or QTC. The linear correlation was weak, but PMI may perhaps be used as an indicator of bone mineral alterations, when PMI values deviate noticeably from the mean PMI of the population.

An analysis of mandibular cortical shape (mandibular cortical index-MCI) was proposed in 1994 [129] as follows: normal cortex, the endosteal margin of the cortex is even and sharp on both sides; mild to moderately eroded cortex, the endosteal margin shows semilunar defects (lacunar resorption) or appears to form endosteal cortical residues; or severely eroded cortex, the cortical layer forms endosteal cortical residues and is clearly porous. Many researchers have used this form of evaluation since then.

The BMD of the lumbar vertebrae was compared to mandibular cortical thickness (MCT) and cortical shape (MCI) categories in 450 postmenopausal women and an increased risk of low vertebral BMD or osteoporosis in those women with a thinner cortical width and/or eroded cortex was found [120]. In another large project named OSTEODENT, a collaboration among five European centers to determine the best radiographic and clinical method for identification of individuals that are at the greatest risk for osteoporosis, Devlin et al. [126] found that MCT has a better efficacy than MCI in detecting osteoporosis, with no evidence for any benefit associated by combining both measurements. Those authors suggested that patients with mandibular cortices <3 mm should be referred for further osteoporosis investigation. A decrease in MCT by 1 mm increased the likelihood of osteopenia or osteoporosis to 43%, taking into consideration the effect of years elapsed since menopause [123, 124].

Most authors agree that the panoramic radiograph could be useful as a simple screening method in the diagnosis of osteoporosis and can provide valuable information on the quality of the jawbone. Dentists have sufficient clinical and radiographic information that enables them to play a significant role in patient screening for osteoporosis [124].

7. Postmenopausal Osteoporosis and Residual Ridge Resorption

Oral bone loss can be divided into bone loss that occurs in periodontal disease and in edentulous areas, also referred to as residual ridge resorption [93]. This is a multi-factorial disease that is the consequence of the anatomic, metabolic, and mechanical history, which may affect denture support, stability, retention, and function. Since several authors have correlated systemic and oral osteoporosis, other research has focused on the relationship between osteoporosis and resorption of residual ridge.

In an early study, Kribbs et al.[132] examined 17 osteoporotic edentulous women and found that the height of the residual ridge was significantly correlated to both total body calcium and mandibular bone mass, indicating a relationship between osteoporosis and resorption of the edentulous alveolar ridge. This was confirmed by Hirai et al. [133], who found that osteoporosis strongly affects reduction of the residual ridge. Authors have suggested that patients with low edentulous residual ridges, osteoporosis should be considered, particularly in women, who deserve special considerations to preserve the underlying structures. Von Wowern and Kollerup [134] verified that symptomatic osteoporosis seems to be a risk factor for residual ridge resorption of the maxillae, but not in the mandible. In contrast, an osteoporotic fracture history was not associated with increased residual ridge resorption in a more recent study [105].

After a literature review in 1996, Klemetti [135] concluded that occlusal forces must be considered as the major cause of residual ridge resorption, because these forces are able to cause rapid and thorough resorption without systemic bone loss. According to Klemetti [135], real osteoporosis does not develop in edentulous jaws until muscular function decreases. Von Wowern [136] also reviewed the literature, and concluded that osteoporosis in the jaws may present a risk for accentuation of alveolar bone loss after wearing full dentures.

Recently, the subject was revisited by Slagter et al. [137]. Due to the different parameters applied in the various studies, in which local factors influencing the degree of residual ridge reduction were not taken into account, no firm conclusions could be drawn regarding the effect of osteoporosis on residual ridge resorption.

8. Estrogens and Orthodontics

There is a gradual increase in the demand for orthodontic services among older patients as a result of the aging population [138], but a few studies regarding the effects of estrogens or estrogen deficiency due to menopause on tooth movements have been performed.

In 2000, Pereira et al. [139] used ovariectomized and non-ovariectomized rats to study tooth movement. After histological analysis, these authors found that estrogen deficiency did not produce alterations in hard dental tissues, but did cause an increase in bone resorption, especially in pressure regions. In studies using a similar experimental model, estrogen deficiency caused rapid orthodontic tooth movement, perhaps due to the further activation of alveolar bone turnover [140, 141]. Orthodontic tooth movement was also influenced by the estrous cycle in rats. In animals that received force principally in estrus, when estrogen levels are lower, the movement was greater than in those that received such force in pro-estrous, when estrogen level peak [142].

Rapid tooth movement is clinically advantageous, but the negative balance of bone metabolism may have a negatively effect on the maintenance of the correction [140, 141]. According to Arslan et al. [141], consolidation therapy in estrogen-deficient patients will probably take longer, and relapse and therapeutic failures will be more common. After a literature review, Sidiropoulou- Chatzigiannis et al. [143] concluded that deviations in bone turnover and consequent periodontal problems may influence the response to orthodontic forces, and these should be taken into consideration when planning the treatment.

Miyajima et al. [138] related a case of orthodontic treatment in a menopausal patient with slow orthodontic tooth movements. However, the patient had been on estrogen therapy for three years, which may have inhibited alveolar bone loss and root resorption. Additional human studies are necessary to determine the effect of the menstrual cycle [142] and estrogen deficiency on orthodontic tooth movement in female patients.

9. Estrogens and Oral Discomfort

Numerous aspects of menopause are universal. Hot flashes, generous perspiration, and atrophic vaginitis are all results of estrogen loss and are experienced by most menopausal women. While the systemic aspects of menopause are well-documented, an understanding of oral discomfort as a part of menopausal complaints is still generally lacking. Oral discomfort involves various complaints, including dry mouth, burning sensations of the tongue or oral mucosa, and changes in taste perception [144]. Diffuse gingival atrophy and oral ulcerations may be included between the clinical characteristics [145].

Several studies regarding this clinical condition have been published. A significantly higher prevalence of oral discomfort in perimenopausal and postmenopausal women than in pre-menopausal women has been reported [146]. Forabosco et al. [145] suggested that oral discomfort may be related to steroid hormone withdrawal only in some postmenopausal women.

Some evidences regarding the influence of estrogen in the oral mucosa and salivary gland have been presented. Seko et al. [147] investigated the possible effect of sex steroid deficiency on the rat oral mucosa and observed a reduction of the epithelium mucosa thickness, mainly in the tongue apex, which is the area most associated with the burning mouth syndrome. Based on an analysis of the proliferative activity of the epithelium, these authors suggested a possible delay in turnover periods, which could induce the thinning of the oral mucosa in ovariectomized rats.

Purushotham et al. [148] investigated specific changes in salivary gland protein synthesis and secretion in response to hormone deficiency caused by ovariectomy of rats. They observed a decline of amylase activity in the parotid as well as the level of the enzyme activity present in the saliva. Epidermal growth factor concentrations were not significantly altered in the submandibular gland, while a decrease was observed in the concentrations in the saliva of ovariectomized rats.

Studies demonstrating estrogen receptors in oral mucosa, as well as in both the major and minor salivary glands, corroborated that steroid receptors are distributed in non-target tissues for estrogen. This finding suggest that mucosal disorders and oral discomfort can be responsive to hormonal treatment [149]. Laine and Leimola-Virtanen [149] proposed that hormone replacement therapy could improve both the quality and the quantity of salivary gland function.

In Sjögren's syndrome almost all patients complain of dry mouth and of dry eyes. These subjective symptoms can be confirmed by objective tests, which may reveal functional impairment of the salivary and lacrimal glands [150]. A possible correlation between gender differences and the extent of inflammation in several mouse models of Sjögren's syndrome have been stablished [151]. Tayim et al. [152] compared the level of estrogen, progesterone, and prolactin in patients with Sjögren's syndrome and healthy controls. However, only significantly higher levels of prolactin were observed among patients compared with controls.

10. Estrogens and Maxillary Bone Repair

Considering that various treatments involving alveolar bone are performed on patients with postmenopausal osteoporosis, it is fundamental to elucidate the structural changes and wound healing processes of alveolar bone in the condition of estrogen-deficient osteoporosis [153].

Several studies regarding the influence of estrogens on the bone wound healing process have been published, and suggest a reduced capacity for bone tissue healing [154-156].

Tanaka et al. [153] demonstrated that acute estrogen deficiency induced by ovariectomy stimulates sustained bone resorption in rats, but has less effect on bone formation. Additionally, these authors found that bone wound healing within extracted alveolar sockets after maxillary molar extraction was not delayed by ovariectomy, but bone support by newly-formed bone mass on the maxillary bone surfaces at the buccal side of the extracted sockets was significantly decreased, due to increased bone resorption. On the other hand, Shimizu et al.[157] demonstrated that new bone formation after maxillary molar extraction is significantly decreased during ovariectomy-induced osteoporosis in rats. According to the authors, ovariectomy stimulates sustained bone resorption, and bone formation and bone resorption both occur at specific sites on alveolar bone surfaces. Hsieh et al. [158] observed that estrogen deficiency can affect alveolar bone turnover following tooth extraction, which may lead to greater residual ridge resorption in postmenopausal women submitted to dental extractions.

The absence of estrogen significantly decreased the gelatinolytic activities and expression of matrix metalloproteinases (MMP) -2 and 9 and types 1 and 3 collagens. Therefore, estrogen deficiency may possible contribute to the delay in alveolar wound healing by interfering with the extracellular matrix turnover [159]. Alveolar bone dynamics induced by traumatic occlusion are also enhanced by estrogen deficiency [160].

Periapical lesions involve recruitment of inflammatory cells, generation of cytokines, elaboration of lytic enzymes, and activation of osteoclasts, which leads to alveolar bone resorption. Due to the effect of estrogen in the bone resorption process, an estrogen deficiency could be suspected as an aggravating factor in apical periodontitis. [161]. Xiong et al. [161] evaluated the impact of estrogen deficiency on bone loss resulting from experimental periapical lesions in rats and found that ovariectomy significantly increased bone loss in the periapical areas of teeth with pulpal exposure.

Zhang et al. [162] observed more severe bone destruction associated with increased expression of receptor activator of nuclear factor kappa B ligand (RANKL) in the periapical lesions of ovariectomized rats than in controls. At the early stage of estrogen deficiency under great osteoclastogenesis, the expression of osteoprotegerin (OPG) in the lesions was also increased, perhaps indicating a protective osteoblastogenesis.

According Lill et al. [156] clinical experience is consistent regarding a possible delay of healing in osteoporosis. To our knowledge, until recently, research concerning the influence of estrogen deficiency in the wound healing of alveolar bone and periapical lesions was not performed in humans.

11. Estrogens and Oral Implants

The impact of osteoporosis on the maxilla and mandible is likely to directly affect the capacity of these bones to integrate endosseous dental implants [163]. Recent studies using animal models have examined the effects of estrogen deficiency or estrogen replacement therapy on the osseointegration of these dental implants.

Yamazaki et al. [164] investigated the reaction of bone tissue after implant insertion in the tibiae of osteopenic rats. The results suggested that a decrease in bone mass causes a decrease in the contact area between implant and bone and may also result in a reduction in the supporting capability of the implant, because of thinning of the surrounding bone trabeculae. However, Motohashi et al. [165] observed that ovariectomy did not seriously affect bone healing after the placement of implants in cortical bone areas, but did reduce the bone contact ratio and the bone in the cancellous bone area.

Estrogen replacement therapy may promote bone healing around implants under the estrogen deficient state in rats. Consequently, this therapy seems to be helpful for the success of dental implants in postmenopausal women [166].

August et al. [163] performed a retrospective study to analyze the rates of osseointegration of endosseous implants in postmenopausal women compared to premenopausal women and male controls. The effect of postmenopausal estrogen status on compromised implant healing was shown in the maxilla, but not in the mandible. Unsupplemented postmenopausal women had the highest failure rate. Although a statistical difference was not reached, estrogen replacement therapy reduced the maxillary failure rate and could improve the implant osseointegration in postmenopausal patients.

Although most studies found in the literature use animal models, it is possible to deduce the importance of careful management of dental implants in patients with postmenopausal osteoporosis. In an attempt to explain the relationship between changes in bone associated with postmenopausal estrogen deficiency and bone wound healing around dental implants, it is necessary to carefully consider alterations in the maxillary bones due to postmenopausal osteoporosis and the effects of occlusion on these tissues [164].

Conclusion

Estrogens affect the oral cavity significantly, but further studies, mainly prospective, are needed to elucidate the extension and molecular mechanisms of those interactions. The knowledge of relevant systemic conditions and risk factors that influence the oral health of women is the responsibility of dentists, who could then perform early diagnosis and treatment of oral diseases or even early referral of patients with suspected systemic involvement for medical treatment.

References

[1] Amar S, Chung KM. Influence of hormonal variation on the periodontium in women. *Periodontol.* 2000. 1994 Oct;6:79-87.

[2] Krejci CB, Bissada NF. Women's health issues and their relationship to periodontitis. *J. Am. Dent. Assoc.* 2002 Mar;133(3):323-9.

[3] Lee W, Cheng M, Chao H, Wang P. The role of selective estrogen receptor modulators on breast cancer: from tamoxifen to raloxifene. Taiwan *J. Obstet. Gynecol.* 2008 Mar;47(1):24-31.

[4] Ku T, Crowe D. Coactivator-mediated estrogen response in human squamous cell carcinoma lines. *J. Endocrinol.* 2007 Apr;193(1):147-55.

[5] Nasser SM, Faquin WC, Dayal Y. Expression of androgen, estrogen, and progesterone receptors in salivary gland tumors. Frequent expression of androgen receptor in a subset of malignant salivary gland tumors. *Am. J. Clin. Pathol.* 2003 Jun;119(6):801-6.

[6] Lamey PJ, Leake RE, Cowan SK, Soutar DS, McGregor IA, McGregor FM. Steroid hormone receptors in human salivary gland tumours. *J. Clin. Pathol.* 1987 May;40(5):532-4.

[7] Pires FR, da Cruz Perez DE, de Almeida OP, Kowalski LP. Estrogen receptor expression in salivary gland mucoepidermoid carcinoma and adenoid cystic carcinoma. *Pathol. Oncol. Res.* 2004;10(3):166-8.

[8] Ozono S, Onozuka M, Sato K, Ito Y. Immunohistochemical localization of estradiol, progesterone, and progesterone receptor in human salivary glands and salivary adenoid cystic carcinomas. *Cell Struct. Funct.* 1992 Jun;17(3):169-75.

[9] Ozono S, Sato K, Ito Y, Kubota N, Hayashi H, Kato H, et al. Immunohistochemical localization of estrogen receptors in the submandibular gland tumors of female rats. *Cell Struct. Funct.* 1994 Oct;19(5):335-40.

[10] Ishida H, Wada K, Masuda T, Okura M, Kohama K, Sano Y, et al. Critical role of estrogen receptor on anoikis and invasion of squamous cell carcinoma. *Cancer Sci.* 2007 May;98(5):636-43.

[11] Suba Z. Gender-related hormonal risk factors for oral cancer. *Pathol. Oncol. Res.* 2007;13(3):195-202.

[12] Yoo HJ, Sepkovic DW, Bradlow HL, Yu GP, Sirilian HV, Schantz SP. Estrogen metabolism as a risk factor for head and neck cancer. *Otolaryngol. Head Neck Surg.* 2001 Mar;124(3):241-7.

[13] Whitaker SB, Bouquot JE, Alimario AE, Whitaker TJ, Jr. Identification and semiquantification of estrogen and progesterone receptors in pyogenic granulomas of pregnancy. *Oral Surg. Oral. Med. Oral. Pathol.* 1994 Dec;78(6):755-60.

[14] Neville BW, Damm DD, Allen CM, Bouquot JE. Oral and maxillofacial pathology. 2nd ed. Philadelphia: W.B. Saunders 2004.

[15] Yuan K, Wing LY, Lin MT. Pathogenetic roles of angiogenic factors in pyogenic granulomas in pregnancy are modulated by female sex hormones. *J. Periodontol.* 2002 Jul;73(7):701-8.

[16] Díaz-Guzmán L, Castellanos-Suárez J. Lesions of the oral mucosa and periodontal disease behavior in pregnant patients. *Med. Oral Patol. Oral Cir. Bucal.* 2004 2004 Nov-Dec;9(5):434-7; 0-3.

[17] Günhan M, Günhan O, Celasun B, Mutlu M, Bostanci H. Estrogen and progesterone receptors in the peripheral giant cell granulomas of the oral cavity. *J. Oral Sci.* 1998 Jun;40(2):57-60.

[18] Aristizabal BH, Clemons KV, Stevens DA, Restrepo A. Morphological transition of Paracoccidioides brasiliensis conidia to yeast cells: in vivo inhibition in females. *Infect. Immun.* 1998 Nov;66(11):5587-91.

[19] Restrepo A, Salazar ME, Cano LE, Stover EP, Feldman D, Stevens DA. Estrogens inhibit mycelium-to-yeast transformation in the fungus Paracoccidioides brasiliensis: implications for resistance of females to paracoccidioidomycosis. *Infect. Immun.* 1984 Nov;46(2):346-53.

[20] Salazar ME, Restrepo A, Stevens DA. Inhibition by estrogens of conidium-to-yeast conversion in the fungus Paracoccidioides brasiliensis. *Infect. Immun.* 1988 Mar;56(3):711-3.

[21] Wada H, Tarumi H, Imazato S, Narimatsu M, Ebisu S. In vitro estrogenicity of resin composites. *J. Dent. Res.* 2004 Mar;83(3):222-6.

[22] Colborn T, vom Saal FS, Soto AM. Developmental effects of endocrine-disrupting chemicals in wildlife and humans. *Environ. Health Perspect.* 1993 Oct;101(5):378-84.

[23] Colborn T. Environmental estrogens: health implications for humans and wildlife. *Environ. Health Perspect.* 1995 Oct;103 Suppl 7:135-6.

[24] Sohoni P, Sumpter JP. Several environmental oestrogens are also anti-androgens. *J. Endocrinol.* 1998 Sep;158(3):327-39.

[25] European Commission. Directorate of general health and consumer protection. Scientific commettee on toxicity eate. Opinion on the results of the risk assessment of bisphenol-A. Human health part. Cas No 80-05-7. Brussels; 2003.

[26] Eliades T, Gioni V, Kletsas D, Athanasiou A, Eliades G. Oestrogenicity of orthodontic adhesive resins. *Eur. J. Orthod.* 2007 Aug;29(4):404-7.

[27] Olea N, Pulgar R, PÃ©rez P, Olea-Serrano F, Rivas A, Novillo-Fertrell A, et al. Estrogenicity of resin-based composites and sealants used in dentistry. *Environ. Health Perspect.* 1996 Mar;104(3):298-305.

[28] Tarumi H, Imazato S, Narimatsu M, Matsuo M, Ebisu S. Estrogenicity of fissure sealants and adhesive resins determined by reporter gene assay. *J. Dent. Res.* 2000 Nov;79(11):1838-43.

[29] Fung EY, Ewoldsen NO, St Germain HA, Jr., Marx DB, Miaw CL, Siew C, et al. Pharmacokinetics of bisphenol A released from a dental sealant. *J. Am. Dent. Assoc.* 2000 Jan;131(1):51-8.

[30] Hashimoto Y, Kawaguchi M, Miyazaki K, Nakamura M. Estrogenic activity of tissue conditioners in vitro. Dent Mater. 2003 Jun;19(4):341-6.

[31] Eliades T, Hiskia A, Eliades G, Athanasiou A. Assessment of bisphenol-A release from orthodontic adhesives. *Am. J. Orthod. Dentofacial. Orthop.* 2007 Jan;131(1):72-5.

[32] Yun KI, Chae CH, Lee CW. Effect of estrogen on the expression of cytokines of the temporomandibular joint cartilage cells of the mouse. *J. Oral. Maxillofac. Surg.* 2008 May;66(5):882-7.

[33] Wang J, Chao Y, Wan Q, Zhu Z. The possible role of estrogen in the incidence of temporomandibular disorders. *Med. Hypotheses.* 2008 Jun.

[34] Min HJ, Lee MJ, Kim JY, Cho SW, Park HD, Lee SI, et al. Alteration of BMP-4 and Runx2 expression patterns in mouse temporomandibular joint after ovariectomy. *Oral Dis.* 2007 Mar;13(2):220-7.

[35] Koidis PT, Zarifi A, Grigoriadou E, Garefis P. Effect of age and sex on craniomandibular disorders. *J. Prosthet. Dent.* 1993 Jan;69(1):93-101.

[36] Abubaker AO, Hebda PC, Gunsolley JN. Effects of sex hormones on protein and collagen content of the temporomandibular joint disc of the rat. J Oral Maxillofac Surg. 1996 Jun;54(6):721-7; discussion 7-8.

[37] Tanaka M, Ejiri S, Nakajima M, Kohno S, Ozawa H. Changes of cancellous bone mass in rat mandibular condyle following ovariectomy. *Bone.* 1999 Sep;25(3):339-47.

[38] Tanaka M, Ejiri S, Kohno S, Ozawa H. The effect of aging and ovariectomy on mandibular condyle in rats. *J. Prosthet. Dent.* 1998 Jun;79(6):685-90.

[39] Tanaka M, Ejiri S, Kohno S, Ozawa H. Region-specific bone mass changes in rat mandibular condyle following ovariectomy. *J. Dent. Res.* 2000 Nov;79(11):1907-13.

[40] Fujita T, Kawata T, Tokimasa C, Tanne K. Influence of oestrogen and androgen on modelling of the mandibular condylar bone in ovariectomized and orchiectomized growing mice. *Arch. Oral. Biol.* 2001 Jan;46(1):57-65.

[41] Craft RM. Modulation of pain by estrogens. *Pain.* 2007 Nov;132 Suppl 1:S3-12.

[42] LeResche L, Saunders K, Von Korff M, Barlow W, Dworkin S. Use of exogenous hormones and risk of temporomandibular disorder pain. *Pain.* 1997 Jan;69(1-2):153-60.

[43] Hatch JP, Rugh JD, Sakai S, Saunders MJ. Is use of exogenous estrogen associated with temporomandibular signs and symptoms? *J. Am. Dent. Assoc.* 2001 Mar;132(3):319-26.

[44] Güncü G, Tözüm T, Cağlayan F. Effects of endogenous sex hormones on the periodontium--review of literature. *Aust. Dent. J.* 2005 Sep;50(3):138-45.

[45] Mascarenhas P, Gapski R, Al-Shammari K, Wang HL. Influence of sex hormones on the periodontium. *J. Clin. Periodontol.* 2003 Aug;30(8):671-81.

[46] Mariotti A. Sex steroid hormones and cell dynamics in the periodontium. *Crit. Rev. Oral. Biol. Med.* 1994;5(1):27-53.

[47] Armitage GC. Development of a classification system for periodontal diseases and conditions. *Ann. Periodontol.* 1999 Dec;4(1):1-6.

[48] Vittek J, Hernandez MR, Wenk EJ, Rappaport SC, Southren AL. Specific estrogen receptors in human gingiva. *J. Clin. Endocrinol. Metab.* 1982 Mar;54(3):608-12.

[49] Tilakaratne A, Soory M, Ranasinghe A, Corea S, Ekanayake S, de Silva M. Effects of hormonal contraceptives on the periodontium, in a population of rural Sri-Lankan women. *J.Clin. Periodonto*l. 2000 Oct;27(10):753-7.

[50] Cao M, Shu L, Li J, Su J, Zhang W, Wang Q, et al. The expression of estrogen receptors and the effects of estrogen on human periodontal ligament cells. Methods and findings in experimental and clinical pharmacology. 2007 Jun;29(5):329-35.

[51] Mealey BL, Moritz AJ. Hormonal influences: effects of diabetes mellitus and endogenous female sex steroid hormones on the periodontium. *Periodontol.* 2000. 2003;32:59-81.

[52] Wojcicki CJ, Harper DS, Robinson PJ. Differences in periodontal disease-associated microorganisms of subgingival plaque in prepubertal, pubertal and postpubertal children. *J. Periodontol.* 1987 Apr;58(4):219-23.

[53] Nakagawa S, Fujii H, Machida Y, Okuda K. A longitudinal study from prepuberty to puberty of gingivitis. Correlation between the occurrence of Prevotella intermedia and sex hormones. *J. Clin. Periodontol.* 1994 Nov;21(10):658-65.

[54] Mombelli A, Gusberti FA, van Oosten MA, Lang NP. Gingival health and gingivitis development during puberty. A 4-year longitudinal study. *J. Clin. Periodontol.* 1989 Aug;16(7):451-6.

[55] Gusberti F, Mombelli A, Lang N, Minder C. Changes in subgingival microbiota during puberty. A 4-year longitudinal study. *J. Clin. Periodontol.* 1990 Nov;17(10):685-92.

[56] Kornman KS, Loesche WJ. Effects of estradiol and progesterone on Bacteroides melaninogenicus and Bacteroides gingivalis. *Infect Immun.* 1982 Jan;35(1):256-63.

[57] Klinger G, Eick S, Pfister W, GrÃ¤ser T, Moore C, Oettel M. Influence of hormonal contraceptives on microbial flora of gingival sulcus. Contraception. 1998 Jun;57(6):381-4.

[58] Lindhe J, AttsfrÃ¶m R. Gingival exudation during the menstrual cycle. *J. Periodontal. Res.* 1967;2(3):194-8.
[59] Holm-Pedersen P, LÃ¶e H. Flow of gingival exudate as related to menstruation and pregnancy. *J. Periodontal Res.* 1967;2(1):13-20.
[60] Machtei EE, Mahler D, Sanduri H, Peled M. The effect of menstrual cycle on periodontal health. *J. Periodontol.* 2004 Mar;75(3):408-12.
[61] Koreeda N, Iwano Y, Kishida M, Otsuka A, Kawamoto A, Sugano N, et al. Periodic exacerbation of gingival inflammation during the menstrual cycle. *J. Oral Sci.* 2005 Sep;47(3):159-64.
[62] Marakoglu I, Gursoy UK, Marakoglu K, Cakmak H, Ataoglu T. Periodontitis as a risk factor for preterm low birth weight. *Yonsei Med J.* 2008 Apr;49(2):200-3.
[63] Jensen J, Liljemark W, Bloomquist C. The effect of female sex hormones on subgingival plaque. *J. Periodontol.* 1981 Oct;52(10):599-602.
[64] Kornman K, Loesche W. The subgingival microbial flora during pregnancy. *J. Periodontal Res.* 1980 Mar;15(2):111-22.
[65] Raber-Durlacher JE, van Steenbergen TJ, Van der Velden U, de Graaff J, Abraham-Inpijn L. Experimental gingivitis during pregnancy and post-partum: clinical, endocrinological, and microbiological aspects. *J. Clin. Periodontol.* 1994 Sep;21(8):549-58.
[66] Yokoyama M, Hinode D, Yoshioka M, Fukui M, Tanabe S, Grenier D, et al. Relationship between Campylobacter rectus and periodontal status during pregnancy. *Oral Microbiol. Immunol.* 2008 Feb;23(1):55-9.
[67] Tilakaratne A, Soory M, Ranasinghe A, Corea S, Ekanayake S, de Silva M. Periodontal disease status during pregnancy and 3 months post-partum, in a rural population of Sri-Lankan women. *J. Clin. Periodontol.* 2000 Oct;27(10):787-92.
[68] Lopatin DE, Kornman KS, Loesche WJ. Modulation of immunoreactivity to periodontal disease-associated microorganisms during pregnancy. *Infect. Immun.* 1980 Jun;28(3):713-8.
[69] L. Experimental gingivitis during pregnancy and post-partum: immunohistochemical aspects. *J. Periodontol.* 1993 Mar;64(3):211-8.
[70] Jonsson R, Howland BE, Bowden GH. Relationships between periodontal health, salivary steroids, and Bacteroides intermedius in males, pregnant and non-pregnant women. *J. Dent. Res.* 1988 Aug;67(8):1062-9.
[71] Pankhurst CL, Waite IM, Hicks KA, Allen Y, Harkness RD. The influence of oral contraceptive therapy on the periodontium--duration of drug therapy. *J. Periodontol.* 1981 Oct;52(10):617-20.
[72] Taichman L, Eklund S. Oral contraceptives and periodontal diseases: rethinking the association based upon analysis of National Health and Nutrition Examination Survey data. *J. Periodontol.* 2005 Aug;76(8):1374-85.
[73] Preshaw PM, Knutsen MA, Mariotti A. Experimental gingivitis in women using oral contraceptives. *J. Dent. Res.* 2001 Nov;80(11):2011-5.
[74] Mullally BH, Coulter WA, Hutchinson JD, Clarke HA. Current oral contraceptive status and periodontitis in young adults. *J. Periodontol.* 2007 Jun;78(6):1031-6.

[75] Friedlander AH. The physiology, medical management and oral implications of menopause. *J. Am. Dent. Assoc.* 2002 Jan;133(1):73-81.

[76] Brennan R, Genco R, Wilding G, Hovey K, Trevisan M, Wactawski-Wende J. Bacterial species in subgingival plaque and oral bone loss in postmenopausal women. *J. Periodontol.* 2007 Jun;78(6):1051-61.

[77] Glickman I QJ. Further observations regarding the effects of ovariectomy upon the tissues of the periodontium. *Journal of Periodontology.* 1960;31(1):31-7.

[78] Kawamoto S, Ejiri S, Nagaoka E, Ozawa H. Effects of oestrogen deficiency on osteoclastogenesis in the rat periodontium. *Arch. Oral Biol.* 2002 Jan;47(1):67-73.

[79] Genant HK, Cooper C, Poor G, Reid I, Ehrlich G, Kanis J, et al. Interim report and recommendations of the World Health Organization Task-Force for Osteoporosis. *Osteoporos .Int.* 1999;10(4):259-64.

[80] Yoshihara A, Seida Y, Hanada N, Miyazaki H. A longitudinal study of the relationship between periodontal disease and bone mineral density in community-dwelling older adults. *J. Clin. Periodontol.* 2004 Aug;31(8):680-4.

[81] Jeffcoat MK, Chesnut CH, 3rd. Systemic osteoporosis and oral bone loss: evidence shows increased risk factors. *J. Am. Dent. Assoc.* 1993 Nov;124(11):49-56.

[82] von Wowern N, Klausen B, Kollerup G. Osteoporosis: a risk factor in periodontal disease. *J. Periodontol.* 1994 Dec;65(12):1134-8.

[83] Payne JB, Reinhardt RA, Nummikoski PV, Patil KD. Longitudinal alveolar bone loss in postmenopausal osteoporotic/osteopenic women. *Osteoporos .Int.* 1999;10(1):34-40.

[84] Tezal M, Wactawski-Wende J, Grossi SG, Ho AW, Dunford R, Genco RJ. The relationship between bone mineral density and periodontitis in postmenopausal women. *J. Periodontol.* 2000 Sep;71(9):1492-8.

[85] Inagaki K, Kurosu Y, Kamiya T, Kondo F, Yoshinari N, Noguchi T, et al. Low metacarpal bone density, tooth loss, and periodontal disease in Japanese women. *J. Dent Res.* 2001 Sep;80(9):1818-22.

[86] Mohammad AR, Hooper DA, Vermilyea SG, Mariotti A, Preshaw PM. An investigation of the relationship between systemic bone density and clinical periodontal status in post-menopausal Asian-American women. *Int. Dent. J.* 2003 Jun;53(3):121-5.

[87] Takaishi Y, Okamoto Y, Ikeo T, Morii H, Takeda M, Hide K, et al. Correlations between periodontitis and loss of mandibular bone in relation to systemic bone changes in postmenopausal Japanese women. *Osteoporos. Int.* 2005 Dec;16(12):1875-82.

[88] Brennan RM, Genco RJ, Hovey KM, Trevisan M, Wactawski-Wende J. Clinical attachment loss, systemic bone density, and subgingival calculus in postmenopausal women. *J. Periodontol.* 2007 Nov;78(11):2104-11.

[89] Kribbs PJ. Comparison of mandibular bone in normal and osteoporotic women. *J. Prosthet. Dent.* 1990 Feb;63(2):218-22.

[90] Elders PJ, Habets LL, Netelenbos JC, van der Linden LW, van der Stelt PF. The relation between periodontitis and systemic bone mass in women between 46 and 55 years of age. *J. Clin. Periodontol.* 1992 Aug;19(7):492-6.

[91] Pilgram TK, Hildebolt CF, Dotson M, Cohen SC, Hauser JF, Kardaris E, et al. Relationships between clinical attachment level and spine and hip bone mineral

density: data from healthy postmenopausal women. *J. Periodontol.* 2002 Mar;73(3):298-301.

[92] Geurs NC, Lewis CE, Jeffcoat MK. Osteoporosis and periodontal disease progression. *Periodontol.* 2000. 2003;32:105-10.

[93] Loza JC, Carpio LC, Dziak R. Osteoporosis and its relationship to oral bone loss. *Curr. Opin. Periodontol.* 1996;3:27-33.

[94] Lerner UH. Inflammation-induced bone remodeling in periodontal disease and the influence of post-menopausal osteoporosis. *J. Dent. Res.* 2006 Jul;85(7):596-607.

[95] Duarte PM, de Assis DR, Casati MZ, Sallum AW, Sallum EA, Nociti FH, Jr. Alendronate may protect against increased periodontitis-related bone loss in estrogen-deficient rats. *J. Periodontol.* 2004 Sep;75(9):1196-202.

[96] Duarte PM, Goncalves PF, Sallum AW, Sallum EA, Casati MZ, Humberto Nociti F, Jr. Effect of an estrogen-deficient state and its therapy on bone loss resulting from an experimental periodontitis in rats. *J. Periodontal. Res.* 2004 Apr;39(2):107-10.

[97] Anbinder AL, Prado Mde A, Spalding M, Balducci I, Carvalho YR, da Rocha RF. Estrogen deficiency and periodontal condition in rats: a radiographic and macroscopic study. *Braz. Dent. J.* 2006;17(3):201-7.

[98] Orrico SR, Goncalves D, Galeazzi ST, Giro G, Takayama L, Pereira RM. The influence of loss of bone mass on induced periodontal disease: a radiographic and densitometric study of female rats. *J. Periodontol.* 2005 Sep;76(9):1436-42.

[99] Klemetti E, Collin HL, Forss H, Markkanen H, Lassila V. Mineral status of skeleton and advanced periodontal disease. J Clin Periodontol. 1994 Mar;21(3):184-8.

[100] [100]Wactawski-Wende J, Grossi SG, Trevisan M, Genco RJ, Tezal M, Dunford RG, et al. The role of osteopenia in oral bone loss and periodontal disease. *J. Periodontol.* 1996 Oct;67(10 Suppl):1076-84.

[101] Krall EA, Garcia RI, Dawson-Hughes B. Increased risk of tooth loss is related to bone loss at the whole body, hip, and spine. *Calcif. Tissue Int.* 1996 Dec;59(6):433-7.

[102] Mohammad AR, Bauer RL, Yeh CK. Spinal bone density and tooth loss in a cohort of postmenopausal women. *Int. J. Prosthodont.* 1997 1997 Jul-Aug;10(4):381-5.

[103] Earnshaw SA, Keating N, Hosking DJ, Chilvers CE, Ravn P, McClung M, et al. Tooth counts do not predict bone mineral density in early postmenopausal Caucasian women. EPIC study group. *Int. J. Epidemiol.* 1998 Jun;27(3):479-83.

[104] Taguchi A, Suei Y, Ohtsuka M, Otani K, Tanimoto K, Hollender LG. Relationship between bone mineral density and tooth loss in elderly Japanese women. *Dentomaxillofac. Radiol.* 1999 Jul;28(4):219-23.

[105] Bollen AM, Taguchi A, Hujoel PP, Hollender LG. Number of teeth and residual alveolar ridge height in subjects with a history of self-reported osteoporotic fractures. *Osteoporos .Int.* 2004 Dec;15(12):970-4.

[106] Inagaki K, Kurosu Y, Yoshinari N, Noguchi T, Krall EA, Garcia RI. Efficacy of periodontal disease and tooth loss to screen for low bone mineral density in Japanese women. *Calcif. Tissue Int.* 2005 Jul;77(1):9-14.

[107] Drozdzowska B, Pluskiewicz W, Michno M. Tooth count in elderly women in relation to their skeletal status. *Maturitas.* 2006 Sep 20;55(2):126-31.

[108] Dervis E. Oral implications of osteoporosis. *Oral Surg Oral Med Oral Pathol Oral. Radiol. Endod.* 2005 Sep;100(3):349-56.

[109] Norderyd OM, Grossi SG, Machtei EE, Zambon JJ, Hausmann E, Dunford RG, et al. Periodontal status of women taking postmenopausal estrogen supplementation. *J. Periodontol.* 1993 Oct;64(10):957-62.

[110] Ronderos M, Jacobs DR, Himes JH, Pihlstrom BL. Associations of periodontal disease with femoral bone mineral density and estrogen replacement therapy: cross-sectional evaluation of US adults from NHANES III. *J. Clin. Periodontol.* 2000 Oct;27(10):778-86.

[111] Reinhardt RA, Payne JB, Maze CA, Patil KD, Gallagher SJ, Mattson JS. Influence of estrogen and osteopenia/osteoporosis on clinical periodontitis in postmenopausal women. *J. Periodontol.* 1999 Aug;70(8):823-8.

[112] Lopez-Marcos JF, Garcia-Valle S, Garcia-Iglesias AA. Periodontal aspects in menopausal women undergoing hormone replacement therapy. *Med. Oral Patol. Oral. Cir Bucal.* 2005 Mar-Apr;10(2):132-41.

[113] Paganini-Hill A. The benefits of estrogen replacement therapy on oral health. The Leisure World cohort. *Arch Intern Med.* 1995 Nov 27;155(21):2325-9.

[114] Grodstein F, Colditz GA, Stampfer MJ. Post-menopausal hormone use and tooth loss: a prospective study. *J. Am. Dent. Assoc.* 1996 Mar;127(3):370-7, quiz 92.

[115] Civitelli R, Pilgram TK, Dotson M, Muckerman J, Lewandowski N, Armamento-Villareal R, et al. Alveolar and postcranial bone density in postmenopausal women receiving hormone/estrogen replacement therapy: a randomized, double-blind, placebo-controlled trial. *Arch. Intern. Med.* 2002 Jun 24;162(12):1409-15.

[116] Taguchi A, Sanada M, Suei Y, Ohtsuka M, Nakamoto T, Lee K, et al. Effect of estrogen use on tooth retention, oral bone height, and oral bone porosity in Japanese postmenopausal women. *Menopause.* 2004 Sep-Oct;11(5):556-62.

[117] Evio S, Tarkkila L, Sorsa T, Furuholm J, Valimaki MJ, Ylikorkala O, et al. Effects of alendronate and hormone replacement therapy, alone and in combination, on saliva, periodontal conditions and gingival crevicular fluid matrix metalloproteinase-8 levels in women with osteoporosis. *Oral Dis.* 2006 Mar;12(2):187-93.

[118] Tarkkila L, Furuholm J, Tiitinen A, Meurman JH. Oral health in perimenopausal and early postmenopausal women from baseline to 2 years of follow-up with reference to hormone replacement therapy. *Clin. Oral Investig.* 2008 Sep;12(3):271-7.

[119] Horner K, Devlin H. The relationship between mandibular bone mineral density and panoramic radiographic measurements. *J. Dent.* 1998 May;26(4):337-43.

[120] Taguchi A, Ohtsuka M, Tsuda M, Nakamoto T, Kodama I, Inagaki K, et al. Risk of vertebral osteoporosis in post-menopausal women with alterations of the mandible. *Dentomaxillofac. Radiol.* 2007 Mar;36(3):143-8.

[121] Bozic M, Ihan Hren N. Osteoporosis and mandibles. *Dentomaxillofac Radiol.* 2006 May;35(3):178-84.

[122] Law AN, Bollen AM, Chen SK. Detecting osteoporosis using dental radiographs: a comparison of four methods. *J. Am. Dent Assoc.* 1996 Dec;127(12):1734-42.

[123] Vlasiadis KZ, Damilakis J, Velegrakis GA, Skouteris CA, Fragouli I, Goumenou A, et al. Relationship between BMD, dental panoramic radiographic findings and

biochemical markers of bone turnover in diagnosis of osteoporosis. *Maturitas.* 2008 Mar 20;59(3):226-33.

[124] Vlasiadis KZ, Skouteris CA, Velegrakis GA, Fragouli I, Neratzoulakis JM, Damilakis J, et al. Mandibular radiomorphometric measurements as indicators of possible osteoporosis in postmenopausal women. *Maturitas.* 2007 Nov 20;58(3):226-35.

[125] Taguchi A, Suei Y, Sanada M, Ohtsuka M, Nakamoto T, Sumida H, et al. Validation of dental panoramic radiography measures for identifying postmenopausal women with spinal osteoporosis. *AJR Am. J. Roentgenol.* 2004 Dec;183(6):1755-60.

[126] Devlin H, Karayianni K, Mitsea A, Jacobs R, Lindh C, van der Stelt P, et al. Diagnosing osteoporosis by using dental panoramic radiographs: the OSTEODENT project. *Oral Surg. Oral Med. Oral Pathol. Oral Radiol. Endod.* 2007 Dec;104(6):821-8.

[127] Cakur B, Sahin A, Dagistan S, Altun O, Caglayan F, Miloglu O, et al. Dental panoramic radiography in the diagnosis of osteoporosis. *J. Int Med. Res.* 2008 Jul-Aug;36(4):792-9.

[128] Taguchi A, Ohtsuka M, Nakamoto T, Naito K, Tsuda M, Kudo Y, et al. Identification of post-menopausal women at risk of osteoporosis by trained general dental practitioners using panoramic radiographs. *Dentomaxillofac. Radiol.* 2007 Mar;36(3):149-54.

[129] Klemetti E, Kolmakov S, Kroger H. Pantomography in assessment of the osteoporosis risk group. *Scand. J. Dent. Res.* 1994 Feb;102(1):68-72.

[130] Klemetti E, Kolmakov S, Heiskanen P, Vainio P, Lassila V. Panoramic mandibular index and bone mineral densities in postmenopausal women. *Oral Surg. Oral Med. Oral Pathol.* 1993 Jun;75(6):774-9.

[131] Benson BW, Prihoda TJ, Glass BJ. Variations in adult cortical bone mass as measured by a panoramic mandibular index. *Oral Surg. Oral Med. Oral Pathol.* 1991 Mar;71(3):349-56.

[132] Kribbs PJ, Chesnut CH, 3rd, Ott SM, Kilcoyne RF. Relationships between mandibular and skeletal bone in an osteoporotic population. *J. Prosthet. Dent.* 1989 Dec;62(6):703-7.

[133] Hirai T, Ishijima T, Hashikawa Y, Yajima T. Osteoporosis and reduction of residual ridge in edentulous patients. *J. Prosthet. Dent.* 1993 Jan;69(1):49-56.

[134] von Wowern N, Kollerup G. Symptomatic osteoporosis: a risk factor for residual ridge reduction of the jaws. *J. Prosthet. Dent.* 1992 May;67(5):656-60.

[135] Klemetti E. A review of residual ridge resorption and bone density. *J. Prosthet. Dent.* 1996 May;75(5):512-4.

[136] von Wowern N. General and oral aspects of osteoporosis: a review. *Clin. Oral Investig.* 2001 Jun;5(2):71-82.

[137] Slagter KW, Raghoebar GM, Vissink A. Osteoporosis and edentulous jaws. *Int. J. Prosthodont.* 2008 Jan-Feb;21(1):19-26.

[138] Miyajima K, Nagahara K, Iizuka T. Orthodontic treatment for a patient after menopause. *The Angle orthodontist.* 1996;66(3):173-8; discussion 9-80.

[139] Pereira AAC, Taveira, L. A. A. Induced tooth movement and ovariectomy: microscopic evaluation. *Rev.FOB.* 2000;8(3/4):1-7.

[140] Yamashiro T, Takano-Yamamoto T. Influences of ovariectomy on experimental tooth movement in the rat. *J. Dent Res.* 2001 Sep;80(9):1858-61.

[141] Arslan SG, Arslan H, Ketani A, Hamamci O. Effects of estrogen deficiency on tooth movement after force application: an experimental study in ovariectomized rats. *Acta odontologica Scandinavica.* 2007 Nov;65(6):319-23.

[142] Haruyama N, Igarashi K, Saeki S, Otsuka-Isoya M, Shinoda H, Mitani H. Estrous-cycle-dependent variation in orthodontic tooth movement. *J. Dent. Res.* 2002 Jun;81(6):406-10.

[143] Sidiropoulou-Chatzigiannis S, Kourtidou M, Tsalikis L. The effect of osteoporosis on periodontal status, alveolar bone and orthodontic tooth movement. A literature review. *J. Int. Acad .Periodontol.* 2007 Jul;9(3):77-84.

[144] Ben Aryeh H, Gottlieb I, Ish-Shalom S, David A, Szargel H, Laufer D. Oral complaints related to menopause. *Maturitas.* 1996 Jul;24(3):185-9.

[145] Forabosco A, Criscuolo M, Coukos G, Uccelli E, Weinstein R, Spinato S, et al. Efficacy of hormone replacement therapy in postmenopausal women with oral discomfort. *Oral Surg. Oral Med .Oral Pathol.* 1992 May;73(5):570-4.

[146]]Wardrop RW, Hailes J, Burger H, Reade PC. Oral discomfort at menopause. *Oral Surg. Oral Med .Oral Pathol.* 1989 May;67(5):535-40.

[147] Seko K, Kagami H, Senga K, Ozeki K, Mizutani H, Ueda M. Effects of ovariectomy and estrogen replacement on rat oral mucosa. *Maturitas.* 2005 Jan;50(1):44-51.

[148] Purushotham KR, Wang PL, Dolce C, Zelles T, Blazsek J, Humphreys-Beher MG. Effects of surgical ovariectomy on rat salivary gland function. *Arch. Oral .Biol.* 1993 Sep;38(9):779-84.

[149]]Laine M, Leimola-Virtanen R. Effect of hormone replacement therapy on salivary flow rate, buffer effect and pH on perimenopausal and postmenopausal women. *Arch. Oral Biol.* 1996 Jan;41(1):91-6.

[150] Delaleu N, Jonsson R, Koller MM. Sjögren's syndrome. *Eur. J. Oral Sci.* 2005 Apr;113(2):101-13.

[151] Toda I, Sullivan BD, Rocha EM, Da Silveira LA, Wickham LA, Sullivan DA. Impact of gender on exocrine gland inflammation in mouse models of Sjögren's syndrome. *Exp. Eye Res.* 1999 Oct;69(4):355-66.

[152] Taiym S, Haghighat N, Al-Hashimi I. A comparison of the hormone levels in patients with Sjogren's syndrome and healthy controls. *Oral Surg. Oral Med. Oral Pathol. Oral Radiol. Endod.* 2004 May;97(5):579-83.

[153] Tanaka S, Shimizu M, Debari K, Furuya R, Kawawa T, Sasaki T. Acute effects of ovariectomy on wound healing of alveolar bone after maxillary molar extraction in aged rats. *Anat. Rec.* 2001 Feb;262(2):203-12.

[154] Junqueira JC, Mancini MN, Carvalho YR, Anbinder AL, Balducci I, Rocha RF. Effects of simvastatin on bone regeneration in the mandibles of ovariectomized rats and on blood cholesterol levels. *J. Oral Sci.* 2002 Dec;44(3-4):117-24.

[155] Pereira MC, Zecchin KG, Campagnoli EB, Jorge J. Ovariectomy delays alveolar wound healing after molar extractions in rats. *J. Oral Maxillofac. Surg.* 2007 Nov;65(11):2248-53.

[156] Lill CA, Hesseln J, Schlegel U, Eckhardt C, Goldhahn J, Schneider E. Biomechanical evaluation of healing in a non-critical defect in a large animal model of osteoporosis. *J. Orthop. Res.* 2003 Sep;21(5):836-42.

[157] Shimizu M, Sasaki T, Ishihara A, Furuya R, Kawawa T. Bone wound healing after maxillary molar extraction in ovariectomized aged rats. *J. Electron. Microsc.* (Tokyo). 1998;47(5):517-26.

[158] Hsieh YD, Devlin H, McCord F. The effect of ovariectomy on the healing tooth socket of the rat. *Arch. Oral Biol.* 1995 Jun;40(6):529-31.

[159] Zecchin KG, Pereira MC, Coletta RD, Graner E, Jorge J. Ovariectomy reduces the gelatinolytic activity and expression of matrix metalloproteinases and collagen in rat molar extraction wounds. *Calcif. Tissue Int.* 2005 Feb;76(2):136-45.

[160] Kawamoto S, Nagaoka E. The effect of oestrogen deficiency on the alveolar bone resorption caused by traumatic occlusion. *J .Oral. Rehabil.* 2000 Jul;27(7):587-94.

[161] Xiong H, Peng B, Wei L, Zhang X, Wang L. Effect of an estrogen-deficient state and alendronate therapy on bone loss resulting from experimental periapical lesions in rats. *J. Endod.* 2007 Nov;33(11):1304-8.

[162] Zhang X, Peng B, Fan M, Bian Z, Chen Z. The effect of estrogen deficiency on receptor activator of nuclear factor kappa B ligand and osteoprotegerin synthesis in periapical lesions induced in rats. *J. Endod.* 2007 Sep;33(9):1053-6.

[163] August M, Chung K, Chang Y, Glowacki J. Influence of estrogen status on endosseous implant osseointegration. J Oral Maxillofac Surg. 2001 Nov;59(11):1285-9; discussion 90-1.

[164] Yamazaki M, Shirota T, Tokugawa Y, Motohashi M, Ohno K, Michi K, et al. Bone reactions to titanium screw implants in ovariectomized animals. *Oral Surg. Oral Med. Oral Pathol. Oral Radiol. Endod.* 1999 Apr;87(4):411-8.

[165] Motohashi M, Shirota T, Tokugawa Y, Ohno K, Michi K, Yamaguchi A. Bone reactions around hydroxyapatite-coated implants in ovariectomized rats. *Oral Surg. Oral Med .Oral Pathol. Oral Radiol. Endod.* 1999 Feb;87(2):145-52.

[166] Qi MC, Zhou XQ, Hu J, Du ZJ, Yang JH, Liu M, et al. Oestrogen replacement therapy promotes bone healing around dental implants in osteoporotic rats. *Int. J. Oral Maxillofac. Surg.* 2004 Apr;33(3):279-85.

In: Estrogens: Production, Functions and Applications ISBN: 978-1-60741-086-7
Editor: James R. Bartos, pp. 215-230

Chapter VIII

Estrogen Effects on Platelets

Mustafa Sahin
Baskent University, Endocrinology and Metabolic Disease Department,
Ankara / Turkey

Introduction:

The randomized, placebo-controlled Women's Health Initiative (WHI) Trial was terminated early because increased risk of breast cancer, thrombosis and cardiovascular disease with hormone replacement therapy were observed (1).

Selective estrogen receptor modulators (SERMs) have been devoleped to decrease the serious side effects of estrogens (2).

Platelets are important mediators of both inflammation and thrombosis. They play a critical role in the pathogenesis of cardiovascular disease (3,4).

Platelets provide the membrane surface for the generation of thrombin and release vasoactive substances. Also, their membrane receptors affect platelet-platelet and platelet-vessel wall interactions. It is possible that the cardiovascular and hemostatic effects of estrogens are mediated, at least in part, through its effects on platelets.

Estrogen Receptors:

Estrogens may influence hemostatic function either with genomic effects on gene expression or via nongenomic rapid effects.

Estrogens and SERMs produce their effects by binding to two estrogen receptors, estrogen receptor α (ERα) and estrogen receptor β (ER β) leading to genomic or nongenomic actions (5-7). Different genes code ER α and ER β. They share considerable sequence identity in their DNA and hormone binding domains; they diverge in their activation domains (6). Both receptors exhibit tissue and cell specific expression (8). ER α is predominantly expressed in testis, breast, uterus, pituitary liver kidney, heart, whereas ER β transcripts predominate in male reproductive tract in tissues such as the cardiovascular system, immune system (9-14). These receptors are also expressed in hematopoietic stem cells (15) endoliocytes (16), mast cells (17-20), T cells (21), thymocytes (22,23), B lymphocyte precursors (24). It appears that ER β has biological roles that are distinct from those of ER α (25).

The biological actions of estrogens are mediated predominantly by nuclear receptors, which belong to the family of ligand-activated nuclear receptors. It is reported that estrogens and SERMs exert tissue-specific effects by regulating unique sets of targets genes through ERα and ER β (26). Estrogens may passively diffuse through plasma membranes and bind to their cognate nuclear receptor protein (27). The estrogen-receptor protein complex modulates transcription of target genes and subsequently their protein synthesis (28).

After activation receptors dimerize to form receptor homodimers or heterodimers, (29) bind to specific DNA response elements, and activate the transcription (30,31). Coregulatory proteins interacts with estrogen receptors to alter transcription of target genes (31). Estrogens may also bind to plasma membrane–associated receptors and acti vate a variety of rapid intracellular signaling pathways (30-32).

Studies Related to Estrogen Effects on Platelet Function:

The role of sex steroid hormones in the regulation of platelet function has been investigated for years, but conflicting results have been reported (33-47).

Platelet aggregation is higher in age-matched women than in men (48,49), aggregation is also enhanced during human pregnancy (50). It has been also found that enhanced platelet fibrinogen binding in luteal phase (25), platelet adhesion to collagen vary by phase of the menstrual cycle (51,52). Platelet function might be modulated by OCs and the female cycle (53). Female platelets are hyperactive compared to male platelets (54, 55). Higher concentrations of estrogen increase platelet reactivity (56). Hormonal deprivation affects ATP, ADP and AMP hydrolysis by platelets and consequently the level of these nucleotides in the circulation (57).

In Framingham Study found that hormone replacement was associated with increased ADP-induced platelet aggregation (58) but in vitro platelet aggregation and ATP release from platelets inhibited by estrogen replacement therapy in postmenopausal women (38,40,59). In vitro adding of 17-β estradiol to platelet inhibit agonist induced platelet aggregation and increase intracellular calcium and release of nitric oxide (39,60-62).

It is reported that platelet function is not impaired by short-term raloxifene therapy at therapeutic dose in patients with postmenopausal osteoporosis (63).

Previous studies have investigated possible mechanisms by which estrogen therapy (ET) alone (64-79), estrogen combined with progesterone (HT) (65-86), tamoxifen (87-95) and raloxifene (95-99) affect hemostasis. In conclusion, all three treatments in our study, estrogen, tamoxifen and raloxifene, produced changes in the hemostatic system favoring thrombosis by increasing levels of coagulation factors and decreasing anticoagulant protein levels (100).

Collective interpretation of studies of the effects of estrogen on platelet functions in humans are confounded by differences in doses and formulations (oral and transdermal) of estrogenic treatments, and differences in the panel of tests used to assess platelet functions. Effects of acute application or nongenomic effects of estrogen on platelet functions are also usually not interpreted relative to the hormonal status of the platelet donor (40, 101-106).

Mechanism of Estrogen Action on Platelets (Figure 1) :

Platelets in the circulation are anucleate cytoplasmic buds of the megakaryocytes. Newly formed platelets contain small amounts of mRNA and endoplasmic reticulum but their ability to synthesize new proteins is limited. Genomic effects of estrogen in platelets would occur only in megakaryocytes as these precursors of platelets contain nuclei, (107). The life of a platelet in the circulation is 10–12 days in humans. So genomic effects of estrogens on megakartocytes will affect platelet pool (108,109). Platelets and their precursors, megakaryocytes, contain both ER α and ER β (40, 110-120 ERβ seems to predominate in circulating platelets (110,111) and is associated to the membranes (101). The location of the receptors within the platelets (extracellular membrane, cytosol or mitochondria) is not well understood (121,122).

Therefore, the presence of estrogen receptors on circulating platelets could initiate nongenomic response to estrogen in the circulation. These concepts are important in order to understand and differentiate the context of acute versus chronic effects of estrogens.

In the absence of a ligand, or in an inactive form, estrogen receptors are associated with a number of heat shock proteins (e.g., hsp70). It has been proposed that receptor-associated proteins keep receptors in a conformation that increases the affinity of the receptor for hormones. (123,124). Differences in expression of estrogen receptors may alter responses of the platelets to exogenous or replaced hormone and thus contribute to increased thrombotic risk. Estrogen can also affect megakaryocyte/platelet function indirectly through other systems; for example, by either changing the threshold of platelet activation or modifying the production of endogenous platelet agonists or inhibitors.

An effect of estrogen on hematopoietic stem cells has been noted for years (125-128).

Many studies provide evidence direct actions of estradiol on the bone marrow and the regulation of bone marrow-derived precursor cells (129-132). Megakaryocytes (MKs) are the bone marrow cells responsible for platelet formation (133). Human studies have also noted marked increases in MK number following estrogen treatment (134-136). In addition to modifying MK number it has become clear that oestrogen has a critical role in platelet formation, as proplatelet production by MKs is initiated by and dependent on autocrine oestrogen synthesis (108). Dr. Nagata and colleagues delineates a genetic mechanism in MK for regulating the formation of blood platelets: The p45 NF-E2 transcription factor turns on 3-hydroxysteroid dehydrogenase gene expression, leading to the synthesis of estradiol and the subsequent activation of proplatelet formation (108). There is intriguing evidence that the platelet content of E2 is higher than the plasma concentration in both males and females (137).

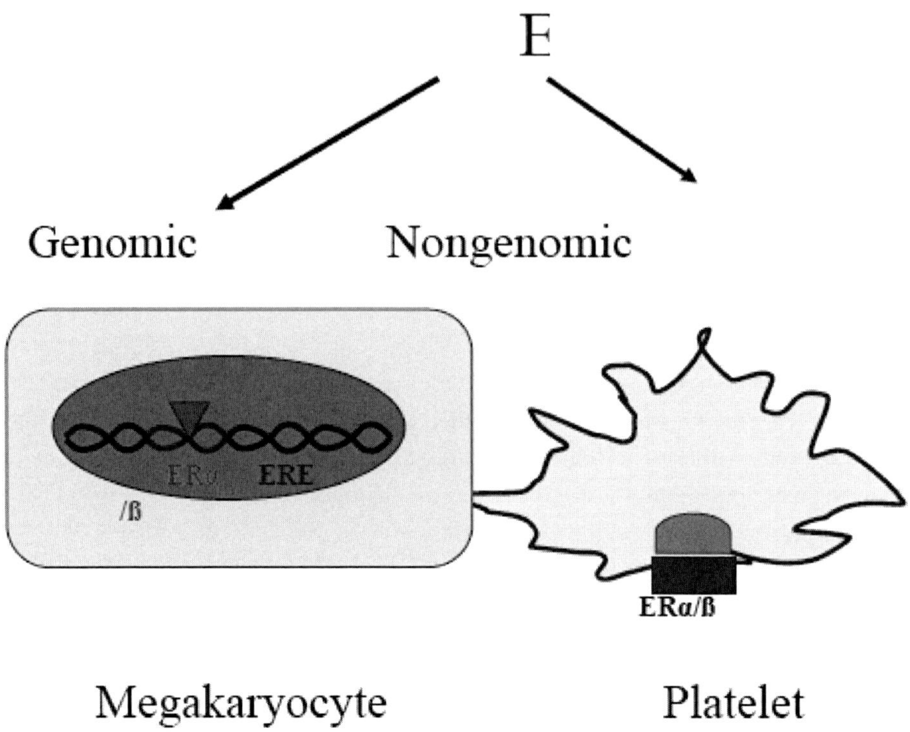

Figure 1. Effects of estrogen on megakaryocyte and platelet, E: Estrogen; ER: Estrogen receptor;ERE: Estrogen response element.

Genomic Effects

Protein products of estrogen-regulated genes that are associated with platelet activity include: prostacyclin synthase, endothelial nitric oxide synthase, and inducible nitric oxide synthase (138). Genes coding for proteins associated with coagulation and fibrinolysis and regulated by estrogen include fibrinogen, protein S, factor VII, PAI, antithrombin III, factor XII and tissue factor (which is also regulated by progestin).(138-141).

The genomic action of sex steroids may directly modulate plasma levels of clotting factors. The use of ethinylestradiol is associated with an increase of plasma concentrations of fibrinogen, plasminogen, factors VII, VIII, X and XIII, but also of coagulation inhibitors such as protein C (142).

Concentrations of platelet-derived growth factor, enzymes such as nitric oxide synthase and MMP-2, and enzyme products such as prostacyclin and 5-hydroxytryptamine increase in lysate of platelets following ovariectomy (40, 116,143). Loss of ovarian hormones by surgical ovariectomy increases platelet aggregation, dense body ATP secretion, and content of factors such as PDGF-BB and matrix metalloproteinase-2 (MMP-2) that affect repair and remodeling of the blood vessel wall (134, 144,145).

Nongenomic

Nongenomic actions of estrogens on platelet functions would be rapid modulate other agonist receptor–coupled activation of platelets. Effects of estrogens that are modulated through the nongenomic signal transduction pathway may also be mechanistically involved in regulating hemostasis. The physiologic consequences of stimulation of membrane receptors would be evident before genomic responses mediated by receptors in megakaryocytes, because platelets turn over in ~10 to 12 days.

One mechanism is through estrogen-receptor α stimulation of nitric oxide, an endothelium-derived product known to reduce platelet aggregation (146-151). Estrogen receptor α, perhaps as a homodimer, is tethered to the cell membrane by striatin in caveoli with nitric oxide synthase (152,153). This mechanism do not require gene transcription. 17β-estradiol–dependent activation of endothelial nitric oxide (NO) synthesis leads to rapid vasodilation, while at the same time inhibiting vascular smooth muscle cell proliferation, leukocyte adhesion, and platelet aggregation, thus contributing to atheroprotection (154-160).

Endothelium-derived nitric oxide is reduced in estrogen receptor α knockout mice but increased with overexpression of the receptor in cultured cells (161-165).

Changes of ion channels are thought to be the cause of the so-called 'activation' of cellular membranes and responsible for the activation of platelets, macrophages and endothelial cells (166). 'Activation' may change the smooth antithrombotic properties of endothelial membranes into the sticky procoagulatory grater-like surfaces that will rapidly induce the activation of the coagulation cascade (167).

It may be hypothesized that. while the genomic effects of steroids may predominantly account for changes in the assembly of the hemostatic factors (factors. inhibitors, substrates). non-genomic effects may predominantly affect the vessel wall and the membranes of platelets and macrophages.

References:

[1] The Writing Group for the Women's Health Initiative. (2002). Risks and benefits of estrogen plus progestin in healthy postmenopausal women: principal results From the Women's Health Initiative randomized controlled trial. Jama *288*, 321-333.

[2] McDonnell, D.P. (2000). Selective estrogen receptor modulators (SERMs): A first step in the development of perfect hormone replacement therapy regimen. J Soc Gynecol Investig *7*, S10-15.

[3] Anderson TJ. (2003) Nitric Oxide, Atherosclerosis and the Clinical Relevance of Endothelial Dysfunction. Heart Failure Rev 8:71–86.

[4] Fitzgerald, D. J. Roy L, Catella F, FitzGerald GA.(1986) Platelet activation in unstable coronary disease. N. Engl. J. Med. 315, 983–989.

[5] Green, S., Walter, P., Kumar, V., Krust, A., Bornert, J.M., Argos, P., and Chambon, P. (1986). Human oestrogen receptor cDNA: sequence, expression and homology to v-erb-A. Nature *320*, 134-139.

[6] Kuiper, G., and Gustafsson, J. (1997). The novel estrogen receptor-beta subtype: potential role in the cell- and promoter-specific actions of estrogens and anti-estrogens. Federation of European Biochemical Societies Letters *410*, 87-90.

[7] Nilsson, S., Makela, S., Treuter, E., Tujague, M., Thomsen, J., Andersson, G., Enmark, E., Pettersson, K., Warner, M., Gustafsson, J.A., 2001. Mechanisms of estrogen action. Physiol. Rev. 81, 1535–1565

[8] O'Lone R, Frith MC, Karlsson EK, Hansen U. (2004) Genomic targets of nuclear estrogen receptors. Mol Endocrinol 18:1859–1875.

[9] Nilsson S, Koehler KF. (2005) Oestrogen receptors and selective oestrogen receptor modulators: Molecular and cellular pharmacology. Basic Clin Pharmacol Toxicol 96:15–25.

[10] Bellido T, Girasole G, Passeri G, Yu XP, Mocharla H, Jilka RL, Notides A, Manolagas SC 1993 Demonstration of estrogen and vitamin D receptors in bone marrow-derived stromal cells: up-regulation of the estrogen receptor by 1,25-dihydroxyvitamin-D_3. Endocrinology 133:553–562

[11] Smithson G, Medina K, Ponting I, Kincade PW 1995 Estrogen suppresses stromal cell-dependent lymphopoiesis in culture. J Immunol 155:3409–3417

[12] Kuiper GG, Enmark E, Pelto-Huikko M, Nilsson S, Gustafsson JA 1996 Cloning of a novel receptor expressed in rat prostate and ovary. Proc Natl Acad Sci USA 93:5925–5930

[13] Couse JF, Lindzey J, Grandien K, Gustafsson JA, Korach KS 1997 Tissue distribution and quantitative analysis of estrogen receptoralphaand estrogen receptorbetamessenger ribonucleic acid in the wild-type and ERalphaknockout mouse. Endocrinology 138:4613–4621

[14] Smithson G, Couse JF, Lubahn DB, Korach KS, Kincade PW 1998 The role of estrogen receptors and androgen receptors in sex steroid regulation of B lymphopoiesis. J Immunol 161:27–34

[15] Zhou, S., Zilberman, Y., Wassermmm, K., Bain, S.D., Sadovsky, Y., Gazit, D., 2001. Estrogen modulates estrogen receptor alpha and beta expression, osteogenic activity, and apoptosis in mesenchymal stem cells (MSCs) of osteoporotic mice. J. Cell. Biochem. 81, 144–155.

[16] Kim-Schulze, S., McGowan, K.A., Hubchak, S.C., Cid, M.C., Martin, M.B., Kleinman, H.K., Greene, G.J., Schnaper, H.W., 1996. Expression of an estrogen receptor by human coronary artery and umbilical vein endothelial cells. Circulation 94, 1402–1407.

[17] Harnish, D.C., Albert, L.M., Leathurby, Y., Eckert, A.M., Ciarletta, A., Kasaian, M.,Keith Jr., J.C., 2004. Beneficial effects of estrogen treatment in the HLAB27 transgenic rat model of inflammatory bowel disease. Am. J. Physiol. Gastrointest. Liver Physiol. 286, G118–G125.

[18] Jiang, Y.A., Zhang, Y.Y., Luo, H.S., Xing, S.F., 2002. Mast cell density and the context of clinicopathological parameters and expression of p185, estrogen receptor, and proliferating cell nuclear antigen in gastric carcinoma. World J. Gastroenterol. 8, 1005–1008.

[19] Nicovani, S., Rudolph, M.I., 2002. Estrogen receptors in mast cells from arterial walls. Biocell 26, 15–24.

[20] Zhao, X.J., McKerr, G., Dong, Z., Higgins, C.A., Carson, J., Yang, Z.Q., Hannigan, B.M., 2001. Expression of oestrogen and progesterone receptors by mast cells alone, but not lymphocytes, macrophages or other immune cells in human upper airways. Thorax 56, 205–211.

[21] Dudley DJ, Chen CL, Mitchell MD, Daynes RA, Araneo BA 1993 Adaptive immune responses during murine pregnancy: pregnancy-induced regulation of lymphokine production by activated T lymphocytes. Am J Obstet Gynecol 168:1155–1163

[22] Muller D, Chen M, Vikingsson A, Hildeman D, Pederson K 1995 Oestrogen influences $CD4^+$ T-lymphocyte activity *in vivo* and *in vitro* in $ß_2$-microglobulin-deficient mice. Immunology 86:162–167

[23] Medina KL, Smithson G, Kincade PW 1993 Suppression of B lymphopoiesis during normal pregnancy. J Exp Med 178:1507–1515

[24] Haruki Y, Seiki K, Enomoto T, Fujii H, Sakabe K 1983 Estrogen receptor in the "non-lymphocytes" in the thymus of the ovariectomized rat. Tokai J Exp Clin Med 8:31–39

[25] Gustafsson JA. (1999) Estrogen receptor beta--a new dimension in estrogen mechanism of action. J Endocrinol.163(3):379-83. Review.

[26] Kian Tee M, Rogatsky I, Tzagarakis-Foster C, Cvoro A, An J, Christy RJ, Yamamoto KR, Leitman DC. (2004) Estradiol and selective estrogen receptor modulators differentially regulate target genes with estrogen receptors alpha and beta. Mol Biol Cell.15(3):1262-72.

[27] Halachmi S, Marden E. Martin G. MacKay H, Abbondanra C, Brown M. (1994) Estrogen receptor-associated proteins: possible mediators of hormone-induced transcription. Science 264: 1455 1458.

[28] Landers JP. Spelsberg TC. (1992) New concepts in steroid hormone action: Transcription factors, proto-oncogenes. and the cascade model for steroid regulation of gene expression. Crit Rev Eukar Gene Express 2: 19.-6.3.

[29] Mendelsohn ME, Karas RH. (1999) The protective effects of estrogen on the cardiovascular system. *N Engl J Med*. 340:1801–1811.

[30] . Meyer MR, Haas E, Barton M. (2006) Gender differences of cardiovascular disease: New perspectives for estrogen receptor signaling. *Hypertension*. 47:1019–1026.

[31] . Mendelsohn ME. (2002) Genomic and nongenomic effects of estrogen in the vasculature. *Am J Cardiol*. 90:3F–6F.

[32] Hayashi T, Yamada K, Esaki T, et al. (1995) Estrogen increases endothelial nitric oxide by a receptormediated system. *Biochem Biophys Res Commun*. 214:847–855.

[33] Elkeles RS, Hampton JR, Mitchell JR. (1968) Effect of oestrogens on human platelet behaviour. Lancet ii:315–318.

[34] Poller L. (1971) Oral contraception and platelet aggregation. Acta Med Scand Suppl 525:197–201.

[35] Altman R, Taboada S, Zielinsky A. (1974) The effect in vitro of the steroidal component of oral contraceptives on platelet aggregation. Experientia 30:1203.

[36] Toy JL, Davies JA, Hancock KW,McNicol GP. (1978) The effects of an increase in endogenous oestrogen on the haemostatic mechanism. Thromb Haemost 39:683–688.

[37] Ishak R, Mohamed AB, Hassan K. (1990) Platelet function studies in women on oral contraceptive pills. Malays J Reprod Health 8:1–4.

[38] Bar J, Tepper R, Fuchs J, Pardo Y, Goldberger S, Ovadia J. (1993) The effect of estrogen replacement therapy on platelet aggregation and adenosine triphosphate release in postmenopausal women. Obstet Gynecol 81:261–264.

[39] Nakano Y, Oshima T, Matsuura H, Kajiyama G, Kambe M. (1998) Effect of 17beta-estradiol on inhibition of platelet aggregation in vitro is mediated by an increase in NO synthesis. Arterioscler Thromb Vasc Biol 18: 961–967.

[40] Nakano Y, Oshima T, Ozono R, Ueda A, Oue Y, Matsuura H, Sanada M, Ohama K, Chayama K, Kambe M. (2002) Estrogen replacement suppresses function of thrombin stimulated platelets by inhibiting Ca(2þ) influx and raising cyclic adenosine monophosphate. Cardiovasc Res 53:634–641.

[41] Seelig MS, Altura BM, Altura BT. (2004) Benefits and risks of sex hormone replacement in postmenopausal women. J Am Coll Nutr 23:482S–496S.

[42] Yasuda Y, Masuda S, Chikuma M, Inoue K, Nagao M, Sasaki R. (1998) Estrogen-dependent production of erythropoietin in uterus and its implication in uterine angiogenesis. *J Biol Chem.* 273:25381–25387.

[43] Bone RC. (1992) Toward an epidemiology and natural history of SIRS (systemic inflammatory response syndrome). JAMA. 268:3452–5.

[44] . McGowan JE Jr, Barnes MW, Finland M. (1975) Bacteremia at Boston City Hospital: occurrence and mortality during 12 selected years (1935–1972), with special reference to hospital-acquired cases. J Infect Dis. 132:316–35.

[45] Angele MK, Schwacha MG, Ayala A, Chaudry IH. (2000) Effect of gender and sex hormones on immune responses following shock. Shock. 14:81–90.

[46] Frink M, Pape HC, van Griensven M, Krettek C, Chaudry IH, Hildebrand F. (2007)Influence of sex and age on MODS and cytokines after multiple injuries. Shock. 27:151–6.

[47] Cuzzocrea S, Mazzon E, Sautebin L, Serraino I, Dugo L, Calabró G, Caputi AP, Maggi A. The protective role of endogenous estrogens in carrageenan-induced lung injury in the rat. Mol Med. 2001;7:478–87.

[48] Haque S F, Matsubayashi H, Izumi S, Sugi T, Arai T, Kondo A, et al. (2001) Sex difference in platelet aggregation detected by new aggregometry using light scattering. Endocr J 48: 33–41.

[49] Kelton J G, Carter C J, Santos A, Hirsh J. (1982) Sex related differences in platelet function: the effect of aspirin. Blood 59: 625–7.

[50] Sheu, J.R Hsiao G, Shen MY, Lin WY, Tzeng CR. (2002) The hyperaggregability of platelets from normal pregnancy is mediated through thromboxane A2 and cyclic AMP pathways. Clin. Lab. Haematol. 24, 121–129

[51] Tarantino, M.D. Kunicki TJ, Nugent DJ. (1994) The estrogen receptor is present in human megakaryocytes. Ann. N.Y. Acad. Sci. 714, 293–296

[52] Jones, S.B. Bylund DB, Rieser CA, Shekim WO, Byer JA, Carr GW. (1983) alpha 2-Adrenergic receptor binding in human platelets: alterations during the menstrual cycle. Clin. Pharmacol. Ther. 34, 90–96

[53] Roell, A., Schueller, P., Schultz, A., Losel, R., Wehling, M., Christ, M. and Feuring, M.(2007)'Effect of oral contraceptives and ovarian cycle on platelet

function',Platelets,18:2,165 — 1709. Anderson TJ. Nitric Oxide, Atherosclerosis and the Clinical Relevance of Endothelial Dysfunction. Heart Failure Rev 2003;8:71–86.

[54] Johnson, M. Ramey E, Ramwell PW.. (1975) Sex and age differences in human platelet aggregation. Nature 253, 355–357

[55] . Faraday, N Goldschmidt-Clermont PJ, Bray PF. (1997) Gender differences in platelet GPIIb-IIIa activation. Thromb. Haemost. 77, 748–754

[56] Rosin, Christiane, Brunner, Markus, Lehr, Stephan, Quehenberger, Peter and Panzer, Simon(2006)'The formation of platelet-leukocyte aggregates varies during the menstrual cycle',Platelets,17:1,61 — 66

[57] .Pochmann, Daniela, Böhmer, Ana Elisa, Bruno, Alessandra Nejar and Sarkis, João J. F.(2005)'Ecto-hydrolysis of adenine nucleotides in rat blood platelets are altered by ovariectomy',Platelets,16:6,334 — 339

[58] . Feng, D. Lindpaintner K, Larson MG et al (1999) Increased platelet aggregability associated with platelet GPIIIa PlA2 polymorphism: the Framingham Offspring Study. Arterioscler. Thromb. Vasc. Biol. 19, 1142–1147

[59] . Bar J, Lahav J, Hod M, Ben-Rafael Z,Weinberger I, Brosens J. (2000) Regulation of platelet aggregation and adenosine triphosphate release in vitro by 17-beta-estradiol and medroxyprogesterone acetate in postmenopausal women. Thromb Haemost 84: 695–700.

[60] Miller M E, Thorpe S L, Dores G M. (1995) Influence of hormones on platelet intracellular calcium. Thromb Res 77: 515–30.

[61] Raman BB, Standley P R, Rajkumar V, Ram J L. (1995) Effects of estradiol and progesterone on platelet calcium responses. Am J Hyperten 8: 197–200.

[62] Boudoulas KD, Cooke GE, Roos CM, Bray PF, Goldschmidt-Clermont PJ. (2001) The PlA polymorphism of glycoprotein IIIa functions as a modifier for the effect of estrogen on platelet aggregation. Arch Pathol Lab Med 125:112–115.

[63] Ertugrul DT, Gürsoy A, Yücel M, Sahin M, Unal A, Pamuk B, Berberoglu Z, Aytürk, S, Tutuncu NB and Demirag NG (2006)'Effects of raloxifene on platelet functions in patients with postmenopausal osteoporosis',Platelets,17:6,351 — 353

[64] Gottsater A, Rendell M, Hulthen UL, Berntorp E, Mattiasson I. (2001) Hormone replacement therapy in healthy postmenopausal women: a randomized, placebo-controlled study of effects on coagulation and fibrinolytic factors. J Intern Med 249(3):237—46.

[65] Luyer MD, Khosla S, Owen WG, Miller VM. (2001) Prospective randomized study of effects of unopposed estrogen replacement therapy on markers of coagulation and inflammation in postmenopausal women. J Clin Endocrinol Metab 86(8):3629—34.

[66] Rabbani LE, Seminario NA, Sciacca RR, Chen HJ, Giardina EG. (2002) Oral conjugated equine estrogen increases plasma von Willebrand factor in postmenopausal women. J Am Coll Cardiol 40(11):1991—9.

[67] Kessler CM, Szymanski LM, Shamsipour Z, Muesing RA, Miller VT, La Rosa JC. (1997) Estrogen replacement therapy and coagulation: relationship to lipid and lipoprotein changes. Obstet Gynecol 89(3):326—31.

[68] Caine YG, Bauer KA, Barzegar S, ten Cate H, Sacks FM, Walsh BW, et al. (1992) Coagulation activation following estrogen administration to postmenopausal women. Thromb Haemost 68(4):392—5.

[69] Post MS, Rosing J, Van Der Mooren MJ, Zweegman S, Van Baal WM, Kenemans P, et al. (2002) Increased resistance to activated protein C after short-term oral hormone replacement therapy in healthy post-menopausal women. Br J Haematol 119(4):1017—23.

[70] Post MS, Hendriks DF, Van Der Mooren MJ, Van Baal WM, Leurs JR, Emeis JJ, et al. (2002) Oral oestradiol/trimegestone replacement reduces procarboxypeptidase U (TAFI): a randomized, placebo-controlled, 12-week study in early postmenopausal women. J Intern Med 251(3):245—51.

[71] van Baal WM, Emeis JJ, van der Mooren MJ, Kessel H, Kenemans P, Stehouwer CD. (2000) Impaired procoagulant-anticoagulant balance during hormone replacement therapy? A randomised, placebo-controlled 12-week study. Thromb Haemost 83(1):29—34.

[72] Koh KK, Mincemoyer R, Bui MN, Csako G, Pucino F, Guetta V, et al.(1997) Effects of hormone-replacement therapy on fibrinolysis in postmenopausal women. N Engl J Med 336(10):683—90.

[73] . Cushman M, Legault C, Barrett-Connor E, Stefanick ML, Kessler C, Judd HL, et al. (1999) Effect of postmenopausal hormones on inflammation-sensitive proteins: the Postmenopausal Estrogen/Progestin Interventions (PEPI) Study. Circulation 100(7):717—22.

[74] . Post MS, van der Mooren MJ, van Baal WM, Blankenstein MA, Merkus HM, Kroeks MV, et al. (2003) Effects of low-dose oral and transdermal estrogen replacement therapy on hemostatic factors in healthy postmenopausal women: a randomized placebo-controlled study. Am J Obstet Gynecol 189(5):1221—7.

[75] Post MS, Christella M, Thomassen LG, van der Mooren MJ, van Baal WM, Rosing J, et al. (2003) Effect of oral and transdermal estrogen replacement therapy on hemostatic variables associated with venous thrombosis: a randomized, placebo-controlled study in postmenopausal women. Arterioscler Thromb Vasc Biol 23(6):1116—21.

[76] Cushman M, Meilahn EN, Psaty BM, Kuller LH, Dobs AS, Tracy RP. (1999) Hormone replacement therapy, inflammation, and hemostasis in elderly women. Arterioscler Thromb Vasc Biol 19(4):893—9.

[77] Cushman M, Psaty BM, Meilahn EN, Dobs AS, Kuller LH. (2001) Postmenopausal hormone therapy and concentrations of protein C and antithrombin in elderly women. Br J Haematol 114(1):162—816.

[78] Lowe GD, Upton MN, Rumley A, McConnachie A, O'Reilly DS, Watt GC. (2001) Different effects of oral and transdermal hormone replacement therapies on factor IX, APC resistance, t-PA, PAI and C-reactive protein—a cross-sectional population survey. Thromb Haemost 86(2):550—6.

[79] Perry W, Wiseman RA. (2002) Combined oral estradiol valeratenorethisterone treatment over 3 years in postmenopausal women: effect on lipids, coagulation factors, haematology and biochemistry. Maturitas 42(2): 157—64.

[80] Salobir BG, Keber I, Vrabic L. (2002) A randomized, placebocontrolled trial of the effects of continuous combined hormone replacement therapy on coagulation and fibrinolytic systems in healthy postmenopausal women. Fertil Steril 78(6):1178—83.

[81] Teede HJ, McGrath BP, Smolich JJ, Malan E, Kotsopoulos D, Liang YL, et al. (2000) Postmenopausal hormone replacement therapy increases coagulation activity and fibrinolysis. Arterioscler Thromb Vasc Biol 20(5): 1404—9.

[82] Scarabin PY, Alhenc-Gelas M, Plu-Bureau G, Taisne P, Agher R, Aiach M. (1997) Effects of oral and transdermal estrogen/progesterone regimens on blood coagulation and fibrinolysis in postmenopausal women. A randomized controlled trial. Arterioscler Thromb Vasc Biol 17(11):3071—8.

[83] Oger E, Alhenc-Gelas M, Lacut K, Blouch MT, Roudaut N, Kerlan V, et al. (2003) SARAH Investigators. Differential effects of oral and transdermal estrogen/progesterone regimens on sensitivity to activated protein C among postmenopausal women: a randomized trial. Arterioscler Thromb Vasc Biol 23(9):1671—6.

[84] Demirol A, Baykal C, Kirazli S, Ayhan A. (2001) Effects of hormone replacement on hemostasis in spontaneous menopause. Menopause 8(2):135—40.

[85] Douketis JD, Gordon M, Johnston M, Julian JA, Adachi JR, Ginsberg JS. (2000) The effects of hormone replacement therapy on thrombin generation, fibrinolysis inhibition, and resistance to activated protein C: prospective cohort study and review of literature. Thromb Res 99(1):25—34.

[86] Love RR, Surawicz TS, Williams EC. (1992) Antithrombin III level, fibrinogen level, and platelet count changes with adjuvant tamoxifen therapy. Arch Intern Med 152(2): 317—20.

[87] Mannucci PM, Bettega D, Chantarangkul V, Tripodi A, Sacchini V, Veronesi U. (1996) Effect of tamoxifen on measure-12 F. Cosman et al. ments of hemostasis in healthy women. Arch Intern Med 156(16):1806—10.

[88] Cushman M, Costantino JP, Tracy RP, Song K, Buckley L, Roberts JD, et al. (2001) Tamoxifen and cardiac risk factors in healthy women: suggestion of an anti-inflammatory effect. Arterioscler Thromb Vasc Biol 21(2):255—61.

[89] Cushman M, Costantino JP, Bovill EG, Wickerham DL, Buckley L, Roberts JD, et al. (2003) Effect of tamoxifen on venous thrombosis risk factors in women without cancer: the Breast Cancer Prevention Trial. Br J Haematol 120(1):109—16.

[90] Jones AL, Powles TJ, Treleaven JG, Burman JF, Nicolson MC, Chung HI, et al. (1992) Haemostatic changes and thromboembolic risk during tamoxifen therapy in normal women. Br J Cancer 66(4):744—7.

[91] Pemberton KD, Melissari E, Kakkar VV. (1993) The influence of tamoxifen in vivo on the main natural anticoagulants and fibrinolysis. Blood Coagul Fibrinolysis 4(6):935—42.

[92] Auger MJ, Mackie MJ. (1988) Effects of tamoxifen on blood coagulation. Cancer 61(7):1316—9.

[93] Cuzick J, Allen D, Baum M, Barrett J, Clark G, Kakkar V, et al. (1992) Long term effects of tamoxifen. Biological effects of TamoxifenWorking Party. Eur J Cancer 29A(1):15—21.

[94] . Bertelli G, Pronzato P, Amoroso D, Cusimano MP, Conte PF, Montagna G, et al. (1988) Adjuvant tamoxifen in primary breast cancer: influence on plasma lipids and antithrombin III levels. Breast Cancer Res Treat 12(3):307—10.

[95] de Valk-de Roo GW, Stehouwer CD, Meijer P, Mijatovic V, Kluft C, Kenemans P, et al. (1999) Both raloxifene and estrogen reduce major cardiovascular risk factors in healthy postmenopausal women: a 2-year, placebo-controlled study. Arterioscler Thromb Vasc Biol 19(12): 2993—3000.

[96] Walsh BW, Kuller LH, Wild RA, Paul S, Farmer M, Lawrence JB, et al. (1988) Effects of raloxifene on serum lipids and coagulation factors in healthy postmenopausal women. JAMA 279(18):1445—51.

[97] Azevedo GD, Franco RF, Baggio MS, Maranhao TM, Ferriani MF, Silva de Sa MF. (2003) Effects of raloxifene therapy on the anticoagulant system in postmenopausal women. Climacteric 6(2):140—5.

[98] Sgarabotto M, Baldini M, Dei Cas A, Manotti C, Luciana Barilli A, Rinaldi M, Benassi L, Bacchi Modena A. (2007) Effects of raloxifene and continuous combined hormone therapy on haemostasis variables: a multicenter, randomized, double-blind study Thromb Res. 119(1):85-91.

[99] Azevedo GD, Franco RF, Baggio MS, Maranhão TM, Sá MF. (2005) Procoagulant state after raloxifene therapy in postmenopausal women. Fertil Steril. 84(6):1680-4.

[100] Cosman F, Baz-Hecht M, Cushman M, Vardy MD, Cruz JD, Nieves JW, Zion M, Lindsay R. (2005) Short-term effects of estrogen, tamoxifen and raloxifene on hemostasis: a randomized-controlled study and review of the literature. Thromb Res. 116(1):1-13.

[101] Tong, M.H. Jiang H, Liu P, Lawson JA, Brass LF, Song WC. (2005) Spontaneous fetal loss caused by placental thrombosis in estrogen sulfotransferase-deficient mice. Nat. Med. 11, 153–159

[102] Silver WP, Keller MP, Teel R, Silver D. (1993) Effects of donor characteristics and platelet in vitro time and temperature on platelet aggregometry. *J Vasc Surg*. 17:726–733.

[103] Miller ME, Dores GM, Thorpe SL, Akerley WL. (1994) Paradoxical influence of estrogenic hormones on platelet-endothelial cell interactions. *Thromb Res*. 74:577–594.

[104] . Dufy B. Vincent JD, Fleury H, du Pasquier P. Gourdji D. Tixier-Vidal A. (1979) Membrane effect of thyrotropin releasing hormone and estrogen shown by intracellular recording from pituitary cells. Science 204: 209-Cl I.

[105] . Halachmi S, Marden E. Martin G. MacKay H, Abbondanra C, Brown M. (1994) Estrogen receptor-associated proteins: possible mediators of hormone-induced transcription. Science 264: 1455 1458.

[106] Landers JP. Spelsberg TC. (1992) New concepts in steroid hormone action: Transcription factors, proto-oncogenes. and the cascade model for steroid regulation of gene expression. Crit Rev Eukar Gene Express 2: 19.-6.3.

[107] White R, Parker M G. (1998) Molecular mechanisms of steroid hormone action. Endocr Relat Cancer 5: 1–14.

[108]. Nagata, Y. Yoshikawa J, Hashimoto A, Yamamoto M, et al. (2003) Proplatelet formation of megakaryocytes is triggered by autocrine-synthesized estradiol. Genes Dev. 17, 2864–2869

[109] McRedmond, J. P., Park, S. D., Reilly, D. F., Coppinger, J. A., Maguire, P. B., Shields, D. C., et al. (2004). Integration of proteomics and genomics in platelets: a profile of platelet proteins and platelet-specific genes. Mol Cell Proteomics 3, 133−144.

[110] Khetawat G, Faraday N, Nealen ML, Vijayan KV, Bolton E, Noga SJ, Bray PF. (2000) Human megakaryocytes and platelets contain the estrogen receptor beta and androgen receptor (AR): Testosterone regulates AR expression. Blood 95:2289–2296.

[111] Jayachandran, M., Mukherjee, R., Steinkamp, T., LaBreche, P., Bracamonte, M. P., Okano, H., et al. (2005). Differential effects of 17b-estradiol, conjugated equine estrogen and raloxifene on mRNA expression, aggregation and secretion in platelets. Am J Physiol: Heart Circ Physiol 288, H2355−H2362

[112] Jayachandran M, Miller VM. (2003) Human platelets contain estrogen receptor, caveolin-1 and estrogen receptor associated proteins. Platelet 14:75–81.

[113]. Miller, V. M., Lewis, D. A., & Barber, D. A. (1999). Gender differences and endothelium-and platelet-derived factors in the coronary circulation. Clin Exper Pharmacol Physiol 26, 132−136.

[114]. Nealen ML, Vijayan KV, Bolton E, Bray PF. (2001) Human platelets contain a glycosylated estrogen receptor beta. Circ Res 88:438–442.

[115] Tarantino, Kunicki TJ, Nugent DJ. (1994) The estrogen receptor is present in human megakaryocytes. Ann. N.Y. Acad. Sci. 714, 293–296

[116]. Bracamonte, M. P., Jayachandran, M., Rud, K. S., & Miller, V. M. (2002). Acute effects of 17b-estradiol on femoral veins from adult, gonadally intact and ovariectomized female pigs. Am J Physiol:Heart Circ Physiol 283, H2389−H2396.

[117] Mendelsohn ME, Zhu Y, O'Neill S. (1991) The 29-kDa proteins phosphorylated in thrombin-activated human platelets are forms of the estrogen receptorrelated 27-kDa heat shock protein. *Proc Natl Acad Sci USA*. 88:11212–11216.

[118] Jayachandran M, Miller VM. (2002) Ovariectomy upregulates expression of estrogen receptors, NOS, and HSPs in porcine platelets. *Am J Physiol Heart Circ Physiol*. 283:H220–H226.

[119] Pirila E, Ramamurthy N, Maisi P, McClain S, et al. (2001) Wound healing in ovariectomized rats: effects of chemically modified tetracycline (CMT-8) and estrogen on matrix metalloproteinases-8, -13 and type I collagen expression. Curr Med Chem. 8:281–94.

[120] Jayachandran M and Miller VM. (2002) *Cardiovascular Health and Disease in Women*. Philadelphia, PA: Harcourt Health Sciences, 207–230

[121] Moriarty K, Kim KH, Bender JR. (2006) Minireview: Estrogen receptor-mediated rapid signaling. *Endocrinology*. 147:5557–5563.

[122] Yang SH, Liu R, Perez EJ, et al. (2004) Mitochondrial localization of estrogen receptor beta. *Proc Natl Acad Sci USA*. 101:4130–4135.

[123] Fliss A E, Benzeno S, Rao J, Caplan A J. (2000) Control of estrogen receptor ligand binding by Hsp90. J Steroid Biochem Mol Biol 72: 223–30.

[124] Knoblauch R, Garabedian J J. (1999) Role for Hsp90-associated cochaperone p23 in estrogen receptor signal transduction. Mol Cell Biol 19: 3748–59.

[125] . Fried W, Tichler T, Dennenberg I, Barone J, Wang F. (1974) Effects of estrogens on hematopoietic stem cells and on hematopoiesis of mice. *J Lab Clin Med.*83:807–815.

[126] Adler SS, Trobough FE. (1978) Effects of estrogen on erythropoiesis and granuloid progenitor cell (CFU-C) proliferation in mice. *J Lab Clin Med.* 91:960–968.

[127] . Pololi-Anagnostou L, Schade S, Anagnostou A. (1981) The effect of estrogens on erythroid stem cells in polycythemic mice. *Mol Cell Endocrinol.* 24:73–84.

[128] Medina KL, Kincade PW. (1994) Pregnancy-related steroids are potential negative regulators of B lymphopoiesis. *Proc Natl Acad Sci U S A.* 91:5382–5386.

[129] Shevde, N.K. and Pike, J.W. (1996) Estrogen modulates the recruitment of myelopoietic cell progenitors in rat through a stromal cell-independent mechanism involving apoptosis. Blood 87, 2683–2692

[130] Masuzawa T, Miyaura C, Onoe Y, Kusano K, Ohta H, Nozawa S, Suda T. (1994) Estrogen deficiency stimulates B lymphopoiesis in mouse bone marrow. *J Clin Invest.* 94:1090–1097.

[131] Jilka RL, Takahashi K, Munshi M, Williams DC, Roberson PK, Manolagas SC. (1998) Loss of estrogen upregulates osteoblastogenesis in the murine bone marrow: evidence for autonomy from factors released during bone resorption. *J Clin Invest.* 101:1942–1949.

[132] . Suenaga R, Evans MJ, Mitamura K, Rider V, Abdou NI. (1998) Peripheral blood T cells and monocytes and B cell lines derived from patients with lupus express estrogen receptor transcripts similar to those of normal cells. *J Rheumatol.* 25:1305–1312.

[133] Perry M, Samuels A, Bird D, Tobias JH. (2000) Effects of high-dose estrogen on murine hematopoietic bone marrow precede those on osteogenesis.Am J Physiol Endocrinol Metab 279:E1159– 65.

[134] Bord, S. Vedi S, Beavan SR, Horner A, Compston JE. (2000) Megakaryocyte population in human bone marrow increases with estrogen treatment: a role in bone remodeling? Bone 27, 397–401

[135] Bord S, Frith E, Ireland DC, Scott MA, Craig JI, Compston JE. (2004) Estrogen stimulates differentiation of megakaryocytes and modulates their expression of estrogen receptors alpha and beta. J Cell Biochem 92:249– 57.

[136] Elam MB, Lipscomb GE, Chesney CM, et al. (1980) Effect of synthetic estrogen on platelet aggregation and vascular release of PGI2-like material in the rabbit. *Prostaglandins.* 20:1039–1051.

[137] Moro, L. Reineri S, Piranda D, Pietrapiana D, Lova P, et al. (2005) Nongenomic effects of 17beta-estradiol in human platelets: potentiation of thrombin-induced aggregation through estrogen receptor beta and Src kinase. Blood 105, 115–121

[138] Mendelsohn ME, Karas, RH. (1994) Estrogen and the blood vessel wall. Curr Opin Cardiol 9:619-26.

[139] Farsetti A, Misti S, Citarella F, Felici A, Andreoli A, Fantoni A, et al. (1995) A molecular basis of estrogen regulation for Hageman Factor XII gene expression. Endocrinology 136:5076-83.

[140] Citarella F, Misti S, Felici A, Aiuti A, La Porta C, Fantoni A. (1993) The 5' sequence of human factor XII gene contains transcription regulatory elements typical of liver-specific, estrogenmodulated genes. Biochim Biophys Acta 1172:197-9.

[141]. Krikum G, Schatz F, Mackman N, Guller S, Lockwood CJ. (1998) Transcription regulation of the tissue factor gene by progestins in human endometrial stromal cells. J Clin Endocrinol Metab 83:926-30.

[142] Berge LN, Hansen J-B, Svensson B, Lyngmo V, Nordoy A. (1990) Female sex hormones and platelet:endothelial interactions Haemostasis 20: 313-320

[143] Bracamonte, M. P., Rud, K. S., Owen, W. G., & Miller, V. M. (2002). Ovariectomy increases mitogens and platelet-induced proliferation of arterial smooth muscle. Am J Physiol Heart Circ Physiol 283, H853–H860.

[144] Jayachandran M and Miller VM. (2002) Ovariectomy upregulates expression of estrogen receptors, NOS, and HSPs in porcine platelets. *Am J Physiol Heart Circ Physiol* 283: H220–H226.

[145]. Jayachandran M, Owen WG, and Miller VM. (2003) Effects of ovariectomy on aggregation, secretion, and metalloproteinases in porcine platelets. *Am J Physiol Heart Circ Physiol* 284: H1679–H1685.

[146] Loscalzo, J. (2001). Nitric oxide insufficiency, platelet activation, and arterial thrombosis. Circ Res 88, 756–762.

[147]. Tanus-Santos, J. E., Desai, M., Deak, L. R., Pezzullo, J. C., Abernethy, D. R., Flockhart, D. A., et al. (2002). Effects of endothelial nitric oxide synthase gene polymorphisms on platelet function, nitric oxide release, and interactions with estradiol. Pharmacogenetics 12, 407–413.

[148] Razandi, M., Pedram, A., Merchenthaler, I., Greene, G. L., & Levin, E. R. (2004). Plasma membrane estrogen receptors exist and functions as dimers. Mol Endocrinol 18, 2854–2865.

[149] Landers JP. Spelsberg TC. (1992) New concepts in steroid hormone action: Transcription factors, proto-oncogenes. and the cascade model for steroid regulation of gene expression. Crit Rev Eukar Gene Express 2: 19.-6.3.

[150] J. Sellés, N. Polini, C. Alvarez and V. Massheimer, (2001) Progesterone and 17 beta-estradiol acutely stimulate nitric oxide synthase activity in rat aorta and inhibit platelet aggregation, *Life Sci.* 69 815–827

[151]. J. Sellés, N. Polini, C. Alvarez and V. Massheimer,(2005) Novel action of estrone on vascular tissue: regulation of NOS and COX activity, *Steroids* 70 251–256.

[152] Lu, Q., Pallas, D. C., Surks, H. K., Baur,W. E., Mendelsohn,M. E., & Karas, R. H. (2004). Striatin assembles a membrane signaling complex necessary for rapid, nongenomic activation of endothelial NO synthase by estrogen receptor a. Proc Natl Acad Sci 101, 17126–17131.

[153] Rubanyi, G. M., Freay, A. D., Kauser, K., Sukovich, D., Burton, G., Lubahn, D. B., et al. (1997). Vascular estrogen receptors and endothelium-derived nitric oxide production in the mouse aorta. Gender difference and the effect of estrogen receptor gene disruption. J Clin Invest 99, 2429–2437.

[154] Simoncini T, Hafezi–Moghadam A, Brazil DP, et al. (2000) Interaction of oestrogen receptor with the regulatory subunit of phosphatidylinositol-3-OH kinase. *Nature*. 407:538–541.

[155] Hayashi T, Esaki T, Sumi D, et al. (2006) Modulating role of estradiol on arginase II expression in hyperlipidemic rabbits as an atheroprotective mechanism. *Proc Natl Acad Sci U S A*. 103:10485–10490.

[156] Vehkavaara S, Silveira A, Hakala-Ala-Pietila T, Virkamaki A, Hovatta O, Hamsten A, et al. (2001) Effects of oral and transdermal estrogen replacement therapy on markers of coagulation, fibrinolysis, inflammation and serum lipids and lipoproteins in postmenopausal women. Thromb Haemost 85(4):619—25.

[157] Hartwig J, Italiano Jr J.(2003) The birth of the platelet. J Thromb Haemost 1:1580– 6

[158] Ikeda H, Takajo Y, Murohara T, Ichiki K, Adachi H, Haramaki N, Katoh A, and Imaizumi T. (2000) Platelet-derived nitric oxide and coronary risk factors. *Hypertension* 35: 904–907.

[159] Mehta JL, Chen LY, Kone BC, Mehta P, and Turner P. (1995) Identification of constitutive and inducible forms of nitric oxide synthase in human platelets. *J Lab Clin Med* 125: 370–377.

[160] Sly MK, Prager MD, Eberhart RC, Jessen ME, and Kulkarni PV. (1995) Inhibition of surface-induced platelet activation by nitric oxide. *ASAIO J* 41: 394–398.

[161] Nilsson, B. O., Ekblad, E., Heine, T., & Gustafsson, J. A. (2000). Increased magnitude of relaxation to oestrogen in aorta from oestrogen receptor beta knock-out mice. J Endocrinol 166, R5−R9.

[162] Darblade, B., Pendaries, C., Krust, A., Dupont, S., Fouque, M. -J., Rami, J., et al. (2002). Estradiol alters nitric oxide production in the mouse aorta through the α-, but not β-, estrogen receptor. Circ Res 90, 413−419.

[163] Chen, Z., Yuhanna, I. S., Galcheva-Gargova, Z., Karas, R. H., Mendelsohn, M. E., & Shaul, P.W. (1999). Estrogen receptor alpha mediates the nongenomic activation of endothelial nitric oxide synthase by estrogen. J Clin Invest 103, 401−406.

[164] Chambliss, K. L., Yuhanna, I. S., Mineo, C., Liu, P. S., German, Z., Sherman, T. S., et al. (2000). Estrogen receptor a and endothelial nitric oxide synthase are organized into a functional signaling module in caveolae. Circ Res 87, E44−E52.

[165] Shaul, P. W. (2000). Novel role of estrogen receptors in vascular endothelium. Semin Perinatol 24, 70−74.

[166] Mann KG, Nesheim ME, Church WR, Haley P, Krishnaswamy S. (1990) Surface-dependent reactions of the vitamin K-dependent enzyme complexes. Blood 1990; 76: 1 - 16.

[167] Barton M. (2001) Postmenopausal oestrogen replacement therapy and atherosclerosis: Can current compounds provide cardiovascular protection? *Expert Opin Investig Drugs*. 10:789–809.

In: Estrogens: Production, Functions and Applications ISBN: 978-1-60741-086-7
Editor: James R. Bartos, pp. 231-273

Chapter IX

The Ligand Binding Domain of the Human Estrogen Receptor Alpha: Mapping and Functions

Yves Jacquot,[ab4] and Guy Leclercq[c]
[a]Université Pierre et Marie Curie-Paris6; CNRS, UMR 7203, "Laboratoire des BioMolécules"; Case courrier 45, 4, place Jussieu, 75252 Paris, France
[b]Ecole Normale Supérieure; CNRS, UMR 7203, "Laboratoire des BioMolécules"; 24, rue Lhomond, 75005 Paris, France
[c]Laboratoire J.-C. Heuson de Cancérologie Mammaire, Université Libre de Bruxelles (U.L.B.), Institut Jules Bordet, 1, rue Héger-Bordet, 1000 Brussels, Belgium

Abstract

The pharmacology of the human Estrogen Receptor α (ERα) depends on a large number of parameters such as post-traductional modifications, nature of ligands and associated ERα conformational changes, intracellular localization of ERα as well as estrogenic pathways that are activated for specific co-regulators recruitment. In this context, a number of amino-acids that constitute the ERα Ligand Binding Domain (LBD) have been shown to play crucial functions. Unfortunately, most data covering these topics are reported in a huge amount of literature not easily accessible to all investigators. We, therefore, attempt to extract essential informations from this literature to constitute a useful database describing the functions ascribed to key residues.

Introduction

Estradiol 17β (E_2), the most important natural estrogen in women, ensures the development of estrogen target tissues (uterus, vagina, breast) as well as the maintenance of secondary sexual characters. This hormone also induces cyclic histological modifications of endometrial tissue associated with the menstrual cycle, allowing various events related to pregnancy (formation of the placenta, implantation). Regulation of plasmatic E_2 level is, indeed, crucial to prepare the uterus for pregnancy and to maintain the fetus within the uterus until delivery. Accordingly, the hypothalamo-pituitary hormones such as the hypothalamic Gonadotrophin Releasing Factor (GnRF), the pituitary Follicle Stimulating Hormone (FSH) and the Luteinizing Hormone (LH) subtlety regulate E_2 production. Physiological features associated with this production are not restricted to the reproductive system. The role of the hormone extends to lipid [1] and bone [2] metabolisms as well as to brain [3] and cardiovascular functions [4].

E_2-mediated processes result from the interaction of the hormone with a specific receptor, the Estrogen Receptor (ER), of which two subtypes have been identified (α and β). Specificity of action of these two ER forms depends upon their intracellular localization (nucleus, cell membrane, cytoplasm, mitochondria, ...) as well as several endogenous factors of which the nature varies among tissues (uterus, breast, bone, blood vessels, brain, ...). Moreover, an intracellular trafficking of ER resulting from conformational / post-translational changes associated with the recruitment of specific proteins named co-activators or co-repressors, amplify or inhibit, respectively, the activation of the receptor [5] (Table 1).

Knowledge of functions associated with ER amino-acids directly implicated in these regulatory mechanisms is necessary to understand all facets of the concept of estrogenicity. It is also required for the design of new strategies specific for Hormone Replacement Therapy (HRT) as well as for the treatment of hormone-dependent tumors. Unfortunately, data accumulated during the last twenty years concerning Structure-Activities Relationships (SAR), extremely helpful for such a task, are reported in a huge chemical / endocrinological literature not easily accessible to all researchers. With the hope to partially palliate this drawback, we present here an overview of SAR data related to the hinge region and the Ligand Binding Domain (LBD) of ERα that mediates the action dictated by the hormone and related molecules. We limit our work to the ERα subtype because it is mainly involved in the development of ER-dependent tumoral pathologies such as breast cancer, which represents the most widespread form of cancer in women. Extensive structural investigations of the ERα LBD also justify our restrictive analysis.

Background

ERα belongs to the intranuclear receptors superfamily [6–8], more precisely the subset for steroidal hormones, i.e progestins, androgens, mineralocorticoids, corticosteroids and estrogens. ERα, as all nuclear receptors, is a transcriptional factor that regulates the expression of specific genes. It is a protein of ~ 66 kDa containing four main functional regions located within six domains: i) an Activation Function 1 (AF-1) enclosed within residues 1 to 180 (domains A / B), ii) a DNA Binding Domain (DBD) corresponding to

4 Corresponding author. Yves Jacquot. Tel: +33-(0)1-44-27-26-78, Fax. +33-(0)1-44-27-38-43; E-Mail: yves.jacquot@upmc.fr.

residues 181 to 262 (domain C), iii) a hinge region corresponding to residues 263 to 302 (domain D) and iv) a Ligand Binding Domain (LBD), that encompasses an Activation Function 2 (AF-2) located between residues 302 to 595 (domains E / F, Figure 1). These domains cooperate to enhance (or to repress) the expression of genes.

Whereas AF-1 activates ERα in a ligand-independent manner, AF-2 is under the control of ligands (estrogen agonists or antagonists). In fact, AF-1 and AF-2, both exposed at the surface of ERα, are platforms appropriate for the recruitment of several co-regulators required for the regulation of transcription [7,8]. Two distinct mechanisms have been described: 1) a **direct** ERα-mediated transcription that results from the direct interaction of liganded receptor / co-regulators complexes with DNA (Figure 2a); 2) an **indirect** ERα-mediated transcription that results from the ability of the membrane form of ERα to enhance transactivation of other transcription factors (Figure 2b).

Table 1. List of co-activators and co-inhibitors that associate with ERα.

Proteins	Binding region	References
Co-activators		
CREB-binding protein family		[5,184-188]
p300/CBP	LBD	[185-190]
p160 family		[5,185-187]
SRC-1 (refers to N-CoA1)	Nter A/B AF1, LBD (H12)	[5,187,191-197]
SRC-2 (refers to N-CoA2/GRIP-1/TIF2)	LBD	[5,192]
SRC-3 (refers to N-CoA3/pCIP/ACTR/AIB1/RAC3/TRAM-1)	LBD	[5,192]
pCIP (refers to AIB1/TRAM-1/ACTR/RAC3/SRC-3)	LBD	[5,186,198,199]
GRIP1 (refers to TIF2/N-CoA2)	AF-2	[5,187,200,201]
TFIIB	AF-1	[5,202]
$hTAF_{II}30$	AF-2a	[5,203]
E6-AP	Hinge region	[5,42,204]
Ada	LBD	[5,205]
RAP46	Hinge region	[5,206]
p68	AF-1	[5,207]
ARA 70	LBD	[5,187,208]
Calmodulin	Hinge region	[5,28,29]
L7/SPA	LBD, hinge region	[5,209]
PBP	LBD	[5,210]
RIP140	AF-2	[5,187,211,212]
SPT6	LBD	[5,213]
SRA	AF-1	[5,214]
SWI/SNF	AF-2, DBD	[5,215,216]
TRIP1/SUG1	AF-2	[5,187,212,217,218]
TRAP220 (refers to TRAP/SMCC/DRIP/ARC)	LBD (F-domain)	[5,185,201,219]
Tip60	LBD	[5,220]
TIF1α	AF-2	[5,217,221]
XBP-1	DBD	[222]
MNAR (PELP1)	LBD	[153,223-225]
PNRC and PNRC2	H4, β-turn	[99,226,227]

Table 1 (Continued).

Co-inhibitors		
N-CoR (refers to CoR/SAP30/SIN3/HDAC2)	LBD	[5,184,186,209,228,229]
SMRT	LBD	[5,184,186,209,212,228-230]
REA	AF-2	[5,229,231]
BRCA1	AF-2	[5,229,232,233]
SHP	AF-2	[5,229,234]
SHARP	DBD, hinge region	[229,235]
SAFB1	DBD, hinge region	[229,236]
LcoR	LBD	[229,237]
DAX-1	AF-2	[229,238]
Smad 4	AF-1	[229,239]
TAF-1β	DBD, hinge region, F domain	[49,229]
TR2	DBD, hinge region, LBD, AF-2	[229,240]
FKHR	LBD	[229,241]
RTA	AF-1	[229,242]
MTA1 and MTA1s	AF-1, DBD, AF-2	[229,243,244]
NSD1	LBD	[229,245]
DP97	LBD/AF-2	[229,246]
COUP-TFI	AF-1, DBD	[229,247,248]

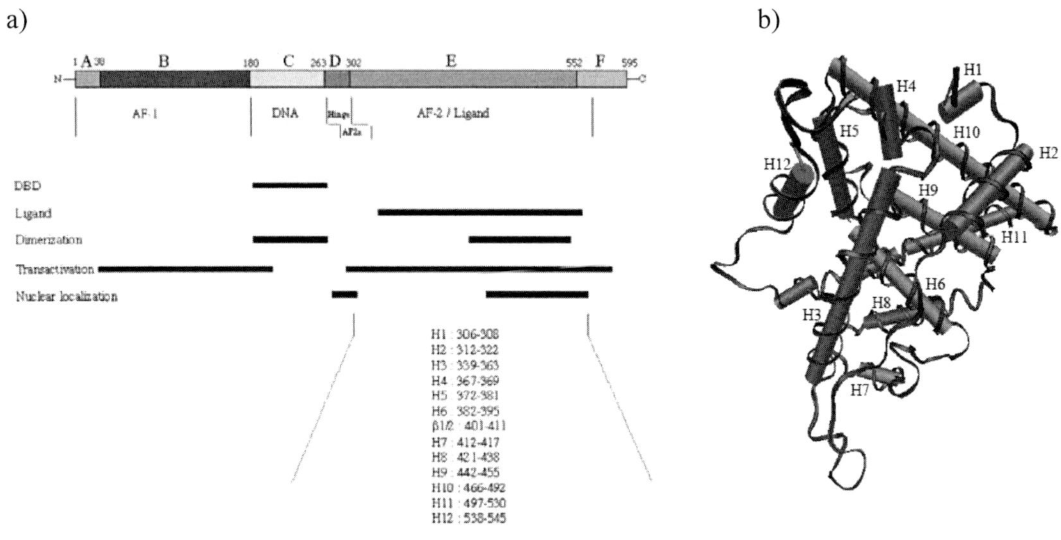

Figure 1. (a) Functional and structural characteristics of ERα (according to the nomenclature supplied by the ExPASy Proteomics Server of Swiss-Prot, code ESR1_HUMAN). (b) Position of helices H1-H12 in the ligand-binding pocket (PDB code: 1ERE [146]). Drawings were made using VMD software [250].

Direct (direct and indirect activation of ER is now recommended to refer to genomic and non-genomic activation, respectively) ERα-mediated transcription is relevant to the intranuclear form of the receptor, which once complexed with E_2, adopts an "active" status with concomitant phosphorylation of surface-exposed serines and / or threonines. Resulting changes of the ERα tertiary structure favors its dimerization as homo- or heterodimers for targeting short DNA segments (termed Estrogen Response Elements, EREs) located in the vicinity of gene promoters (Figure 2). In contrast, the membrane form of ERα associates with other membrane receptors, especially those for growth factors, to activate MAPK cascades that ultimately induce biological responses through the stimulation of oncogenic transcription factors such as *c-fos*, *c-jun*, or *c-myc*. Together, these pathways induce cell proliferation, cell morphogenesis differentiation, cell specialization, survival or programmed cell death (apoptosis).

Delineation and Structure of D and E Domains – Function of Erα Residues

1) D-Domain (Hinge-Region, Residues 263-302)

Arg-263 and Lys-302 delimit a hinge region that separates the A / B (AF-1) and C domains from the LBD (E domain). This region contains an autonomous Activation Function AF-2a for a basal constitutive transcriptional activity. Accordingly, it is particularly subjected to post-traductional modifications (acetylation or SUMOylation / ubiquitination) to regulate not only ERα-mediated transcription but also the trafficking and the turnover of the receptor. Accordingly, this region also contributes to the recruitment of the E6-AP ubiquitine ligase, calmodulin and Hsp-70.

Lys-266, Lys-268 and Lys-299 of the hinge region are acetylated by the p300 histone acetylase (Table 1) in a ligand-dependent (Lys-266 and 268) or ligand-independent (Lys-299) manner to facilitate interaction of ERα with EREs [9,10]. Lysines 266 and 268 are also subjected to SUMO (Small Ubiquitin-like MOdifier) ligation in a ligand-dependent manner to facilitate the nuclear transport of ERα and its interaction with protein kinases [11]. SUMOylation is, in fact, a three-step enzymatic process that necessitates a labile thioester bond on the εNH_2 group of lysines often embedded in a ψKxE motif. At first, an E1 activating enzyme transiently activates the SUMO protein, which is subsequently transferred to an E2 conjugating enzyme. Final covalent linkage of SUMO to ERα requires the SUMO-1 E3 ligases PIAS1 and PIAS3 [11,12].

Ubiquitination, as SUMOylation, is a three steps process that directs ERα to intracellular compartments, to regulate its turnover, degradation (polyubiquitination), endocytosis (mono-ubiquitination), and interactions with DNA and protein kinases. Thus, an E1 enzyme activates ubiquitin, which is transferred in as second step to the E2 conjugating enzyme Ubc4. Finally, 26S proteasome targeting is mediated by ubiquitin E3 ligases such as CHIP, Mdm2 and E6-AP. Proteasome 26S is a multi-enzymatic complex shaped in a cylinder structure in which ubiquitinated proteins enter to suffer attacks from trypsin-like, chemotrypsin-like and glutamyl protease-like activities (Figure 3) [13–20]. Implication of lysines 266, 268 and 299 in these regulatory processes confer to the latter a great importance in the mechanism of action of ERα. In this regard, it should be stressed that a K299R mutation has been detected in patients with psychiatric diseases [21], suggesting that this residue play an important function in the brain.

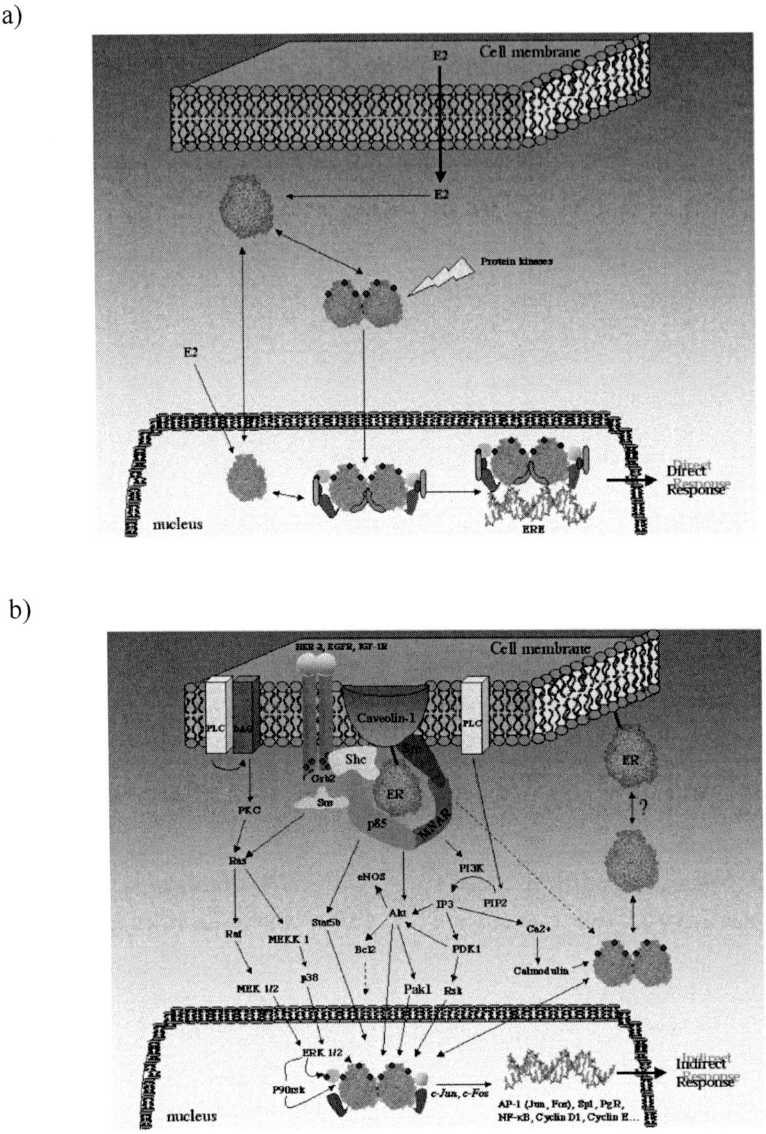

Figure 2. ERα-mediated transcription. The upper panel (a) refers to the direct interaction of the activated dimeric form of the receptor with EREs. The lower panel (b) refers to the activation of various signal transduction pathways initiated at the membrane by the receptor; these pathways lead to activation of transcription factors others than ERα. AP-1, activating protein 1; Bcl2, B cell lymphoma 2; DAG, diacylglycerol; EGFR, endothelial growing factor receptor; eNOS, endothelial nitric oxide synthase; ER, estrogen receptor α; ERK, extracellular-signal regulated protein kinase; Grb-2, growth factor receptor-bound protein 2; HER-2, human epidermal growth factor receptor-2; IP3, inositol triphosphate; MEK, extracellular signal regulated kinase; MEKK, extracellular signal regulated kinase kinase; MNAR, modulator of indirect activity of estrogen receptor; NF-κB, nuclear factor kappa 2; p85, active subunit of phosphatidylinositol-3-kinase; P90rsk, p90 ribosomal S6 kinase; Pak1, p21 activated kinase; PDK1, pyruvate dehydrogenase kinase isoenzyme 1; PgR, progesterone receptor; PI3K, phospahtidylinositol-3-kinase; PIP2, phosphatidylinositol-3-biphosphate; PKC, protein kinase C; PLC, phospholipase C; Sos, son of sevenless; Stat5b, signal transducer and activator of transcription 5b.

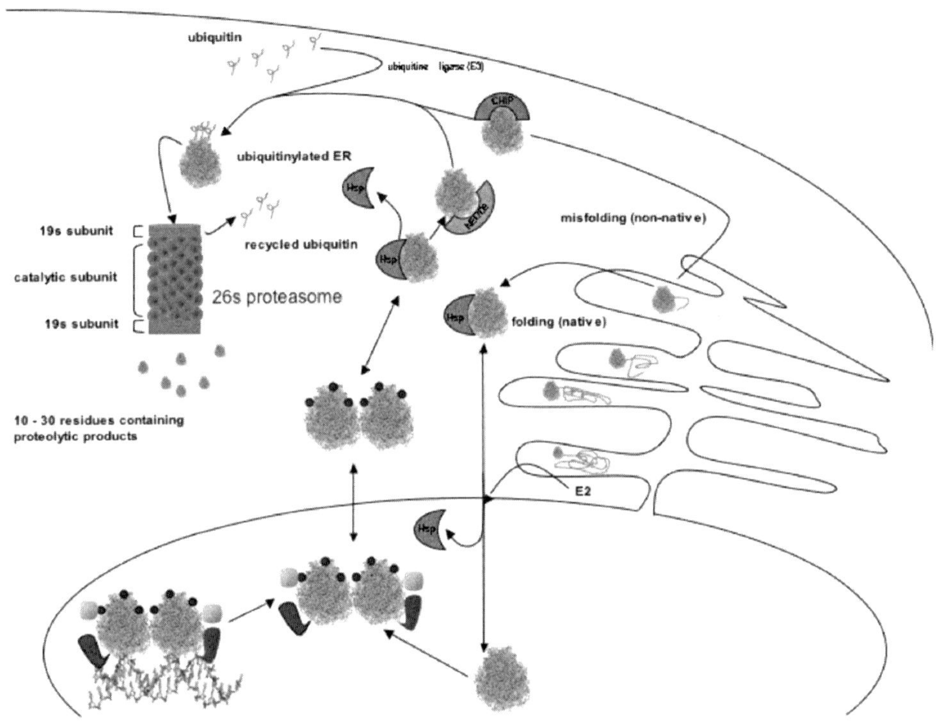

Figure 3. Degradation of ERα by 26S proteasome. After its maturation, the newly synthesized ERα interacts with Hsp to acquire its ligand binding form. This native receptor enters into the nucleus to induce transcription. In case of misfolding, ERα is ubiquitinated by the E3-ubiquitin ligase CHIP [19] to be immediately degraded by the 26S proteasome. Likewise, after estrogenic response, ERα translocates into the cytoplasmic compartment where it transiently interacts with Hsp, then with a E3 ubiquitin-ligase to direct it into the 26S proteasome. ER, estrogen receptor α; Hsp, heat shock protein; NEDD8, neural precursor cell expressed, developmentally down-regulated 8 (a ubiquitin-like protein required for proteasome-mediated degradation of ERα / antiestrogen complex [251]); CHIP, carboxy terminus of Hsc70 interacting protein.

Substitution of *Leu-296* by a proline that significantly decreases ERα transactivation has been found in breast tumors [22–24]. Inappropriate ubiquitination / SUMOylation affecting the recruitment of kinases as well as ERα turnover may be at the origin of this deleterious effect. In this regard, it should be stressed that *Ser-294* is a constituent of an xSPx consensus motif ($P_{293}SPL_{296}$) appropriate for proline-directed protein kinases (as Ser-104, Ser-106 and Ser-118, A / B domain) even if it is not a major site of phosphorylation [25].

Ile-298 as well as the $K_{299}RSKK_{303}$ motif (third Nuclear Localization Signal NLS [26]) are key determinants for ERα association with calmodulin, a calcium-binding protein that enhances ERα-mediated transcription [27,28] (Table 1). Complexion of calmodulin to its binding site ($P_{295}LMIKRSKKNSLALSLTADQMVS_{317}$) decreases the capacity of ERα to bind E_2 while it enhances its ability to interact with EREs, as does also acetylation of Lys-266 and 268.

Properties described here over are in favor of an important role of the whole hinge region in ERE-dependent transcription [29-33]. They also introduce the concept that structural changes occuring at this level orient ERα in distinct activating pathways appropriate for transcription mediated by the receptor itself or other transcription factors with which it cooperates [34,35]. The ability of tamoxifen to decrease the stability of the ERα / calmodulin complex is in agreement with this concept [36] since this antiestrogen inhibits ERE-dependent transcription while it favors AP-1 transactivation. Hence, if calmodulin steers ERα towards an ERE-dependent or independent mechanism, alterations as well as partial proteolysis of the receptor that affects calmodulin binding (presence of a motif for proteolysis [37–39] in this binding site) would logically strongly modify its transactivation profile; such alterations may perhaps also influence intracellular location of ERα as provoked by SUMOylation of Lys-299, which is implied in its nuclear transport [11].

2) E domain

The LBD (E domain), defined from Lys-302 to Pro-552, encompasses about half of the ERα. It contains 12 helices (H1 to H12, Figure 1) forming an E_2-binding pocket that accepts a huge panel of agonists and antagonists. In fact, the binding of such ligands induces deep conformational changes that modify the surface of the receptor, allowing recruitment of specific co-activators and co-inhibitors, including enzymes for post-translational modifications (methylation, acetylation, phosphorylation, ubiquitination, SUMOylation, ...).

Lys-302, which belongs to a polyproline-II (PPII)-containing sequence (residues 301 – 311) located at the N-terminal extremity of the LBD [40], participates to inter- and intramolecular interactions as commonly observed with PPII regions [41]. Moreover, this residue enhances the recruitment of calmodulin [27-34,42] and E6AP [42] (Table 1), both known to modulate ERα transactivation. In this regard, acetylation of Lys-302 may influence ERα activity by provoking a switch from a calmodulin-dependent to a calmodulin-independent mechanism [27]. Moreover, agonist-induced transcription as well as constitutive transcription relevant to AF-2a expression seems to be under the control of this lysine. Interestingly, K302R mutation enhances estrogen-induced transcription without changing ERα activation [10], suggesting that the PPII-containing region around Lys-302 is functionally independent from the MAPK-binding domain of the receptor. Hence, this residue may selectively modulate the efficiency of estrogen-mediated processes as well as related co-regulators recruitment [10,11,43]. Strikingly, the influence of Lys-302 on ERα sensitivity towards ligands would depend on the presence of polar or charged groups. Free Lys-302 may indeed maintain ERα in an inactive conformation by interacting with residues of a co-regulator binding groove delimited by Asp-369, Glu-470 and Arg-477, compromising thereby the recruitment of such co-regulators [40].

Lys-303, that just precedes H1, is important for ERα transactivation. It belongs to the PPII-containing region strongly implicated in calmodulin binding and SUMOylation [29–36]. The fact that this residue is also subjected to acetylation [10] suggests a prominent role in the mechanism of action of the receptor [22]. Accordingly, a mutant K303R (Table 2) has been reported to enhance phosphorylation of Ser-305 and the recruitment of the co-activators

SRC1 and SRC2 (Table 1) at low estrogen levels. Remarkably, this mutation, which does not affect the interaction of ERα with DNA [22], has been detected in one third of grade III breast tumors as well as mixed lobular / ductal carcinomas, introducing the concept of its implication in the development of breast cancer (this mutation is totally absent in Japanese women, usually less susceptible to develop breast cancer than Western counterparts) [23,44–46]. It may also affect the ERα turnover rate since the $K_{299}RSKK_{303}$ motif is particularly sensitive to SUMOylation, ubiquitination, proteasome-dependent and trypsin proteolysis [38,43,47].

Table 2. ER mutations related to emergence of hormone-dependent tumors

Mutant	Possible Effect	References
L296P	Lack of recognition of E3 ubiquitin ligase or other co-regulatory proteins Decrease of responsiveness (at low level of E_2) and of ER degradation / Accumulation of ER	[22–24]
K303R	Lack of stabilization of ER/ligand complexes Increase of the activation of the ligand-independent pathways	[22,44–46]
S309F	Changes of conformation to confer resistance to tamoxifen Decrease of responsiveness for estrogenicity (at low level of E_2) and antiestrogenicity (in the presence of tamoxifen)	[22,249]
D351Y	Lack of recruitment of co-repressors Insufficient recognition of tamoxifen	[22,79,90]
E353V	Inefficient recognition of tamoxifen by ER	[22,23,72,73]
E396V	Decrease of responsiveness for estrogenicity (at low level of E_2)	[22]
K531E	Lack of control of the AF-1	[23,143]
Y537N	Lack of dimerization and of interaction with ERE Increase of the activation of indirect pathways	[23,26,78,148–156]

In fact, ERα activation is silenced by Lys-303 acetylation, a process reversed by the protein pp32 [48] (an intranuclear acidic protein which plays a role in self-renewing cell population [49]) and TAF-1β (a co-activator) [50].

In contrast, *Ser-305* phosphorylation sensitizes ERα to agonists by preventing Lys-303 acetylation [12]. This phosphorylation enhances the interaction of the receptor with promoters of target genes without increasing its dimerization. Moreover, it provokes conformational changes appropriate for AF-2 exposition and subsequent AF-1 activation [51]. Inclusion of Ser-305 within a KxxS consensus motif ($K_{302}KNS_{305}$) suggests the implication of the p21-activated kinase-1 (Pak1) [52]. However, Phosphatidyl-Inositol 3-Kinase (PI3K) / Akt and PKA seem also to operate to induce rapid responses through mechanisms initiated at the membrane (Figure 2b) [43,53–58]. In this regard, it should be stressed that phosphorylation of Ser-305 by PKA confers resistance to tamoxifen by affecting the conformational stability of ERα upon (anti)estrogen binding [54].

A. Helix H1 (Residues 306-308), Helix H2 (Residues 312-322) and Region Between H2 and H3 (Residues 323-338)

Helix H1 displays strong similarities with the hinge-region (D domain). Principally structured in a polyproline II (PPII) conformation, it contains a motif for calmodulin recruitment (residues 295-311) and is subject to phosphorylation (H2 residues as well as the region flanked by H2 and H3). Moreover, it contributes to the recruitment of co-activators at AF-1 and AF-2. At least, it is also a component of a suspected second ligand-binding pocket.

The region between the residues Leu-306 and Thr-311 participates to the recruitment of calmodulin [27-33] and other co-regulators required for ERα transactivation. Substitution of Ser-309 by a phenylalanine confers resistance to tamoxifen despite a decrease of transactivation at low dose of E_2 [22]. Under E_2 stimulation, *Thr-311* is specifically phosphorylated by a kinase associated to p38 MAPK to induce transcription and nuclear export of the receptor [59]. Accordingly, amino-acids *Pro-324* and *Pro-325*, located in the neighborhood of the AF-2 co-activator-binding region most probably control the recruitment of activators [40,60]. Finally, *Ile-326* and *Leu-327*, included within this region, participate to the topology of a suspected second estrogen-binding pocket [61]. These two amino-acids could play a role in ligand selectivity between α or β ER subtypes since they correspond to two of the four residues of this pocket that differ between both receptors. Interestingly, the 335-338 region (RPFS) encompasses a xRxxSx consensus motif, which is the signature of a calmodulin-dependent protein kinase cognate domain [25].

B. Helix H3 (Residues 339-363)

H3 encompasses key-residues required for the interaction of ligands with the E_2-binding pocket. It is of prime importance for the stabilization of active / inactive conformations adopted by ERα.

Met-343, Leu-345, Leu-346, Thr-347 and Leu-349 attract the phenolic A ring of E_2 principally through hydrophobic contacts. In fact, ERα ligands could be classified in two main classes, both containing a phenolic ring that mimics the role played by this phenolic A ring: type I that refer to linear planar molecules and type II that refer to angular molecules (Figure 4).

According to modeling studies, *Glu-353* and *Arg-394* participate to hydrogen interactions with the phenolic hydroxyl common to these two classes of ligands (Figure 5) [62–71]. Among 17β-OH steroidal hormones, Glu-353 selects phenol-containing molecules (A ring) leading to estrogen / androgen discrimination [64]. Note that the mutant E353V affects E_2-induced transcription without affecting DNA-binding [22] (Table 2). This mutation has been found in some tamoxifen-resistant breast tumors [22,23,72,73], suggesting that this residue is important for the antineoplasic activity of the drug (Table 2). Thr-347 is an additional screening determinant: it constitutes a selective anchoring point for type II estrogens, as shown with diphenolic imidazolines and piperazines [62,74,75]. This residue is also structurally and functionally active in tamoxifen-induced antagonism by participating to the formation of the "neck" of a channel in which engulfs the basic side chain of the drug responsible for its antiestrogenicity (Figure 6) [65].

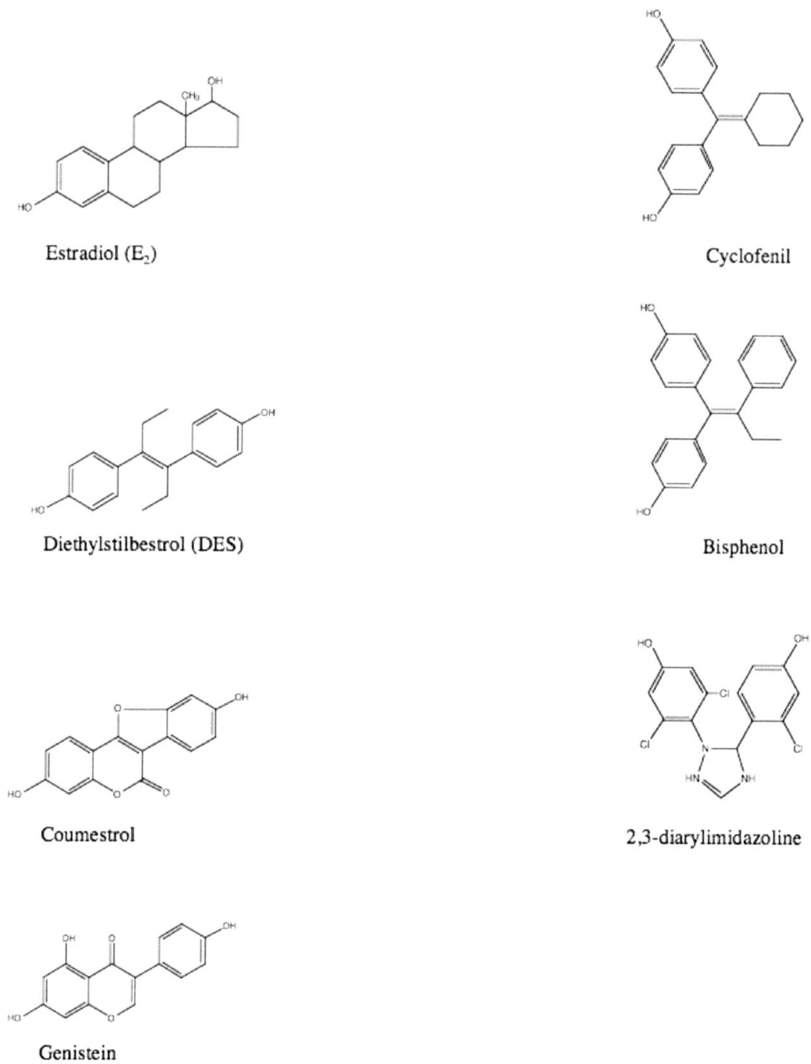

Figure 4. Examples of type I and type II ligands.

Massive amount of data concerns *Asp-351*. Under the exposure to tamoxifen and related partial antagonists / agonists, ERα is stabilized in an inactive conformation [63,65,76–78] in which the negative charge of Asp-351 is neutralized (Figure 6) [23,63,65,72,75,79–92]. This neutralization provoked by the tertiary amino group of the side chain of the drug weakens the recruitment of co-activators such as SRC-1 or GRIP-1 [65,76–78,83–88] while it enhances the recruitment of the co-repressors N-Cor and SMART [90] (Table 1). Loss of ERα transactivation when the Asp-351 is substituted by a lysine or an arginine confirms the importance of the anionic character of this residue for estrogenicity [78]. In agreement with this view, a D351G (or D351A) mutation affects the stimulatory effect of E_2 and silences the agonistic activity of tamoxifen, most probably through affecting AF-1-dependent mechanisms [78,92]. In contrast, the D351Y mutation increases the estrogenicity displayed by tamoxifen [90] (Table 2).

Several residues located between *Leu-354* and *Ala-361* belong to the binding domain for co-regulators (i.e CBP, p160 co-activators and the co-repressors N-Cor and PNRC, Table 1) [63,93–99]. This domain corresponds to a region packed against a hydrophobic groove located between H3 and H5 (Figure 7) [10], in which Val-376 and Leu-379 engulf in the absence of co-activators [65,100]. This co-activator binding pocket may constitute a promising target to control ERα-dependent transcription [94,95,98,101].

Lys-362, with the participation of H12 residues (Glu-542, Met-543 and Leu-544) facilitates to the capture of the C-terminal carboxylate of p160 co-activators [78] and allows the latters to "corkscrew" along their binding site, more particularly within a hydrophobic cleft delimited by H3, H4 and H5 [65,78,91,93,100-103]. Moreover, Lys-362 and Glu-542 form a charge clamp that interacts with a dipole induced by the α-helical conformation adopted by most of p160-co-activator LxxLL motifs of co-activators [63,65,66,78,94]. Accordingly, K362D mutation partially abolishes the recruitment of CBP [97].

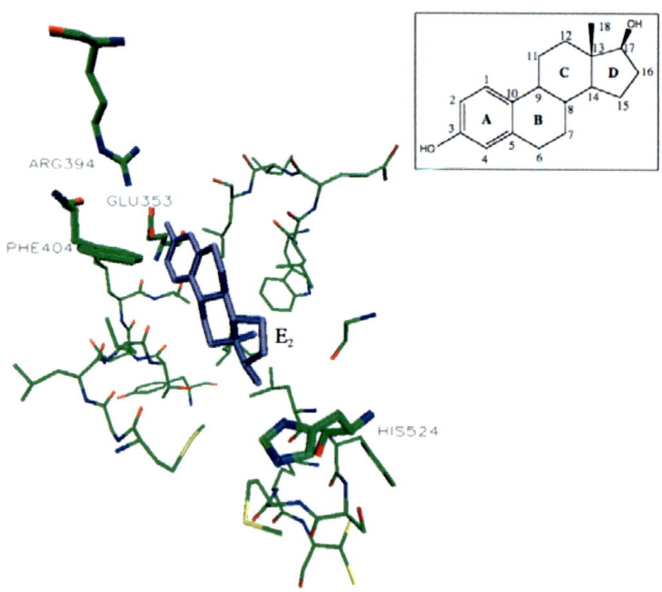

Figure 5. Interaction of E_2 within the ligand-binding region (PDB code: 1ERE [146]). Fundamental residues Glu-353, Arg-394, Phe-404 and His-524 are in bold. Drawing was made using VMD software [250].

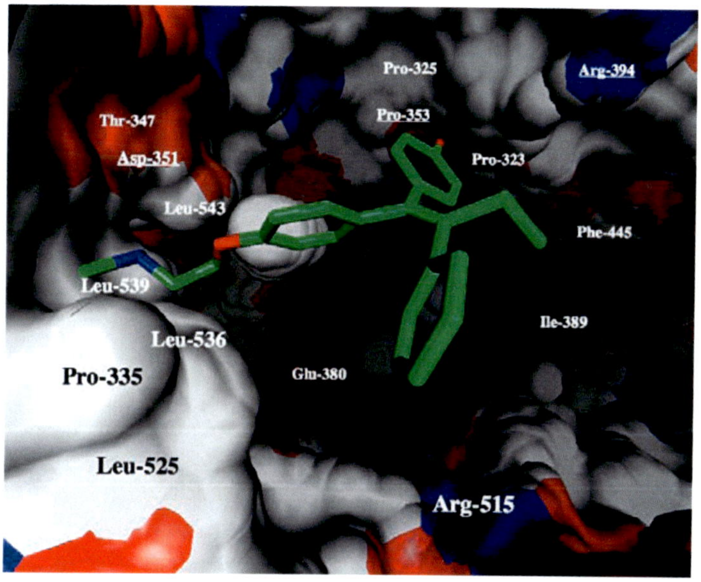

Figure 6. Interaction of tamoxifen within the E_2-binding pocket. The "neck" channel of the LBD in which engulfs the side chain of the compound is delimited by Pro-335, Leu-536, Leu-539 and Leu-543. Tamoxifen is colored in green, apolar residues in white, polar and acidic residues in red and basic residues in blue (PDB code: 3ERT [63]). Drawing was made using VMD software [250].

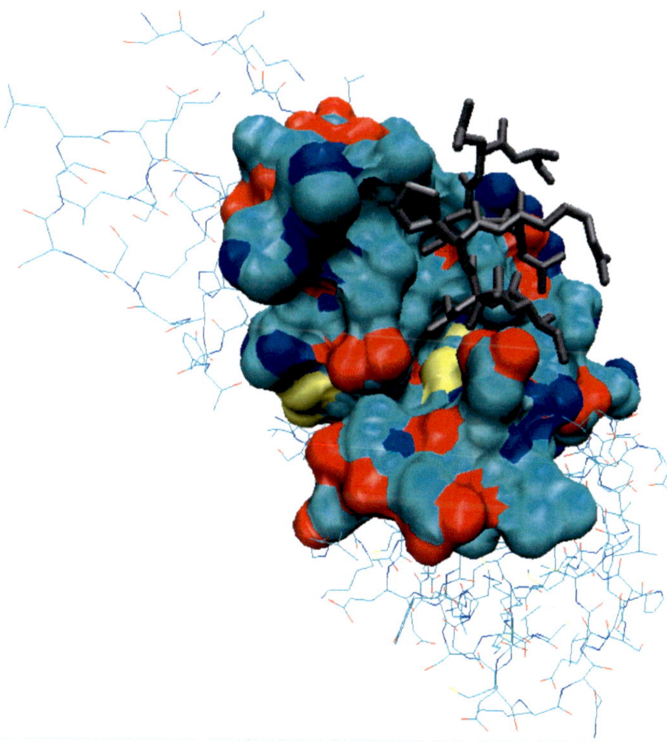

Figure 7. LxxLL co-activator binding-site. The figure refers to the interaction of the KILHRLLND motif of the coactivator TIF2 (in grey) with this site (PDB code: 1GWQ [96]). Drawings were made using VMD software [250].

C. The Type II β Turn (Residues 363-366) and the Helix H4 (Residues 367-370)

A flexible region located between H3 and H4 appears to be important for interactions between ERα and the C-terminal proline-rich region of PNRC co-activator [99]. In fact, a type II β-turn of this part of the receptor [40] corresponds to a platform for the recruitment of the latters as well as intramolecular interactions with the calmodulin-binding domain (Figure 8) [32,33]. This type II β-turn is followed by a short one-turn α helix (H4) that seems to participate to these interactions [40].

Val-364, that directly follows the residue at the C-terminal tail of H3, is involved in the interaction of LxxLL motifs of p160 co-activators with ERα [95]. It is also required for folding and conformational stabilization of the receptor [19,103].

As described for various residues of H3, *Phe-367* and *Val-368* orient H4 to the surface of ERα through widening the hydrophobic groove located between H3 and H5 to the surface of the receptor [63,93–95]. Hence, implication of these residues in the recruitment of p160 as well as the orientation of H12 in its agonist position seems likely [65,100].

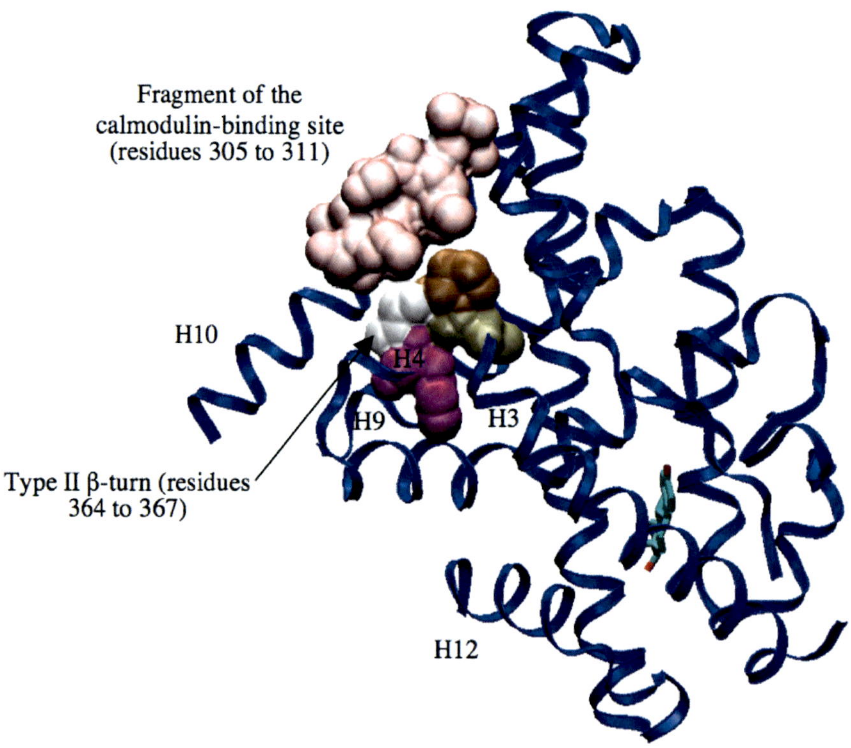

Figure 8. Intramolecular interactions between the calmodulin-binding site (in pink) and the type IIβ turn-containing region defined by the residues $V_{364}PGF_{367}$ (Val in khaki, Pro in brown, Gly in white and Phe in magenta, PDB code: 1ERE [146]). Drawings were made using VMD software [250].

D. Helix H5 (Residues 372-381)

As illustrated for H3, H4 and the type II β-turn, H5 contributes to the stabilization of H12 in an appropriate position to recruit co-activators. Moreover, several residues of H5 implicated in the stability of ERα / ligand complexes favor discrimination between agonists and partial (ant)agonists.

As *Phe-367* and *Val-368, Leu-372* and *Val-376* participate to the widening of the hydrophobic co-regulator binding groove, located between H3 and H5, in which H12 engulfs. This helix is stabilized in this groove [65,100,101] through hydrogen contacts with Leu-372 and Tyr-537 as well as van der Waals interactions with Leu-540 (Figure 9 and Figure 10) [63,65]. Accordingly, L372A and V376A mutations significantly decrease the interaction of ERα with the N-CoR co-repressor when it is exposed to tamoxifen [98]. Similarly, V376D totally abolishes the association of ERα with CBP in the presence of E_2 [97].

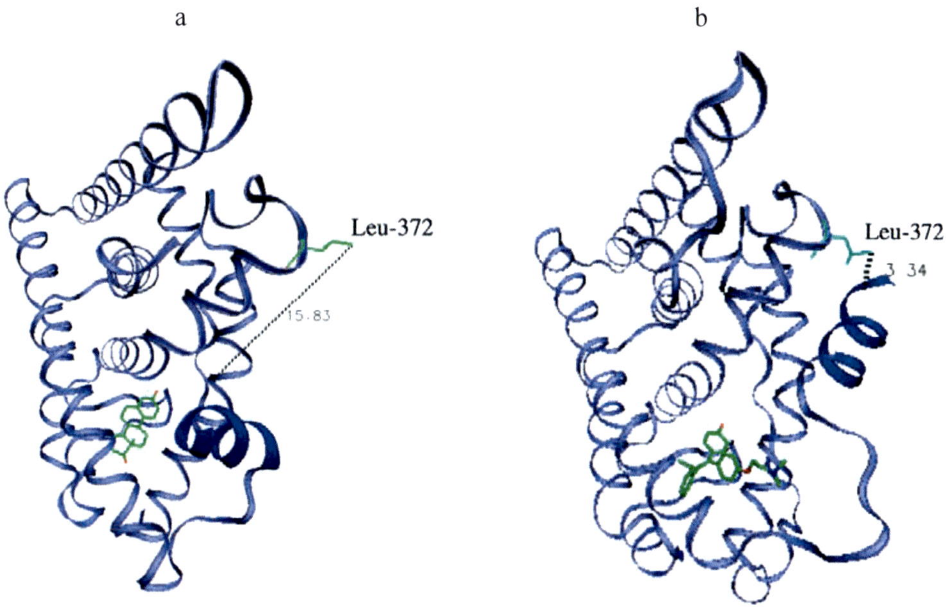

Figure 9. Role of Leu-372 in the spatial stabilization of helix H12 when ERα is complexed with a) E_2 (PDB code: 1ERE [146]) or b) tamoxifen (PDB code: 3ERT [63]). Distance between Leu-372 and H12: ~ 15.83 Å in the presence of E_2 and ~ 3.34 Å in the presence of tamoxifen. Drawings were made using VMD software [250].

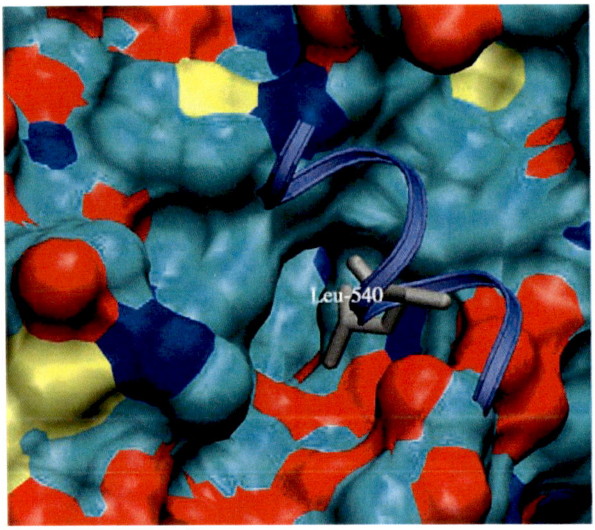

Figure 10. Orientation of Leu-540 of helix H12 in direction of the hydrophobic groove in which LxxLL motif of co-regulators motifs engulf (PDB code: 1ERE [146]). Drawing was made using VMD software [250].

The ability of *Glu-380* to discriminate between agonistic and antagonistic structural determinants of partial (ant)agonists provides mechanistic data related to the potency of these compounds to activate AP-1 sites [104–108]. Indeed, following the activation of specific mitogen-activated and stress-activated kinases, co-activators associate with DNA regions involved in transcription mediated by the proto-oncogenes *c-fos* and *c-jun* [107,109]. Implication of ERα in the activation of these transduction pathways is important in normal cells; they also participate to oncogenic transformation as well as tumor progression [105-109]. On the other hand, the negative charge shared by Glu-380 controls the kinetics of ligand-dependent transactivation since the mutated E380Q ERα requires less times than the wild ERα to achieve an optimal maximal transcription under exposure to E_2, without affecting capacity of its binding pocket to capture the hormone [110]. This mutant confers also ligand-independent transactivation potency since it triggers a high constitutive activity.

Cys-381 participates to the stabilization of H12 [111] in a position appropriate for the insertion of LxxLL motifs (SRC-2, Table 1) [95]. Moreover, this residue constitutes an alternative covalent anchoring point for tamoxifen aziridine, an alkylating derivative of tamoxifen that normally associates with ERα through covalent linkage at Cys-572 [112,113]. At least, it should be stressed that Cys-381 interacts with heavy metals (especially cadmium [114] and rhenium carbonyl organometallic complexes [115], giving rise to estrogenic responses) and is implicated in the activation of ERα by nitrites [116].

E. Helix H6 (Residues 382-395)

Located in the vicinity of the ligand-binding pocket, H6 regulates interactions between ligands and ERα. It also facilitates to the expression of the antagonistic activity of partials antiestrogens.

Amino-acids extending from Leu-387 to Leu-391 encompasses *Glu-353* and are in the neighborhood of *Arg-394,* two residues directly implicated in the interaction of the phenolic ring of E_2 with the receptor (Glu-353, Arg-394 and a molecule of water constitute a triumvirate determinant of a hydrogen bonding region). These residues attract type I and type II ligands within the E_2 binding pocket, favoring their anchorage within the latter. Leu-387 acts, through van der Waals contacts, as a "pincer-like" in a restricted polar cavity of this pocket [62,63,66,117] while Arg-394 operates in a larger polar region [62,63,65-68]. Note also that *Leu-384, Ile-386* and *Leu-387* have been reported to participate to the selectivity of ERα and β for ligands by modifying the topology of their binding site. In this context, it is noteworthy that Leu-384 is replaced by a methionine in ERβ, reducing the size of this cavity (390 $Å^3$ for the hERβ and 490 $Å^3$ for the hERα) [61,62,64,66,91,117].

Several residues of H6 are devoted to co-regulators recruitment. In this aim, *Trp-393* favors the recruitment of LxxLL motifs in an alternative binding-site, located at the opposite face of the conventional LxxLL interacting region [60].

F. The Antiparallel β-Hairpin (Residues 401-411), the Helix H7 (Residues 412-417), the Helix H8 (Residues 421-438)

The 400 – 444 region encompasses four different conformational entities: i) an antiparallel β-hairpin composed by two β strands S1 and S2 (residues 401-411), ii) a short helix containing only six residues (helix H7, residues 412 – 417), iii) helix H8 (residues 422 – 438) and iv) a flexible region that extends from residues 439 to 441. The antiparallel β-hairpin appears crucial in the stabilization of the A-ring of E_2 within the ligand-binding pocket. Moreover, H7 displays some discriminative properties for type I / II ligands and H8 is a solvent-exposed helix (located at the ERα surface) implied in the homo- or hetero-dimerization of the receptor.

Gly-400 in front of the antiparallel β-hairpin seems to be important for AP-1 dependent transcription since it contributes to the potent agonist activity of tamoxifen [23,79,92,117,118].

Phe-404 stabilizes ERα / ligand complexes through π-π contacts with the phenolic ring that interacts with Glu-353 and Arg-394 [61,63,66,117]. In fact, this residue, with the participation of Ala-350, Leu-387 and Leu-391, constitutes a stabilizing hydrophobic quartet (Figure 5) [67].

Implication of *Cys-417* in ligand anchorage seems likely since this residue constitutes a potential nucleophilic site for the covalent binding of 17α-(haloacetamidoalkyl) E_2 [119,120]). Proximity of Cys-417 and H3 is reflected in the C417S mutant in which conformation changes observed with partial (ant)agonists are recorded, due to a significant displacement of H3 [111]. As expected, this change modifies the selectivity of the LBD for type I / II ligands [67,111,121]. At least, this cysteine may orient some ligands to ERα rather than ERβ since it is substituted by an isoleucine in the latter [61].

G. Helix H9 (residues 442-455)

H9 is subject to important functional features since it participates to the structure of a suspected second ligand-binding pocket as well as to the targeting of ERα to the plasma membrane.

The domain that extends from *Gln-441 to Glu-444* and that localizes within the region of a suspected second ligand-binding pocket [61], delineates an alternative site for co-activators recruitment, at a face opposite to the conventional LxxLL binding region [60].

Phe-445 is one of the four residues of this second binding pocket (Ile-326, Leu-327, Leu-384, Phe-445) that differs between α and β ER subtypes, suggesting a role in ligand binding selectivity of these receptors [61].

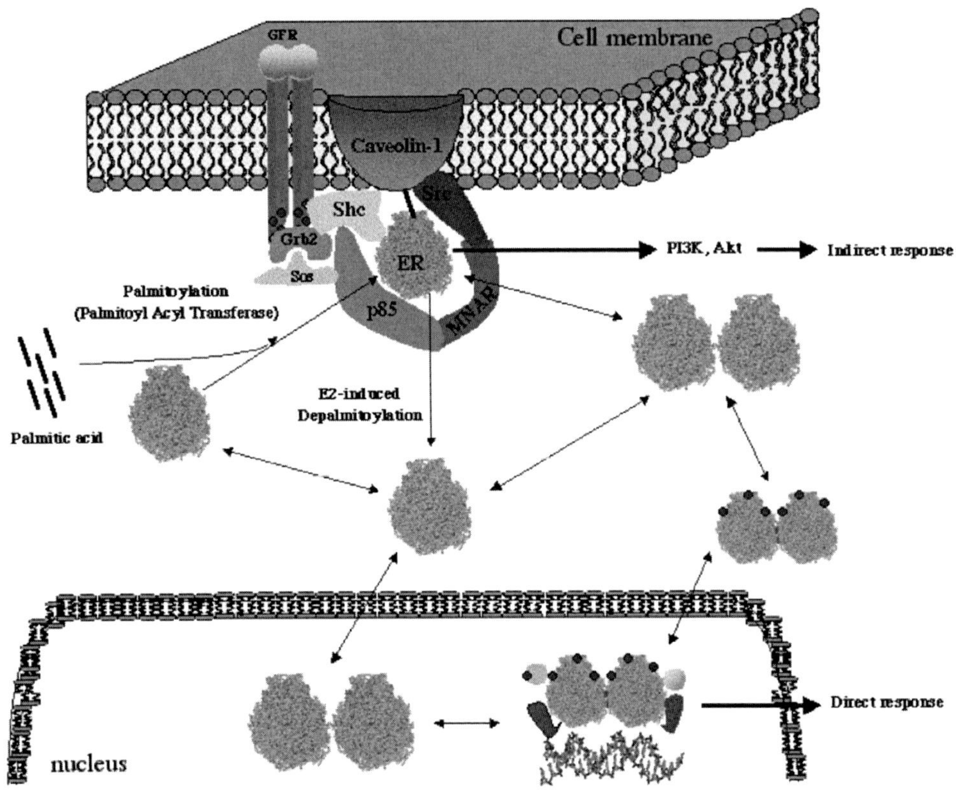

Figure 11. Proposed mechanisms for signal transduction pathways initiated by ERα at the membrane. A Palmitoyl-Acetyl Transferase (PAT) catalyzes the linkage of palmitic acid to a surface-exposed cysteine of the receptor (Cys-447). When palmitoylated, ERα associates with caveolin1, Src, MNAR, p85, Grb2 / Sos and Shc to activate PI3K / Akt pathways. Even if the mechanisms underlying ERα palmitoylation are not entirely elucidated, palmitoylation of ERα seems to be hormone-dependent.

Cys-447 is a target for palmitoylation, a post-traductional modification required for the location of ER onto the membrane. In fact, Cys-447 is a solvent accessible residue close to a hydrophobic patch (a leucine zipper) and a hydrophilic lysine (Lys-449) [122]. Palmitoylated ERα interacts with the scaffolding plasma membrane protein caveolin-1 [123,124] to rapidly activate E_2-mediated processes through PKC, PI3K / Akt or MAPK pathways (Figure 11)

[125,126]. Cys-447 is also important for the folding and stability of the nuclear form of the receptor [19,127]. Finally, it contributes to the interaction of ERα with heavy metals [114].

H. Helix 10 (Residues 466-492) and Helix 11 (Residues 497-530)

The region between H9 and H11 participates to hetero- and homo-dimerization of ERα, as does H8 [66]. It also regulates the binding of type I / II ligands despite a modest role in transcription. Finally, the 525-530 region is a very flexible loop regulating intramolecular interactions between AF-1 and AF-2 sites

Remarkably, 14 to 16% of solvent-exposed residues of H10 - H11 are implied in ERα dimerization [66] and most probably, in its ability to recruit co-regulators, as shown for Leu-504 [98] and Leu-507 [23]. Several amino-acids of this region may also play a role in ligand binding selectivity, as evidenced for Leu-509 [65], *Met-481 and Leu-384* [71].

Arg-515, His-516, Lys-520 (and Asn-532) play a role in tamoxifen association and related activity [128]. These residues confer activation potency under nitrite exposure as does Cys-381 [116]. Finally, interaction of ERα with heavy metals able to induce transcription is stabilized by *Met-522* [114,129,130].

Gly-521 stabilizes type I ligands within the LBD [62,63,112,128,131–134]. *His-524* (as Glu-353, Arg-394 and Phe-404) is an additional residue for the anchorage of these ligands through an interaction with the hydrogen of the 17β hydroxyl of the steroidal hormone or the corresponding phenolic hydroxyl of their non-steroidal counterparts [62,63,65–68]. This hydrogen bond network, that implies also Glu-339, Glu-419 and Lys-531, keeps H3 and H11 in close contact provided that His-524 is under its ε tautomeric form. Actually, this tautomeric effect prevents the ligand to escape from the binding cavity [135]. The strength of the interaction of the ligand with His-524 influences estrogenicity. For example, the interaction of apigenin and genistein are significantly weaker than that described for E_2, explaining the weak binding affinity and estrogenicity displayed by these two phytoestrogens [136]. Moreover, orientation of His-524 depends on the ability of the ligand to interact with Met-343 and Met-421. In this regard, it has been highlighted that pure steroidal agonists are more effective than SERMs, an observation that may be also related to the attraction of the latter by Asp-351, which provokes their displacement in the direction of Glu-353 and Arg-394 with concomitant decrease of interaction with His-524 [137].

Leu-525 and *Tyr-526* both stabilize type I / II ligands within the E_2-binding pocket, contributing to their ability to induce transcription [62,127,128,131]. *Met-528* and *Cys-530* produce a same effect by enhancing hydrophobic contacts with the D-ring of steroids or the related phenolic ring of their non-steroidal counterparts. At least, Met-528 located on the border of the LBD, participates to ERα folding as well as to ligand discrimination [128].

Lys-529 and Cys-530 are enclosed within a KCK motif (amino-acids Lys-529 / Cys-530 / *Lys-531*) corresponding to a highly flexible loop [98]. They contribute to transcription by causing the association of the 525-530 region with AF-1 [98,128]. This association results from salt bridges between an ELE motif (Glu-22 / Leu-23 / Glu-24) with this KCK motif. On the other hand, Cys-530 plays a fundamental role in ERα trafficking [23,126,138] and constitutes a potential nucleophilic site appropriate for covalent links with various alkylating ligands, i.e 17α-(haloacetamidoalkyl) E_2, ketononestrol aziridine and tamoxifen aziridine [91,112,113,119,120,126,139-142].

At least, it should be stressed that the C-terminal tail of H11 (also called H11a), flanked by two unstructured domains and corresponding to a one turn 3,10 helix, contributes to AF-2 flexibility, allowing intramolecular interactions within the receptor [40,89].

I. The 531-537 Intermediary Region

The 531-537 region that directly follows the helix H11a induces AP-1 transcription through interaction with AF-1. Strikingly, this part of ERα is important for rapid activation of transduction pathways induced by the agonist core of partial (anti)estrogens.

Occurrence of metastatic breast cancers seems to increase when *Lys-531* is mutated into a glutamate [23,143]. In addition, *Asn-532* may be involved in activation of ERα by nitrite [116].

Pro-535 and *Leu-536* contribute to the expression of the agonistic activity of tamoxifen (AP-1 mediated transcription). In the ligand-binding pocket, the isopropyl side-chain of Leu-536 is orientated to form, with Leu-540 (Figure 10) and Leu-541, a hydrophobic cluster [63,65,111,144–146]. As shown with raloxifene and tamoxifen, this side chain may orient in distinct directions to allow specific responses dictated by the ligands [65]. In this context, it should be noted that the mutant L536P confers a high constitutive activity to the receptor, which may be abrogated by (anti)estrogens. A constitutive recruitment of SRC-1 may explain these properties [147].

j. Helix H12 (residues 538 - 545)

The helix H12, located in the C-terminal tail of the LBD, is a well-structured element of prime importance for transcription since its orientation is ligand-dependent (Figure 9 and Figure 12) [66]. Moreover, residues in the N-terminal tail of H12 appear crucial for interactions with co-activators or co-inhibitors [89].

Located at the N-terminal extremity of H12, *Tyr-537* stabilizes ERα / ligand complexes by generating a hydrogen bond with Asn-348 (helix H3). In fact, the Tyr-537 regulates the kinetic of the ligand association with ERα, influencing thereby receptor dimerization [140,144,148,149]. It has been shown that H12 is spatially oriented to confer a "close" (state II, ligand-bound) or an "open" (state III, ligand free) conformation to ERα, appropriate for enhancing or silencing transcription, respectively [66,78,148-162].

a) b)

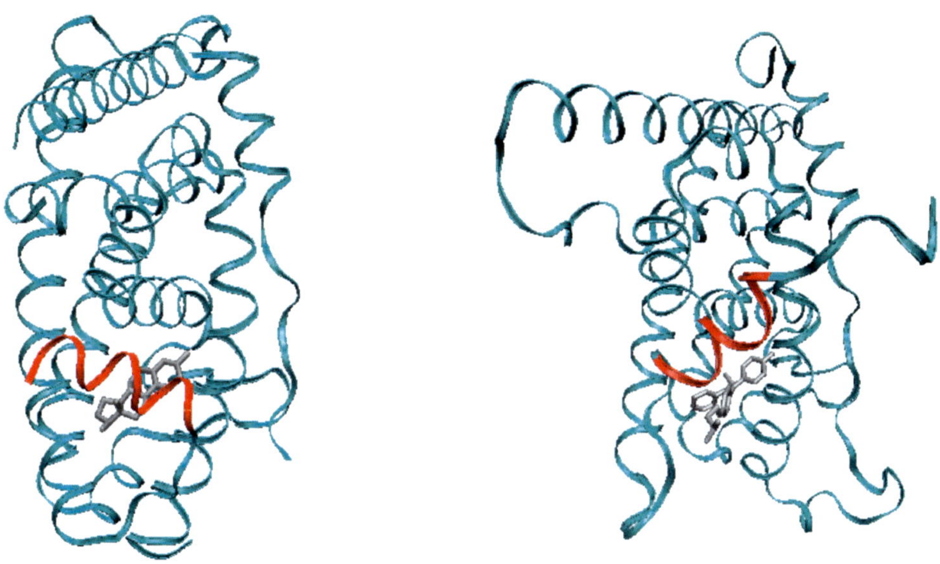

Figure 12. Orientation of helix H12 when ERα is complexed with (a) E2 (PDB code: 1ERE [146]) or (b) tamoxifen (PDB code: 3ERT [63]). The ligand is in gray and H12 in red. Drawings were made using VMD software [250].

Interestingly, the receptor mutant Y537S confers a collapsed status (state I) to the unliganded ERα as well as an unusual open form appropriate for ligand exchanges [149]. The absence of interaction between Tyr-537 and Asp-351 appears crucial for the recruitment of co-activators such as SRC-1: when it does not occur, ERα adopts an active "open" form [78,128,140,145–149,161]. Moreover, several studies revealed that Tyr-537 is a site of phosphorylation required for the activation of protein kinase-dependent (Src) ERα pathways [23,150,151,153]. Remarkably, this phosphorylation process is analogous to the one occuring with Src-2 homology 2 (SH2) domains, suggesting that H8-H12 delineate a potential intramolecular SH2-like domain. Accordingly, the pTyr-537 interacts in a ligand-independent manner with the SH2 domain of the p160$^{c\text{-}src}$ kinase and with the participation of the proline-, glutamic acid-, and leucine-rich protein MNAR (Table 1), a modulator of indirect action of estrogen receptor that favores ERα dimerization and ERE association [23,145,149–156]. Thus, the Tyr-537 seems to constitute a molecular link between direct / indirect pathways. In this regard, an Y537N mutation (Table 2) has been found in patients with tamoxifen-resistant tumors whereas Y537S and Y537A mutations are mainly recorded in patients with endometrial cancers [23,145,148,161,162].

Asp-538 is required for AF1-dependent activation, provided that Asp-351 is free and H12 orientates in such a way that AF2 is silenced [93]. In fact, the Asp-538, as Tyr-537, Met-543, Leu-536, 540 and 544, engulfs in the shallow depression in which fit p160 co-activators when ERα is in its "active" state [94,95].

In contrast, *Leu-539* is crucial for AF-2 activation. Although AF-2 site belongs to a depression in which co-activators dock [67], Leu-539 interferes with the recruitment of LxxLL motifs [92,96,163] as well as with PNRC (Table 1) [99]. In this regard, the mutant

L539A abrogates AF-2 by preventing interactions between H12 and co-activators [23,98,149,164].

Leu-540 acts slightly differently than the residues just described above: it is a prominent residue for the sealing of ligands within their E_2 binding pocket [65]. Moreover, this leucine regulates estrogenic activity of partial (anti)estrogens, suggesting that it is of prime importance for AP-1 transcriptions [165-168]. Indeed, L540Q and L540A mutations enhance the agonist activity of these compounds. L540Q mutation induces also apoptosis by provoking the increase of Bax (a protein that determines cell death or cell survival after apoptosis stimuli) and phosphorylation of p38 MAPK [169].

Glu-542 contributes to ERα transactivation by interacting with p160 [65,66,92,96] and PNRC [99]. Remarkably, this residue is a member of the charge clamp that aligned with Lys-362 in such a way that it interacts with the dipole formed by the helical LxxLL motif of co-regulators [67,102].

Interestingly, some regions of ERα containing leucine-rich motifs have been reported to mimic the function of such LxxLL motifs by fitting within the co-activator binding groove in the absence of co-activators (Figure 13). Accordingly, Leu-540 plays a role of prime importance in the stabilization of the H12 in its "inactive" position [63,65,66,111,145]. Note, in this context, that the side chain of the lysine 362 makes hydrogen contacts with the *Met-543* and *Leu-544* to cap the C-terminal extremity of H12 for preventing recruitment of co-activators [65,163]. At least, *His-547* has been shown to be implicated in nitrite activation of ERα as Cys-381, His-516, Lys-520, Lys-529 and Asn-547 [116].

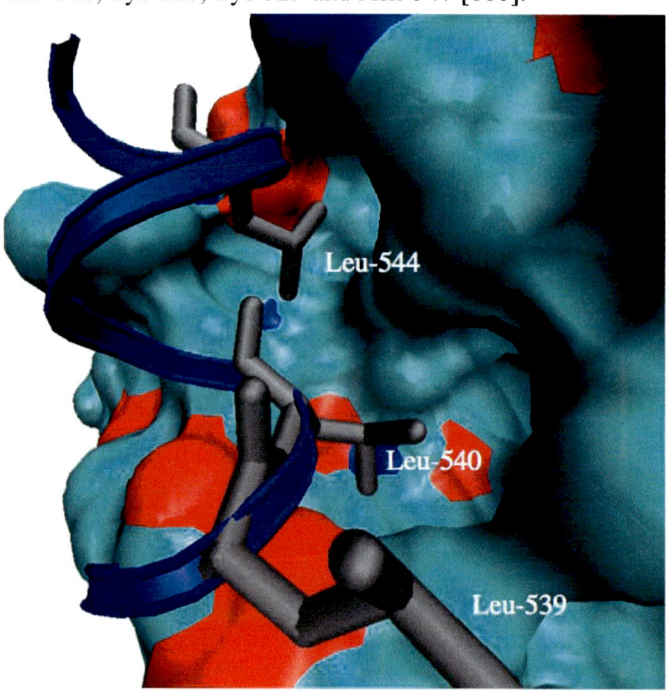

Figure 13. Insertion of the $L_{539}LLEML_{544}$ motif of H12 within the co-activator binding groove when ERα is complexed with tamoxifen (PDB code: 3ERT [63]). H12 is in blue, the leucines 539, 540 and 544 in grey. Drawings were made using VMD software [250].

3) Domain F (Residues 555 - 595)

This domain regulates the activity of partial (ant)agonists, probably by promoting the association of ERα with the co-repressor TATA-binding protein-associated factor 1β (TAF-1β) [49,170,171] or the selective transcription factor 1 (Sp1) [172]. In contrast, when ERα is exposed to E_2, it inhibits the interaction of the LBD with the co-repressor RIP140 (Table 1) [173]. Thus, F-domain is important to control the recruitment of various ERα partners [174,175].

The F-domain also controls ERα homo-dimerization [176]. It stabilizes ERα / co-activator complexes in such a way that the related spatial positioning of H12 is not sufficient to explain the agonism and antagonism of ligands [177,178]. Accordingly, a dynamic view of this domain should be taken into account. The finding of an alteration of tamoxifen-induced antagonism when it is truncated or mutated accredits this view [179,180].

This part of ERα is also subject to post-translational modifications such as O-glycosylation, O-phosphorylation or N-acetylation, suggesting that it contributes to ERα degradation, trafficking, and transcription [47,181].

```
10         20         30         40         50         60
MTMTLHTKAS GMALLHQIQG NELEPLNRPQ LKIPLERPLG EVYLDSSKPA VYNYPEGAAY

        70         80         90        100        110        120
EFNAAAAANA QVYGQTGLPY GPGSEAAAFG SNGLGGFPPL NSVSPSPLML LHPPPQLSPF

       130        140        150        160        170        180
LQPHGQQVPY YLENEPSGYT VREAGPPAFY RPNSDNRRQG GRERLASTND KGSMAMESAK

       190        200        210        220        230        240
ETRYCAVCND YASGYHYGVW SCEGCKAFFK RSIQGHNDYM CPATNQCTID KNRRKSCQAC

       250        260        270        280        290        300
RLRKCYEVGM MKGGIRKDRR GGRMLKHKRQ RDDGEGRGEV GSAGDMRAAN LWPSPLMIKR

       310        320        330        340        350        360
SKKNSLALSL TADQMVSALL DAEPPILYSE YDPTRPFSEA SMMGLLTNLA DRELVHMINW

       370        380        390        400        410        420
AKRVPGFVDL TLHDQVHLLE CAWLEILMIG LVWRSMEHPG KLLFAPNLLL DRNQGKCVEG

       430        440        450        460        470        480
MVEIFDMLLA TSSRFRMMNL QGEEFVCLKS IILLNSGVYT FLSSTLKSLE EKDHIHRVLD

       490        500        510        520        530        540
KITDTLIHLM AKAGLTLQQQ HQRLAQLLLI LSHIRHMSNK GMEHLYSMKC KNVVPLYDLL

       550        560        570        580        590
LEMLDAHRLH APTSRGGASV EETDQSHLAT AGSTSSHSLQ KYYITGEAEG FPATV
```

Acetylation
Acetylation + SUMOylation + ubiquitination
Phosphorylation
SUMOylation
Phosphorylation + acetylation
Palmitoylation
Glycozylation + acetylation

Figure 14. Residues of ERα subject to post-translational modifications.

Note in this regard that *Thr-574* is a component of a proline (P) – glutamate (E) – serine (S) – threonine (T) proteolytic signal sequence (PEST) [182] that could be subject to post-translational modifications.

Conclusion

The present review highlights the extremely high complexity of the cross-talk mechanisms to which ERα, ligands and co-activators contribute. In fact, each residue of the LBD (Figure 14) may participate in such a complex network. The functions of a large number of these residues being still unknown (only ~ 30% of the primary sequence of the Hinge / LBD regions have been investigated), pursuit of the systematic delineation of ERα appears, therefore, as an absolute requirement for a better knowledge of its functioning, emergence of tumors and resistance towards antitumoral therapeutics. Unidentified partners in the jungle of steroid receptors may most likely emerge from this work, as recently highlighted by Rosenfeld *et al.* [183]. Assessment of molecular mechanisms generating hormone-dependent cancers seems also of prime importance for the development of new therapeutic strategies as well as for the design of new drugs.

References

[1] Tikkanen, M.J.; Vihma, V.; Jauhiainen, M.; Höckerstedt, A.; Helisten, H.; Kaamanen, M. Lipoprotein-associated estrogens. *Cardiovasc. Res.*, 2002 56, 184 – 188.

[2] Compston, J.E. Sex steroids and bone. *Physiol. Rev.*, 2001 81, 419 – 447.

[3] Garcia-Segura, L.M.; Azcoitia, I.; DonCarlos, L.L. Neuroprotection by estradiol. *Pr ogress Neurobiol.*, 2001 63, 29 – 60.

[4] Farhat, M.Y.; Lavigne, M.C.; Ramwell, P.W. The vascular protective effects of estrogen. *FASEB J.*, 1996 10, 615 – 624.

[5] Klinge, CM. Estrogen receptor interaction with co-activators and co-repressors. *Steroids*, 2000 65, 227 – 251.

[6] Kumar, R.; Thompson, E.B. The structure of the nuclear hormone receptors. *Steroids*, 1999 64, 310 – 319.

[7] Agarwal, M.K. Analysis of steroid receptor domains with the aid of antihormones. *Int. J. Biochem.*, 1994 6, 341 – 350.

[8] Tsai, M.-J.; O'Malley, B.W. Molecular mechanisms of action of steroid / thyroid receptor superfamily members. *Annu. Rev. Biochem.*, 1994 63, 451 – 486.

[9] Kim; M.Y.; Woo, E.M.; Chong, Y.T.E.; Homenko, D.R.; Kraus, W.L. Acetylation of estrogen receptor α by p300 at lysines 266 and 268 enhances the deoxyribonucleic acid binding and transactivation activities of the receptor. *Molec. Endocrinol.*, 2006 20, 1479 – 1493.

[10] Wang, C; Fu, M.; Angeletti, R.H.; Siconolfi-Baez, L.; Reutens, A.T.; Albanese, C.; Lisanti, M.P.; Katzenellenbogen, B.S.; Kato, S.; Hopp, T.; Fuqua, S.A.W.; Lopez, G.N.; Kushner, P.J.; Pestell, R.G. Direct acetylation of the estrogen receptor α hinge region by p300 regulates transactivation and hormone sensitivity. *J. Biol. Chem.*, 2001 276, 18375 – 18383.

[11] Sentis, S.; Le Romancer, M.; Bianchin, C.; Rostan, M.-C.; Corbo, L. Sumoylation of the estrogen receptor α hinge region regulates its transcriptional activity. *Molec. Endocrinol.*, 2005 19, 2671 – 2684.

[12] Faus, H.; Haendler, B. Post-translational modifications of steroid receptors. *Biomed. Pharmacother.*, 2006 60, 520 – 528.
[13] El Khissiin, A.; Leclercq, G. Implication of proteasome in estrogen receptor degradation. *FEBS. Lett.*, 1999 448, 160-166.
[14] Nawaz, Z.; Lonard, D.M.; Dennis, A.P.; Smith, C.L.; O'Malley, B.W. Proteasome-dependent degradation of the human estrogen receptor. *Proc. Nat. Acad. Sci. USA*, 1999 65, 1858-1862.
[15] Ohta, T.; Fukuda, M. Ubiquitin and breast cancer. *Oncogene*, 2004 23, 2079-2088.
[16] Stenoien, D.L.; Patel, K.; Mancini, M.G.; Dutertre, M.; Smith, C.L.; O'Malley, B.W.; Mancini, M.A. FRAP reveals that mobility of oestrogen receptor-α is ligand- and proteasome-dependent. *Nat. Cell Biol.*, 2001 3, 15-23.
[17] Laïos, I.; Journe, F.; Nonclercq, D.; Vidal, D.S.; Toillon, R.-A.; Laurent, G.; Leclercq, G. Role of the proteasome in the regulation of estrogen receptor α turnover and function in MCF-7 breast carcinoma cells. *J. Steroid Biochem. Molec. Biol.*, 2005 94, 347-359.
[18] Wijayaratne, A.L.; McDonnell, D.P. The human estrogen receptor-α is a ubiquitinated protein whose stability is affected differentially by agonists, antagonists, and selective estrogen receptor modulators. *J. Biol. Chem.*, 2001 276, 35684-35692.
[19] Tateishi, Y.; Kawabe, Y.-I.; Chiba, T.; Murata, S.; Ichikawa, K.; Murayama, A.; Tanaka, K.; Baba, T.; Kato, S.; Yanagisawa, J. Ligand-dependent switching of ubiquitin-proteasome pathways for estrogen receptor. *EMBO J.*, 2004 23, 4813-4823.
[20] Kinyamu, H.K.; Chen, J.; Archer, T.K. Linking the ubiquitin-proteasome pathway to chromatin remodeling / modification by nuclear receptors. *J. Molec. Endocrinol.*, 2005 34, 281-297.
[21] Feng, J.; Yan, J.; Michaud, S.; Craddock, N.; Jones, I.R.; Cook Jr E.H.; Goldman, D.; Heston, L.L.; Peltonen, L.; Delisi, L.E.; Sommer, S.S. Scanning of estrogen receptor α (ERα) and thyroid hormone receptor α (TRα) genes in patients with psychiatric diseases: four missense mutations identified in ERα gene. *Am. J. Med. Genet.*, 2001 105, 369 – 374.
[22] Komagata, S.; Nakajima, M.; Tsuchiya, Y.; Katoh, M.; Kizu, R.; Kyo, S.; Yokoi, T. Decreased responsiveness of naturally occuring mutants of human estrogen receptor α to estrogens and antiestrogens. *J. Steroid Biochem. Molec. Biol.*, 2006 100, 79-86.
[23] McGuire, W.L.; Chamnes, G.C.; Fuqua, S.A. Abnormal estrogen receptor in clinical breast cancer. *J. Steroid Biochem. Molec. Biol.*, 1992 43, 243 – 247.
[24] Herynk, M.H.; Fuqua, S.A.W. Estrogen receptor mutations in human disease. *Endocrine Rev.*, 2004 25, 869 – 898.
[25] Le Goff, P.; Montano, M.M.; Schodin, D.J.; Katzenellenbogen, B.S. Phosphorylation of the human estrogen receptor. *J. Biol. Chem.*, 1994 269, 4458 – 4466.
[26] Pierrat, B.; Heery, D.M.; Chambon, P.; Losson, R. A highly conserved region in the hormone-binding domain of the human estrogen receptor functions as an efficient transactivation domain in yeast. *Gene*, 1994 143, 193 – 200.
[27] Li, L.; Li, Z.; Sacks, D.B. The transcriptional activity of estrogen receptor-α is dependent on Ca^{2+} / calmodulin. *J. Biol. Chem.*, 2005 280, 13097 – 13104.

[28] Li, L.; Sacks, D.B. Functional interactions between calmodulin and estrogen receptor-α. *Cell. Signal.*, 2007 19, 439 – 443.

[29] Gallo, D.; Jacquemotte, F.; Cleeren, A.; Laïos, I.; Hadiy, S.; Rowlands, M.G.; Caille, O.; Nonclercq, D.; Laurent, G.; Jacquot, Y.; Leclercq, G. Calmodulin-independent, agonistic properties of a peptide containing the calmodulin binding site of estrogen receptor α. *Molec. Cell. Endocrinol.*, 2007 268, 37 – 49.

[30] Gallo, D.; Jacquot, Y.; Cleeren, A.; Jacquemotte, F.; Laïos, I.; Laurent, G.; Leclercq, G. Molecular basis of agonistic activity of ERα17p, a synthetic peptide corresponding to a sequence located at the N-terminal part of the estrogen receptor α ligand binding domain. *Lett. Drug Design Discov.*, 2007 4, 346 – 355.

[31] Gallo, D.; Haddad, I.; Duvilliers, H.; Jacquemotte, F.; Laïos, I.; Laurent, G.; Jacquot, Y.; Vinh, J.; Leclercq, G. Trophic effect in MCF-7 cells of ERα17p, a peptide corresponding to a platform regulary motif of the estrogen receptor α - Underlying mechanisms. *J. Steroid Biochem. Molec. Biol.*, 2008 109, 138 – 149.

[32] Gallo, D.; Leclercq, G.; Jacquot, Y. The N-terminal Part of the ligand-binding domain of the human estrogen receptor α: A new target for estrogen disruptors. In "Medicinal Chemistry Research Progress", Ed. Nova Science Publishers. 2008 (*in press*).

[33] Gallo, D.; Jacquot, Y.; Laurent, G.; Leclercq, G. Calmodulin, a regulatory partner of the estrogen receptor alpha in breast cancer. *Molec. Cell. Endocrinol.*, 2008 291, 20-26.

[34] Bouhoute, A.; Leclercq, G. Modulation of estradiol and DNA binding to estrogen receptor upon association with calmodulin. *Biochem. Biophys. Res. Commun.*, 1995 208, 748 – 755.

[35] Björnström, L.; Sjöberg, M. Mechanisms of estrogen receptor signaling: convergence of genomic and non-genomic actions of target genes. *Molec. Endocrinol.*, 2005 19, 833 – 842.

[36] Bouhoute, A.; Leclercq, G. Estradiol derivatives bearing the side-chain of tamoxifen antagonize the association between the estrogen receptor and calmodulin. *Biochem. Pharmacol.*, 1994 47, 748 – 751.

[37] Melchior, F.; Schergaut, M.; Pichler, A. SUMO: ligases, isopeptidases and nuclear pores. *Trends Biochem. Sci.*, 2003 28, 612 - 618.

[38] Seielstad, D.A.; Carlson, K.E.; Kushner, P.J.; Greene, G.L.; Katzenellenbogen, J.A. Analysis of the structural core of the human estrogen receptor ligand binding domain by selective proteolysis / mass spectrometic analysis. *Biochemistry*, 1995 34, 12605 – 12615.

[39] Ylikomi, T.; Bocquel, M.T.; Berry, M.; Gronemeyer, H.; Chambon, P. Cooperation of proto-signals for nuclear accumulation of estrogen and progesterone receptors. *EMBO J.*, 1992 11, 3681 – 3694.

[40] Jacquot, Y.; Gallo, D.; Leclercq, G. Estrogen receptor alpha – Identification by a modeling approach of a potential polyproline II recognizing domain within the AF2 region of the receptor that would play a role of prime importance in its mechanism of action. *J. Steroid. Biochem. Molec. Biol.*, 2007 104, 1-10.

[41] Cubellis, M.V.; Caillez, F.; Blundell, T.L.; Lovell, S.C. Properties of polyproline II, a secondary structure element implicated in protein-protein interactions. *Proteins*, 2005 58, 880-892.

[42] Li, L.; Li, Z.; Howley, P.M.; Sacks, D.B. E6AP and calmodulin reciprocally regulate estrogen receptor stability. *J. Biol. Chem.*, 2006 281, 1978 – 1985.

[43] Berry, N.B.; Fan, M.; Nephew, K.P. Estrogen receptor-α hinge-region lysines 302 and 303 regulate estrogen receptor degradation by the proteasome. *Molec. Endocrinol.*, 2008 22, 1535-1551.

[44] Fuqua, S.A.; Wiltschke, C.; Zhang, Q.X.; Borg, A.; Castles, C.G.; Friedrichs, W.E; Hopp, T.; Hilsenbeck, S.; Mohsin, S.; O'Connell, P.; Allred, D.C. A hypersensitive estrogen receptor-α mutation in premalignant breast lesions. *Cancer Res.*, 2000 60, 4026 – 4029.

[45] Zhang, Z.; Yamashita, H.; Toyama, T.; Omoto, Y.; Sugiura, H.; Hara, Y.; Haruki, N.; Kobayashi, S.; Iwase, H. Estrogen receptor α mutation (A-to-G transition at nucleotide 908) is not found in different types of breast lesions from Japanese women. *Breast Cancer*, 2003 10, 70 – 73.

[46] Conway, K.; Parrish, E.; Edmiston, S.N.; Tolbert, D.; Tse, C.-K., Geradts, J.; Livasy, C.A.; Singh, H.; Newman, B.; Millikn, R.C. The estrogen receptor-α A908G (K303R) mutation occurs at a low frequency in invasive breast tumors: results from a population-based study. *Breast Cancer Res.*, 2005 7, R871 – R880.

[47] Leclercq, G. Molecular forms of the estrogen receptor in breast cancer. *J. Steroid Biochem. Molec. Biol.*, 2002 80, 259 – 272.

[48] Chen, T.H.; Brody, J.R.; Romantsev, F.E.; Yu, J.G.; Kayler, A.E.; Voneiff, E.; Kuhajda, F.P.; Pasternack, G.R. Structure of pp32, an acidic nuclear protein which inhibits oncogene-induced formation of transformed foci. *Molec. Biol. Cell.* 1996 12, 2045-2056.

[49] Loven, M.A.; Davis, R.E.; Curtis, C.D.; Muster, N.; Yates, J.R.; Nardulli, A.M. A novel estrogen receptor alpha-associated protein alters receptor – deoxyribonucleic acid interactions and represses receptor-mediated transcription. *Molec. Endocrinol.*, 2004 18, 2649 – 2659.

[50] Loven, M.A.; Muster, N.; Yates, J.R.; Nardulli, A.M. A novel estrogen receptor alpha-associated protein, template-activating factor Ibeta, inhibits acetylation and transactivation. *Molec. Endocrinol.*, 2003 17, 67-78.

[51] Tharakan, R.; Lepont, P.; Singleton, D.; Kumar, R.; Khan, S. Phosphorylation of estrogen receptor alpha, serine residue 305 enhances activity. *Molec. Cell. Endocrinol.*, 2008 (in press)

[52] Wang, R.A.; Mazumdar, A.; Vadlamudi, R.K.; Kumar, R. p21-activated kinase 1 phosphorylates and transactivates estrogen receptor α and promotes hyperplasia in mammary epithelium. *EMBO J.*, 2002 21, 5437 – 5447.

[53] Zubairy, S.; Cui, Y.; Fuqua, S.A. The K303R estrogen receptor alpha breast cancer mutant generates a new Akt kinase site. *Proc. Am. Assoc. Cancer Res.*, 2004 45, 659.

[54] Michalides, R.; Griekspoor, A.; Balkenende, A.; Verwoerd, D.; Janssen, L.; Jalink, K.; Floore, A.; Velds, A.; van't Veer, L.; Neef, J.S, J. Tamoxifen resistance by a conformational arrest of the estrogen receptor α after PKA activation in breast cancer. *Cancer Cell*, 2004 5, 597 – 605.

[55] Migliaccio, A.; Domenico, M.Di.; Castoria, G.; de Falco, A.; Bontempo, P.; Nola, E.; Auricchio, F. Tyrosine kinase/p21^{ras}/MAP-kinase pathway activation by estradiol-receptor complex in MCF-7 cells. *EMBO J.*, 1996 15, 1292-1300.

[56] Simoncini, T.; Rabkin, E.; Liao, J.K. Molecular basis of cell membrane estrogen receptor interaction with phosphatidylinositol 3-kinase in endothelial cells. *Artherioscler. Thromb. Vasc. Biol.*, 2003 23, 198-203.

[57] Norman, A.W.; Mizwicki, M.T.; Norman, D.P.G. Steroid-hormone rapid actions, membrane receptors and a conformational ensemble model. *Nature Rev.*, 2004 3, 27-41.

[58] Revankar, C.M.; Cimino, D.F.; Sklar, L.A.; Arterburn, J.B.; Prossnitz, E.R. A transmembrane intracellular estrogen receptor mediates rapid cell signaling. *Science*, 2005 307, 1625-1630.

[59] Lee, H.; Bai, W. Regulation of estrogen receptor nuclear export by ligand-induced and p38-mediated receptor phosphorylation. *Molec. Cell. Biol.*, 2002 22, 5835 – 5845.

[60] Kong, E.H.; Heldring, N.; Gustafsson, J.-Å.; Treuter, E.; Hubbard, R.E.; Pike, A.C.W. Delineation of a unique protein-protein interaction site on the surface of the estrogen receptor. *Proc. Natl. Acad. Sci. USA*, 2005 102, 3593 – 3598.

[61] van Hoorn, W.P. Identification of a second binding site in the estrogen receptor. *J. Med. Chem.* 2002 45, 584 – 589.

[62] Kekenes-Huskey, P.M.; Muegge, I.; von Rauch, M.; Gust, R.; Knapp, E.-W. A molecular docking study of estrogenically active compounds with 1,2-diarylethane and 1,2-diarylethene pharmacophores. *Bioorg. Med. Chem.*, 2004 12, 6527 – 6537.

[63] Shiau, A.K.; Barstad, D.; Loria, P.M.; Cheng, L.; Kushner, P.J.; Agard, D.A.; Greene, G.L. The structural basis of estrogen receptor / coactivator recognition and the antagonism of this interaction by tamoxifen. *Cell*, 1998 95, 927 – 937.

[64] Ekena, E.; Katzenellenbogen, J.A.; Katzenellenbogen, B.S. Determinants of ligand specificity of estrogen receptor-α: estrogen *versus* androgen discrimination. *J. Biol. Chem.*, 1998 273, 693 – 699.

[65] Pike, A.C.W.; Brzozowski, A.M.; Hubbard, R.E.; Bonn, T.; Thorsell, A.-G.; Engström, O.; Ljunggren, J.; Gustafsson, J.-Å.; Carlquist, M. Structure of the ligand-binding domain of oestrogen receptor beta in the presence of a partial agonist and a full antagonist. *EMBO J.*, 1999 78, 4608 – 4618.

[66] Pike, A.C.W.; Brzozowski, M.; Hubbard, R.E. A structural biologist's view of the oestrogen receptor. *J. Steroid Biochem. Molec. Biol.*, 2000 74, 261 – 268.

[67] England, G.M.; Bilimoria, M.M.; Chen, Z.; Assikis, V.J.; Muenzner, H.D.; Jordan, V.G. Characterization of a point mutation in the hormone binding domain of the estrogen receptor from an estrogen-independent tumor. *Int. J. Oncol.*, 1998 12, 981 – 986.

[68] Jacquot, Y.; Rojas, C.; Refouvelet, B.; Robert, J.-F.; Leclercq, G.; Xicluna, A. Recent advances in the development of phytoestrogens and derivatives: an update of the promising perspectives in the prevention of postmenopausal diseases. *Mini-Rev. Med. Chem.*, 2003 3, 387 – 400.

[69] Fang, H.; Tong, W.; Shi, L.M.; Blair, R.; Perkins, R.; Branham, W.; Hass, B.S.; Xie, Q.; Dial, S.L.; Moland, C.L.; Sheehan, M. Structure – activity relationships for a large

diverse set of natural, synthetic, and environmental estrogens. *Chem. Res. Toxicol.*, 2001 14, 280 – 294.

[70] Klopman, G.; Chakravarti, S.K. Structure – activity relationship study of a diverse set of estrogen receptor ligands (I) using MultiCASE expert system. *Chemosphere*, 2003 51, 445 – 459.

[71] Matthews, J.B.; Clemons, J.H.; Zacharewski, T.R., P. Reciprocal mutagenesis between human α(L349, M528) and rainbow trout (M317, I496) estrogen receptor residues demonstrates their importance in ligand binding and gene expression at different temperatures. *Molec. Cell. Endocrinol.*, 2001 183, 127 – 139.

[72] Karnik, P.S.; Kulkarni, S.; Liu, X.P.; Budd, G.T.; Bukowski, R.M. Estrogen receptor mutations in tamoxifen-resistant breast cancer. *Cancer Res.*, 1994 54, 349 – 353.

[73] Garcia, T.; Sanchez, M.; Cox, J.L.; Shaw, P.A.; Ross, J.B.; Lehrer, S.; Schachter, B. Identification of a variant form of the human estrogen receptor with an amino acid replacement. *Nucleic Acids Res.*, 1989 17, 8364.

[74] von Rauch, M.; Schlenk, M.; Gust, R. Effects of C2-alkylation, N-alkylation, and N,N'-dialkylation on the stability and estrogen receptor interaction of (4*R*,5*S*) / (4*S*,5*R*)-4,5-bis(4-hydroxyphenyl)-2-imidazolines. *J. Med. Chem.*, 2004 47, 915 – 927.

[75] Laïos, I.; Cleeren, A.; Leclercq, G.; Nonclercq, D.; Laurent, G.; Schlenk, M.; Wellner, A.; Gust, R. Effects of (R,S)/(S,R)-4,5-bis(2-chloro-4-hydroxyphenyl)-2-imidazolines and (R,S)/(S,R)-2,3-bis(2-chloro-4-hydroxyphenyl)piperazines on estrogen receptor alpha level and transcriptional activity in MCF-7 cells. *Biochem. Pharmacol.*, 2007 74, 1029-1038.

[76] Lieberman, M.E.; Gorski, J.; Jordan, V.C. An estrogen receptor model to describe the regulation of prolactin synthesis by antiestrogens in vitro. *J. Biol. Chem.*, 1983 258, 4741 – 4745.

[77] Tate, A.C.; Greene, G.L.; DeSombre, E.R.; Jensen, E.V.; Jordan, V.C. Differences between estrogen- and antiestrogen receptor complexes from human breast tumors identified with an antibody raised against the estrogen receptor. *Cancer Res.*, 1984 44, 1012 – 1018.

[78] Kim, J.H.; Lee, M.H.; Kim, B.J.; Kim, J.H.; Han, S.J.; Kim, H.Y.; Stallcup, R. Role of aspartate 351 in transactivation and active conformation of estrogen receptor α. *J. Molec. Endocrinol.*, 2005 35, 449 – 464.

[79] Catherino, W.H.; Wolf, D.M.; Jordan, W.C. A naturally occurring estrogen receptor mutation results in increased estrogenicity of a tamoxifen analog. *Molec. Endocrinol.*, 1995 9, 1053 – 1063.

[80] Murphy, L.C.; Dotzlaw, H.; Leygue, E.; Douglas, D.; Coutts, A.; Watson, P.H. Estrogen receptor variants and mutations. *J. Steroid Biochem. Molec. Biol.*, 1997 62, 363 – 372.

[81] Levenson, A.S.; Catherino, W.H.; Jordan, V.C. Estrogenic activity is increased for an antiestrogen by a natural mutation of the estrogen receptor. *J. Steroid Biochem. Molec. Biol.*, 1997 60, 261 – 268.

[82] Roodi, N.; Bailey, R.; Kao, W.-Y.; Verrier, C.S.; Yee, C.J.; Dupont, W.D.; Parl, F.F. Estrogen receptor gene analysis in estrogen receptor-positive and receptor-negative primary breast cancer. *J. Natl. Cancer Inst.*, 1995 87, 446 – 451.

[83] Liu, H.; Park, W.-C.; Bentrem, D.J.; McKian, K.P.; De Los Reyes, A.; Loweth, J.A.; MacGregor Schafer, J.; Zapf, J.W.; Jordan, V.C. Structure-function relationships of the raloxifene-estrogen receptor-α complex for regulating transforming growth factor-α expression in breast cancer cells. *J. Biol. Chem.*, 2002 277, 9189 – 9198.

[84] Jordan, V.C. Antiestrogenic action of raloxifene and tamoxifen: today and tomorrow. *J. Natl. Cancer Inst.*, 1998 90, 967 – 971.

[85] Wolf, D.M.; Jordan, V.C. The estrogen receptor from a tamoxifen stimulated MCF-7 tumor variant contains a point of mutation in the ligand binding domain. *Breast Cancer Res. Treat.*, 1994 31, 129 – 138.

[86] Grese, T.A; Sluka, J.P.; Bryant, H.U.; Cullinan, G.J.; Glasebrook, A.L.; Jones, C.D.; Matsumoto, K.; Palkowitz, A.D.; Sato, M.; Termine, J.D.; Winter, M.A.; Yang, N.N.; Dodge, J.A. Molecular determinants of tissue selectivity in estrogen receptor modulators. *Proc. Natl. Acad. Sci. USA.*, 1997 94, 14105 – 14110.

[87] Levenson, A.S.; Jordan, V.C. The key to the antiestrogenic mechanism of raloxifene is amino acid 351 (aspartate) in the estrogen receptor, *Cancer Res.*, 1998 58, 1872 – 1875.

[88] Levenson, A.S.; Tonetti, D.A.; Jordan, V.C. The estrogen-like effect of 4-hydroxytamoxifen on induction of transforming growth factor alpha mRNA in MDA-MB-231 breast cancer cells stably expressing the estrogen receptor. *Br. J. Cancer*, 1998 77, 1812 – 1819.

[89] Zhao, C.; Abrams, J.; Skafar, D.F. Targeted mutation of key residues at the start of helix 12 in the hERα ligand-binding domain identifies the role of hydrogen-bonding and hydrophobic interactions in the activity of the protein. *J. Steroid Biochem. Molec. Biol.*, 2006 98, 1 – 11.

[90] Yamamoto, Y.; Wada, O.; Suzawa, M.; Yogiashi, Y.; Yano, T.; Kato, S.; Yanagisawa, J. The tamoxifen-responsive estrogen receptor α mutant D351Y shows reduced tamoxifen-dependent interaction with corepressor complexes. *J. Biol. Chem.*, 2001 276, 42684 – 42691.

[91] Pike, A.C.W.; Brzozowski, A.M.; Walton, J.; Hubbard, R.E.; Bonn, T.; Gustafsson, J.-Å.; Carlquist, M. Structural aspects of agonism and antagonism in the oestrogen receptor. *Biochem. Soc. Trans.*, 2000 28, 396 – 400.

[92] MacGregor Schafer, J.; Liu, H.; Bentrem, D.J.; Zapf, J.W.; Craig Jordan, V. Allosteric silencing of activating function 1 in the 4-hydroxytamoxifen estrogen receptor complex is induced by substituting glycine for aspartate at amino acid 351. *Cancer Res.*, 2000 60, 5097 – 5105.

[93] Bentrem, D.; Fox, J.E.; Pearce, S.T.; Liu, H.; Pappas, S.; Kupfer, D.; Zapf, J.W.; Jordan, V.C. Distinct molecular conformations of the estrogen receptor α complex exploited by environmental estrogens. *Cancer Res.*, 2003 63, 7490 – 7496.

[94] Rodriguez, A.L.; Tamrazi, A.; Collins, M.L.; Katzenellenbogen, J.A. Design, synthesis, and in vitro biological evaluation of small molecule inhibitors of estrogen receptor α coactivator binding. *J. Med. Chem.*, 2004 47, 600 – 611.

[95] Geistlinger, T.R.; McReynolds, A.C.; Guy, R.K. Ligand-selective inhibition of the interaction of steroid receptor coactivators and estrogen receptor isoforms. *Chem. Biol.*, 2004 11, 273 – 281.

[96] Wärnmark, A.; Treuter, E.; Gustafsson, J.-Å.; Hubbard, R.E.; Brzozowski, A.M.; Pike, A.C.W. Interaction of transcriptional intermediary factor 2 nuclear receptor box peptides with the coactivator binding site of estrogen receptor α. *J. Biol. Chem.*, 2002 277, 21862 – 21868.

[97] Jaber, B.M.; Gao, T.; Huang, L.; Karmakar, S.; Smith, C.L. The pure estrogen receptor antagonist ICI 182,780 promotes a novel interaction of estrogen receptor-α with the 3',5'-cyclic adenosine monophosphate response element-binding protein-binding protein / p300 coactivators. *Molec. Endocrinol.*, 2006 20, 2695 – 2710.

[98] Métivier, R.; Stark, A.; Flouriot, G.; Hübner, M.R.; Brand, H.; Penot, G.; Manu, D.; Denger, S.; Reid, G.; Kos, M.; Russel, R.B.; Kah, O.; Pakdel, F.; Gannon, F. A dynamic structural model for estrogen receptor-α activation by ligands, emphasizing the role of interactions between distant A and E domains. *Molec. Cell.*, 2002 10, 1019 – 1032.

[99] Zhou, D.; Ye, J.J.; Li, Y.; Lui, K.; Chen, S. The molecular basis of the interaction between the proline-rich SH3-binding motif of PNRC and estrogen receptor alpha. *Nucleic Acids Res.*, 2006 34, 5974 – 5986.

[100] Feng, W.J.; Ribeiro, R.C.J.; Wagner, Nguyen, H.; Aprilleti, J.W. Hormone-dependent coactivator binding to a hydrophobic cleft on nuclear receptors. *Science*, 1998 280, 1747 – 1749.

[101] Estébanez-Perpiná, E.; Arnold, A.A.; Nguyen, P.; Delgado Rodriguez, E.; Mar, E.; Bateman, R.; Pallai, P.; Shokat, K.M.; Baxter, J.D.; Guy, K.; Webb, P.; Fletterick, R.J. A surface of the androgen receptor that alloserically regulates coactivator binding. *Proc. Natl. Acad. Sci. USA*, 2007 104, 16074 – 16079.

[102] Kong, E.H.; Pike, A.C.W.; Hubbard, R.E. Structure and mechanism of the oestrogen receptor. *Biochem. Soc. Trans.*, 2003 31, 56 – 59.

[103] McInerney, E.M.; Ince, B.A.; Shapiro, D.J.; Katzenellenbogen, B.S. A transcriptionally active estrogen receptor mutant is a novel type of dominant negative inhibitor of estrogen action. *Molec. Endocrinol.*, 1996 10, 1519 – 1526.

[104] Kushner, P.J.; Agard, D.A.; Greene, G.L.; Scanlan, T.S.; Shiau, A.K.; Uht, R.M.; Webb, P. Estrogen receptor pathways to AP-1. *J. Steroid Biochem. Molec. Biol.*, 2000 74, 311-317.

[105] Awasthi, S.; Daverey, A.; Dwivedi, A. Modulation of AP-1 mediated estrogenic response by ormeloxifene in rat uterus. *J. Steroid Biochem. Molec. Biol.*, 2007 104, 208-214.

[106] Ludes-Meyers, J.H.; Liu, Y.; Muñoz-Medellin, D.; Hilsenbeck, S.G.; Brown, P.H. AP-1 blockade inhibits the growth of normal and malignant breast cells. *Oncogene*, 2001 20, 2771-2780.

[107] Smith, L.M.; Wise, S.C.; Hendricks, D.T.; Sabichi, A.L.; Bos, T.; Reddy, P.; Brown, P.H.; Birrer, M.J. cJun overexpression in MCF-7 breast cancer cells produces a tumorigenic, invasive and hormone resistant phenotype. *Breast Cancer Res.*, 1999 18, 6063-6070.

[108] Daschner, P.J.; Ciolino, H.P.; Plouzek, C.A.; Yeh, G.C. Increased AP-1 activity in drug resistant human breast cancer MCF-7 cells. *Breast Cancer Res. Treat.*, 1999 53, 229-240.

[109] Langer, S.; Singer, C.F.; Hudelist, G.; Dampier, B.; Kaserer, K.; Vinatzer, U.; Pehamberger, H.; Zielinski, C.; Kubista, E.; Schreibner, M. Jun and Fos family protein expression in human breast cancer: correlation of protein expression and clinicopathological parameters. *Eur. J. Gynecol. Oncol.*, 2006 27, 345-352.

[110] Pakdel, F.; Reese, J.C.; Katzenellenbogen, B.S. Identification of charged residues in an N-terminal portion of the hormone-binding domain of the human-estrogen receptor important in transcriptional activity of the receptor. *Molec. Endocrinol.*, 1993 7, 1408-1417.

[111] Gangloff, M.; Ruff, M.; Eiler, S.; Duclaud, S.; Wurtz, J.-M.; Moras, D. Crystal structure of a mutant hERα ligand-binding domain reveals key structural features for the mechanism of partial agonism. *J. Biol. Chem.*, 2001 276, 15059 – 15065.

[112] Katzenellenbogen, B.S.; Fang, H.; Ince, B.A.; Pakdel, F.; Reese, J.C.; Wooge, C.H.; Wrenn, C.K. Estrogen receptors: ligand discrimination and antiestrogen action. *Breast Cancer Res. Treat.*, 1993 27, 17 – 26.

[113] Reese, J.J.; Wooge, C.H.; Katzenellenbogen, B.S. Identification of two cysteines closely positioned in the ligand-binding pocket of the human estrogen receptor: roles in ligand binding and transcriptional activation. *Molec. Endocrinol.*, 1992 6, 2160 – 2166.

[114] Stoica, A.; Katzenellenbogen, B.S.; Martin, M.B. Activation of estrogen receptor-alpha by the heavy metal cadmium. *Molec. Endocrinol.*, 2000 14, 545 – 553.

[115] Top, S.; El Haffa, H.; Vessières, A.; Quivy, J.; Vaissermann, J.; Hughes, D.W.; McGlinchey, M.J.; Mornon, J.-P.; Thoreau, E.; Jaouen, G. Rhenium carbonyl complexes of β-estradiol derivatives with high affinity for the estradiol receptor: An approach to selective organometallic radiopharmaceuticals. *J. Am. Chem. Soc.*, 1995 117, 8372 – 8380.

[116] Veselik, D.J.; Divekar, S.; Dakshanamurthy, S.; Storchan, G.B.; Turner, J.M.A.; Graham, K.L.; Huang, L.; Stoica, A.; Martin, M.B. Activation of estrogen receptor-α by the anion nitrite. *Cancer Res.*, 2008 68, 3950-3958.

[117] Gallinari, P.; Lahm, A.; Koch, U.; Paolini, C.; Nardi, M.C.; Roscilli, G.; Kinzel, O.; Fattori, D.; Muraglia, E.; Toniatti, S.; Cortese, R.; De Francesco, R.; Ciliberto, G. A functionally orthogonal estrogen receptor-based transcription switch specifically induced by a nonsteroid synthetic ligand. *Chem. Biol.*, 2005 12, 883 – 893.

[118] Jiang, S.Y.; Parker, C.J.; Jordan, V.C. A model to describe how a point mutation of the estrogen receptor alters the structure-function relationship of antiestrogens. *Breast Cancer Res. Treat.*, 1993 26, 139 – 147.

[119] Aliau, S.; El Garrouj, D.; Yasri, A.; Katzenellenbogen, B.S.; Borgna, J.-L. 17α-(haloacetamidoalkyl)estradiols alkylate the human estrogen receptor at cysteine residues 417 and 530. *Biochemistry*, 1997 36, 5861 – 5867.

[120] Mattras, H.; Aliau, S.; Demey, E.; Poncet, J.; Borgna, J.-L. Mass spectrometry identification of covalent attachment sites of two related estrogenic ligands on human estrogen receptor α. *J. Steroid Biochem. Molec. Biol.*, 2006 98, 236 – 247.

[121] Bhat, R.A.; Stauffer, B.; Unwalla, R.J.; Xu, Z.; Harris, H.A.; Komm, B.S. Molecular determinants of ERα and ERβ involved in selectivity of 16α-iodo-17β estradiol. *J. Steroid Biochem. Molec. Biol.*, 2004 88, 17 – 26.

[122] Acconcia, F.; Bocedi, A.; Ascenzi, P.; Marino, M. Does palmitoylation target estrogen receptors to plasma membrane caveolae? IUBM Life, 2003 55,33-35.

[123] Marino, M.; Ascenzi, P.; Acconcia, F. S-palmitoylation modulates estrogen receptor-α localization and functions. *Steroids*, 2006 71, 298 – 303.

[124] Marino, M.; Ascenzi, P.; Bocedi, A.; Spisni, E.; Tomasi, V.; Trentalance, A.; Visca, P.; Maino, M. Palmitoylation-dependent estrogen receptor α membrane localization: regulation by 17β-estradiol. *Molec. Biol. Cell*, 2006 16, 231 – 237.

[125] Acconcia, F.; Ascenzi, P.; Fabozzi, G.; Visca, P.; Marino, M. S-palmitoyaltion modulates human estrogen receptor-α functions. *Biochem. Biophys. Res. Comm.*, 2004 316, 878 – 883.

[126] Reese, J.C.; Katzenellenbogen, B. Mutagenesis of cysteines in the hormone binding domain of the human estrogen receptor. *J. Biol. Chem.*, 1991 266, 10880 – 10887.

[127] Reese, J.C.; Katzenellenbogen, B.S. Characterization of a temperature-sensitive mutant in the hormone binding domain of the human estrogen receptor. Studies in cell extracts and intact cells and their implications for hormone-dependent transcriptional activation. *J. Biol. Chem.*, 1992 267, 9868 – 9873.

[128] Ekena, K.; Weis, K.E.; Katzenellenbogen, J.A.; Katzenellenbogen, B.S. Different residues of the human estrogen receptor are involved in the recognition of structurally diverse estrogens and antiestrogens. *J. Biol. Chem.*, 1997 272, 5069 – 5075.

[129] Maaroufi, Y.; Cleeren, A.; Leclercq, G. Inhibition of estradiol binding to its receptor by the cupric ion. *J. Biol. Inorg. Chem.*, 1998 3, 508-514.

[130] Martin, M.B.; Reiter, R.; Pham, T.; Avellanet, Y.R.; Camara, J.; Lahm, M.; Pentecost, E.; Pratap, K.; Gilmore, B.A.; Divekar, S.; Dagata, R.S.; Bull, J.L.; Stoica, A. Estrogen-like activity of metals in MCF-7 breast cancer cells. *Endocrinology*, 2003 144, 2425-2436.

[131] Ekena, K.; Weis, K.E.; Katzenellenbogen, J.A.; Katzenellenbogen, B.S. Identification of amino acids in the hormone binding domain of the human estrogen receptor important in estrogen binding. *J. Biol. Chem.*, 1996 271, 20053 – 20059.

[132] Danielian, P.S.; White, R.; Hoare, S.A.; Fawell, S.E.; Parker, M.G. Identification of residues in estrogen receptor that confer differential sensitivity to estrogen and hydroxytamoxifen. *Molec. Endocrinol.*, 1993 7, 232 – 240.

[133] Littlewood, T.D.; Hancock, D.C.; Danielian, P.S.; Parker, M.G.; Evan, G.I. A modified oestrogen receptor ligand-binding domain as an improved switch for the regulation of heterologous proteins. *Nucleic Acids Res.*, 1995 23, 1686 – 1690.

[134] Paulmurugan, R.; Tamrazi, A.; Katzenellenbogen, J.A.; Katzenellenbogen, B.S.; Gambhir, S.S. A human estrogen receptor (ER)α mutation with differential responsiveness to non steroidal ligands: novel approaches for studying mechanism of ER action. *Molec. Endocrinol.*, 2008 22, 1552-1564.

[135] Celik, L.; Lund, J.D.D.; Schiott, B. Conformational dynamics of the estrogen receptor α: molecular dynamics simulations of the influence of binding site structure on protein dynamics. *Biochemistry*, 2007 46, 1743-1758.

[136] Seo, H.-S.; DeNardo, D.G.; Jacquot, Y.; Laïos, I.; Salazar Vidal, D.; Rojas Zambrana, C.; Leclercq, G.; Brown, P.H. Stimulatory effect of genistein and apigenin on the

growth of breast cancer cells correlates with their ability to activate ER alpha. *Breast Cancer Res. Treat.*, 2006 99, 121 – 134.

[137] Aliau, S.; Mattras, H.; Richard, E.; Bonnafous, J.-C.; Borgna, J.-L. Differential interactions of estrogens and antiestrogens at the 17β-hydroxyl or counterpart hydroxyl with histidine 524 of the human estrogen receptor α. *Biochemistry*, 2002 41, 7979 – 7988.

[138] Leclercq, G.; Lacroix, M.; Laïos, I.; Laurent, G. Estrogen receptor alpha: impact of ligands on intracellular shuttling and turnover rate in breast cancer cells. *Curr. Cancer Drugs Targets*, 2006 6, 561 571.

[139] Aliau, S.; Mattras, H.; Borgna, J.-L. Identification of covalent attachment site of antiestrogenic estradiol 11β-derivatives on human estrogen receptor α ligand-binding domain. *J. Steroid Biochem. Molec. Biol.*, 2006 98, 111 – 121.

[140] Yudt, M.R.; Vorojeikina, D.V.; Zhong, L.; Skafar, D.F.; Sasson, F.; Gasiewicz, T.A.; Notides, A.C. Function of estrogen receptor tyrosine 537 in hormone binding, DNA binding, and transactivation. *Biochemistry*, 1999 38, 14146 – 14156.

[141] Harlow, K.W.; Smith, D.N.; Katzenellenbogen, J.A.; Greene, G.L.; Katzenellenbogen, B.S. Identification of cysteine 530 as the covalent attachment site of an affinity-labeling estrogen (ketononestrol aziridine) and antiestrogen (tamoxifen aziridine) in the human estrogen receptor. *J. Biol. Chem.*, 1989 264, 17476 – 17485.

[142] Aliau, S.; Mattras, H.; Richard, E.; Borgna, J.L. Cysteine 530 of the human estrogen receptor α is the main covalent attachment site of 11β-(aziridinylalkoxy-phenyl)estradiols. *Biochemistry*, 1999 38, 14752 – 14762.

[143] Zhang, Q.X.; Borg, A.; Wolf D.M.; Oesterreich, S.; Fuqua, S.A. An estrogen receptor mutant with strong hormone-independent activity from a mestastatic breast cancer. *Cancer Res.*, 1997 57, 1244 – 1249.

[144] Zhao, C.; Koide, A.; Abrams, J.; Deighton-Collins, S.; Martinez, A.; Schwartz, J.A.; Koide, S.; Skafar, D.F. Mutation of Leu-536 in human estrogen receptor-α alters the coupling between ligand binding, transcription activation, and receptor conformation. *J. Biol. Chem.*, 2003 278, 27278 – 27286.

[145] Skafar, D.F. Formation of a powerful capping motif corresponding to start of helix "H12" in agonist-bound estrogen receptor-α contributes to increased constitutive activity of the protein. *Cell Biochem. Biophys.*, 2000 33, 53 – 62.

[146] Brzozowski, A.M.; Pike, A.C.W.; Dauter, Z.; Hubbard, R.E.; Bonn, T.; Engstrom, O.; Ohman, L.; Greene, G.L.; Gustafsson, J.-Å.; Carlquist, M. Molecular basis of agonism and antagonism in the oestrogen receptor. *Nature*, 1997 389, 753 – 758.

[147] Eng, F.C.S.; Lee, H.S.; Ferrara, J.; Willson, T.M.; White, J.H. Probing the structure and function of the estrogen receptor ligand binding domain by analysis of mutants with altered transactivation characteristics. *Molec. Cell. Biol.*, 1997 17, 4644 – 4653.

[148] Zhong, L.; Skafar, D.F. Mutations of Tyrosine 537 in the human estrogen receptor-α selectively alter the receptor's affinity for estradiol and the kinetics of the interaction. *Biochemistry*, 41 2002, 4209 – 4217.

[149] Carlson, K.E.; Choi, I.; Gee, A.; Katzenellenbogen, B.S.; Katzenellenbogen, J.A. Altered ligand binding properties and enhanced stability of a constitutively active

estrogen receptor: evidence that an open pocket conformation is required for ligand interaction. *Biochemistry*, 1997 36, 14897 – 14905.

[150] Arnold, S.F.; Melamed, M.; Vorojeikina, D.P.; Notides, A.C.; Sasson, S. Estradiol-binding mechanism and binding capacity of the human estrogen receptor is regulated by tyrosine phosphorylation. *Molec. Endocrinol.*, 1997 11, 48 – 53.

[151] Arnold, S.F.; Notides, A.C. An antiestrogen: a phosphotyrosyl peptide that blocks dimerization of the human estrogen receptor. *Proc. Natl. Acad. Sci. USA*, 1995 92, 7475 – 7479.

[152] Migliaccio, A.; Piccolo, D.; Castoria, G.; Di domenico, M.; Bilancio, A.; Lombardi, M.; Gong, W.; Beato, M.; Auricchio, F. Activation of the Src / p21ras / Erk pathway by progesterone receptor via cross-talk with estrogen. *EMBO J.*, 1998 17, 2008 – 2018.

[153] Barletta, F.; Wong, C.-W.; McNally, C.; Komm, B.S.; Katzenellenbogen, B.; Cheskis, B. Characterization of the interactions of estrogen receptor and MNAR in the activation of cSRC. *Molec. Endocrinol.*, 2004 18, 1096 – 1108.

[154] Tremblay, G.B.; Tremblay, A.; Labrie, F.; Giguere, V. Ligand-independent activation of the estrogen receptors α and β by mutations of a conserved tyrosine can be abolished by antiestrogens. *Cancer Res.*, 1998 58, 877 – 881.

[155] Migliaccio, A.; Castoria, G.; Di Domenico, M.; de Falco, A.; Bilancio, A.; Lombardi, M.; Barone, M.V.; Ametrano, D.; Zannini, M.S.; Abbondanza, C.; Auricchio, F. Steroid-induced androgen receptor-oestradiol receptor β-Src complex triggers prostate cancer cell proliferation. *EMBO J.*, 2000 19, 5406 – 5417.

[156] Arnold, S.F.; Vorojeikina, D.P.; Notides, A.C. Phosphorylation of tyrosine 537 on the human estrogen receptor is required for binding to an estrogen response element. *J. Biol. Chem.*, 1995 270, 30205 – 30212.

[157] Auricchio, F.; Migliaccio, A.; Castoria, C.; Rotondi, A.; Lastoria, S. Direct evidence of in vitro phosphorylation dephosphorylation of the estradiol-17β receptor. Role of Ca^{2+}-calmodulin in the activation of hormone binding sites. *J. Steroid Biochem.*, 1985 20, 31 – 35.

[158] McGee, T.D.; Edwards, J.; Roitberg, A.E. Preliminary molecular dynamics simulations of the estrogen receptor alpha ligand binding domain from antagonist to apo. *Int. J. Environ. Res. Public Health.*, 2008 5, 111-114.

[159] Arnold, S.F.; Obourn, J.D.; Jaffe, H. Notides, A.C. Phosphorylation of the human estrogen receptor on tyrosine 537 in vivo and by Src family tyrosine kinases in vitro. *Molec. Endocrinol.*, 1995 9, 24 – 33.

[160] Lannigan, D.A. Estrogen receptor phosphorylation. *Steroids*, 2003 68, 1 – 9.

[161] Weis, K.E.; Ekena, K.; Thomas, J.A.; Lazennec, G.; Katzenellenbogen, B.S. Constitutively active human estrogen receptors containing amino acid substitutions for tyrosine 537 in the receptor protein. *Molec. Endocrinol.*, 1996 10, 1388 – 1398.

[162] Kohler, M.F.; Berkholz, A.; Risinger, J.I.; Elbendary, A.; Boyd, J.; Berchuck, A. Mutational analysis of the estrogen-receptor gene in endometrial carcinoma. *Obstet. Gynecol.*, 1995 86, 33 – 37.

[163] Voegel, J.J.; Heine, M.J.S.; Zechel, C.; Chambon, P.; Gronemeyer, H. TIF2, a 160 kDa transcriptional mediator for the ligand-dependent activation function AF-2 of nuclear receptors. *EMBO J.*, 1996 15, 3667 – 3675.

[164] Tremblay, A.; Tremblay, G.B.; Labrie, E.; Giguère, V. Ligand-independent recruitment of SRC-1 by estrogen receptor through phosphorylation of activation function AF-1. *Molec. Cell*, 1999 3, 513 – 519.

[165] Wrenn, CK; Katzenellenbogen, B.S. Structure-function analysis of the hormone binding domain of the human estrogen receptor by region-specific mutagenesis and phenotypic screening in yeast. *J. Biol. Chem.*, 1993 268, 24089 – 24098.

[166] Ince, B.A.; Zhuang, Y.; Wrenn, C.K.; Shapiro, D.J.; Katzenellenbogen, B.S. Powerful dominant negative mutants of the human estrogen receptor. *J. Biol. Chem.*, 1993 268, 14026 – 14032.

[167] Montano, M.M.; Ekena, M.; Krueger, K.D.; Keller, A.L.; Katzenellenbogen, B.S. Human estrogen receptor ligand activity inversion mutants: receptors that interpret antiestrogens as estrogens and estrogens as antiestrogens and discriminate among different antiestrogens. *Molec. Endocrinol.* 1996 10, 230 – 242.

[168] Ince, B.A.; Schodin, D.J.; Shapiro, D.J.; Katzenellenbogen, B.S. Repression of endogenous estrogen receptor activity in MCF-7 human breast cancer cells by dominant negative estrogen receptors. *Endocrinology*, 1995 136, 3194 – 3199.

[169] Lee, E.J.; Jakacka, M.; Duan, W.R.; Chien, P.Y.; Martinson, F.; Gehm, B.D.; Jameson, J.L. Adenovirus-directed expression of dominant negative estrogen receptor induces apoptosis in breast cancer cells and regression of tumors in nude mice. *Molec. Biol.*, 2001 7, 773 – 782.

[170] Montano, M.M.; Muller, V.; Trobaugh, A.; Katzenellenbogen, B.S. The carboxy-terminal F domain of the human estrogen receptor: role in the transcriptional activity of the receptor and the effectiveness of antiestrogens as estrogen antagonists. *Molec. Endocrinol.*, 1995 9, 814-825.

[171] Schwartz, J.A.; Zhong, L.; Deighton-Collins, S.; Zhao, C.; Skafar, D.F. Mutations targeted to a predicted helix in the extreme carboxyl-terminal region of the human estrogen receptor-α alter its response to estradiol and 4-hydroxytamoxifen. *J. Biol. Chem.*, 2002 277, 13202-13209.

[172] Kim, K.; Thu, N.; Saville, B.; Safe, S. Domains of estrogen receptor α (ERα) required for ERα/Sp1-mediated activation of GC-rich promoters by estrogens and antiestrogens in breast cancer cells. *Molec. Endocrinol.*, 2003 17, 804-817.

[173] Peters, G.A.; Khan, S.A. Estrogen receptor domains E and F: role in dimerization and interaction with coactivator RIP-140. *Molec. Endocrinol.*, 1999 13, 286-296.

[174] Koide, A.; Abbatiello, S.; Rothgery, L.; Koide, S. Probing protein conformational changes in living cells by using designer binding proteins: Application to the estrogen receptor. *Proc. Natl. Acad. Sci. USA*, 2002 99, 1253-1258.

[175] Koide, A.; Zhao, C.; Naganuma, M.; Abrams, J.; Deighton-Collins, S.; Skafar, D.F.; Koide, S. Identification of regions within the F domain of the human estrogen receptor α that are important for modulating transactivation and protein-protein interactions. *Molec. Endocrinol.*, 2007 21, 829-842.

[176] Yang, J.; Singleton, D.W.; Shaughnessy, E.A.; Khan, S.A. The F-domain of estrogen receptor-alpha inhibits ligand-induced receptor dimerization. *Molec. Cell. Endocrinol.*, 2008 (*in press*).

[177] Puigserver, P.; Wu, Z.; Park, C.W.; Graves, R.; Wright, M.; Spiegelman, B.M. A cold-inducible coactivator of nuclear receptors linked to adaptive thermogenesis. *Cell*, 1998 92, 829 – 839.

[178] Puigserver, P.; Spiegelman, B.M. Peroxisome proliferator-activated receptor-gamma coactivator 1 alpha (PGC-1 alpha): transcriptional coactivator and metabolic regulator. *Endocrinol. Rev.*, 2003 24, 78 – 90.

[179] Nichols, M.; Rientjes, J.M.J.; Stewart, A.F. Different positioning of the ligand-binding domain helix 12 and the F domain of the estrogen receptor accounts for functional differences between agonists and antagonists. *EMBO J.*, 1998 17, 765-773.

[180] Kojetin, D.J.; Burris, T.P.; Jensen, E.V.; Khan, S.A. Implications of the binding of tamoxifen to the coactivator recognition site of the estrogen receptor. *Endocrine-Related Cancer*, 2008 (*in press*).

[181] Jiang, M.S.; Hart, G.W. A subpopulation of estrogen receptors are modified by O-linked *N*-acetylglucosamine. *J. Biol. Chem.*, 1997 272, 2421 – 2428.

[182] Rechsteiner, M.; Rogers, S.W. PEST sequences and regulation by proteolysis. *Trends Biochem. Sci.*, 1996 21, 267 – 271.

[183] Rosenfeld, M.G.; Lunyak, V.V.; Glass, C.K. Sensors and signals: a coactivator/corepressor/epigenetic code for integrating signal-dependent programs of transcriptional response. *Genes Dev.*, 2006 20, 1405-1428.

[184] Kraus, W.L.; Kadonaga, J.T. P300 and estrogen receptor cooperatively activate transcription via differential enhancement of initiation and reinitiation. *Genes Dev.*, 1998 12, 331-342.

[185] Nilsson, S.; Mäkelä, S.; Treuter, E.; Tujague, M.; Thomsen, J.; Andersson, G.; Enmark, E.; Petterson, K.; Warner, M.; Gustafsson, J.-Å. Mechanisms of estrogen action. *Physiol. Rev.*, 2001 81, 1535-1565.

[186] Horwitz, K.B.; Jackson, T.A.; Bain, D.L.; Richer, J.K.; Takimoto, G.S.; Tung, L. Nuclear receptor coactivators and corepressors. *Molec. Endocrinol.*, 1996 10, 1167-1177.

[187] Glass, C.K.; Rose, D.W.; Rosenfeld, M.G. Nuclear receptor coactivators. *Curr. Opin. Cell Biol.*, 1997 9, 222-232.

[188] McKenna, N.J.; Xu, J.; Nawaz, Z.; Tsai, S.Y.; Tsai, M.-J.; O'Malley, B.W. Nuclear receptor coactivators: multiple enzyme, multiple complexes, multiple functions. *J. Steroid. Biochem. Molec. Biol.*, 1999 69, 3-12.

[189] Chakravarti, D.; LaMorte, V.; Nelson, M.; Nakajima, T.; Schulman, I.; Juguilon, H.; Montminy, M.; Evans, R. Role of CBP/P300 in nuclear receptor signalling. *Nature*, 1996 383, 99-103.

[190] Hanstein, B.; Eckner, R.; DiRenzo, J.; Halachmi, S.; Liu, H.; Searcy, B.; Kurokawa, R.; Brown, M. p300 is a component of an estrogen receptor coactivator complex. *Proc. Natl. Acad. Sci. USA*, 1996 93, 11540-11545.

[191] Onate, S.A.;Tsai, S.Y.; Tsai, M.-J.; O'Malley, B.W. Sequence and characterization of a coactivator for the steroid hormone receptor superfamily. *Science*, 1995 270, 1354-1357.

[192] Kamei, Y.; Xu, L.; Heinzel, T.; Torchia, J.; Kurokawa, R.; Gloss, B.; Lin, S.C.; Heyman, R.A.; Rose, D.W.; Glass, C.K.; Rosenfled, M.G. A CBP integrator complex

mediates transcriptional activation and AP-1 inhibition by nuclear receptor coactivator. *Cell*, 1996 85, 403-414.

[193] Takeshita, A.; Yen, P.M.; Misiti, S.; Cardona, G.R.; Liu, Y.; Chin, W.W. Molecular cloning and properties of a full-length putative thyroid hormone receptor coactivator. *Endocrinology*, 1996 137, 3594-3597.

[194] McInerney, E.M.; Rose, D.W.; Flynn, S.E.; Westin, S.; Mullen, T.-M.; Krones, A.; Inostroza, J.; Torchia, J.; Notle, R.T.; Assa-Munt, N.; Milburn, M.V.; Glass, C.K.; Rosenfeld, M.G. Determinants of coactivator LXXLL motif specificity in nuclear receptor transcriptional activation. *Gene Dev.*, 1998 12, 3357-3368.

[195] McKenna, N.J.; Lanz, R.B.; O'Malley, B.W. Nuclear receptor coregulators: cellular and molecular biology. *Endocr. Rev.*, 1999 20, 321-344.

[196] Bramlett, K.S.; Wu, Y.; Burris, T.P. Ligands specificy coactivator nuclear receptor (NR) box affinity for estrogen receptor subtypes. *Molec. Endocrinol.*, 2001 15, 909-922.

[197] Schwartz, J.A.; Brooks, S.C. Changes in the structure of the ligand or substitutions to AF2 residues in the estrogen receptor make independent contributions to coactivator sensitivity by SRC-1. *J. Steroid. Biochem. Molec. Biol.*, 1998 67, 223-232.

[198] Torchia, J.; Rose, D.W.; Inostroza, J.; Kamei, Y.; Westin, S.; Glass, C.K.; Rosenfeld, M.G. The transcriptional co-activator p/CIP binds CBP and mediates nuclear-receptor function. *Nature*, 1997 387, 677-684.

[199] Anzick, S.L.; Kononen, J.; Walker, R.L.; Azorsa, D.O.; Tanner, M.M.; Guan, X.Y.; Sauter, G.; Kallioniemi, O.P.; Trent, J.M.; Meltzer, P.S. AIB1, a steroid receptor coactivator amplified in breast and ovarian cancer. *Science*, 1997 277, 965-968.

[200] Hong, H.; Kohli, K.; Trivedi, A.; Johnson, D.L.; Stallcup, M.R. GRIP1, a novel mouse protein that serves as a transcriptional coactivator in yeast for the hormone binding domains of steroid receptors. *Proc. Natl. Acad. Sci. USA*, 1996 93, 4948-4952.

[201] Hong, H.; Kohli, K.; Garabedian, M.; Stallcup, M. GRIP1, a transcriptional coactivator for the AF-2 transactivation domain of steroid, thyroid, retinoid, and vitamin D receptors. *Molec. Cell. Biol.*, 1997 17, 2735-2744.

[202] Ing, N.H.; Beekman, J.M.; Tsai, S.Y.; Tsai, M.-J.; O'Malley, B.W. Members of the steroid hormone receptor superfamily interact with TFIIB (S300-II). *J. Biol. Chem.*, 1992 267, 17617-17623.

[203] Jacq, X.; Brou, C.; Lutz, Y.; Davidson, I.; Chambon, P.; Tora, L. Human TAFII30 is present in a distinct TFIID complex and is required for transcriptional activation by the estrogen receptor. *Cell*, 1994 79, 107-117.

[204] Nawaz, Z.; Lonard, D.M.; Smith, C.L.; Lev-Lehman, E.; Tsai, S.Y.; Tsai, M.-J.; O'Malley, B.W.The Angelman syndrome-associated protein, E6-AP, is a co-activator for the nuclear hormone receptor superfamily. *Molec. Cell. Biol.*, 1999 19, 1182-1189.

[205] vom Baur, E.; Harbers, M.; Um, S.J.; Benecke, A.; Chambon, P.; Losson, R. The yeast Ada complex mediates the ligand-dependent activation function AF-2 of retinoid X and estrogen receptors. *Genes Dev.*, 1998 12, 1278-1289.

[206] Zeiner, M.; Gehring, U. A protein that interacts with members of the nuclear hormone receptor family: identification of cDNA cloning. *Proc. Natl. Acad. Sci. USA*, 1995 92, 11465-11469.

[207] Endoh, H.; Maruyama, K.; Masuhiro, Y.; Kobayashi, Y.; Goto, M.; Tai, H.; Yanagisawa, J.; Metzger, D.; Hashimoto, S.; Kato, S. Purification and identification of p68 RNA helicase acting as a transcriptional co-activator specific for the activation function 1 of human estrogen receptor alpha. *Molec. Cell. Biol.*, 1999 19, 5363-5372.

[208] Yeh, S.; Chang, C. Cloning and characterization of a specific co-activator, ARA70, for the androgen receptor in human prostate cells. *Proc. Natl. Acad. Sci. USA*, 1997 93, 5517-5521.

[209] Jackson, T.A.; Richer, J.K.; Bain, D.L.; Takimoto, G.S.; Tung, I.; Horwitz, K.B. The partial agonist activity of antagonist-occupied steroid receptors is controlled by a novel hinge domain-binding co-activator L7/SPA and the co-repressors N-CoR or SMRT. *Molec. Endocrinol.*, 1997 11, 693-705.

[210] Zhu, Y.; Qi, C.; Jain, S. Amplification and overexpression of peroxisome proliferator-activated receptor binding protein (PBP/PPARBP) gene in breast cancer. *Proc. Natl. Acad. Sci. USA*, 1999 96, 10848-10853.

[211] Cavailles, V.; Dauvois, S.; L'Horset, F.; Lopez, G.; Hoarc, S.; Kushner, P.J.; Parker, M.G. Nuclear receptor RIP 140 modulates transcriptional activation by the estrogen receptor. *EMBO J.*, 1995 14, 3741-3751.

[212] Treuter, E.; Albrektsen, T.; Johansson, L.; Leers, J.; Gustafsson, J.-Å. A regulatory role of RIP-140 in nuclear receptor activation. *Molec. Endocrinol.*, 1998 12, 864-881.

[213] Baniahmad, C.; Nawaz, Z.; Baniahmad, A.; Gleeson, M.A.G.; Tsai, M.-J.; O'Malley, B.W. Enhancement of human estrogen receptor activity by SPT6: a potential co-activator. *Molec. Endocrinol.*, 1995 9, 34-43.

[214] Lanz, R.B.; McKenna, N.J.; Onate, S.A.; Albrecht, U.; Wong, J.; Tsai, S.Y.; Tsai, M.-J.; O'Malley, B.W. A steroid receptor co-activator, SRA, functions as an RNA and is present in an SRC-1 complex. *Cell*, 1999 97, 17-27.

[215] Yoshinaga, S.K.; Peterson, C.L.; Herskowitz, I.; Yamamoto, K.R. Roles of SWI1, SWI2, and SWI3 proteins for transcriptional enhancement by steroid receptors. *Science*, 1992 258, 1598-1604.

[216] Belandia, B.; Orford, R.L.; Hurst, H.C.; Parker, M.G. Targeting of SWI/SNF chromatin remodelling complexes to estrogen-responsive genes. *EMBO J.*, 2002 21, 4094-4103.

[217] vom Baur, E.; Zechel, C.; Heery, D.; Heine, M.J.; Garnier, J.M.; Vivat, V.; Le Douarin, B.; Gronemeyer, H.; Chambon, P.; Losson, R. Differential ligand-dependent interactions between the AF-2 activating domain of the nuclear receptors and the putative transcriptional intermediary factors mSUG1 and TIF1. *EMBO J.*, 1996 15, 110-124.

[218] Masuyama, H.; Hiramatsu, Y. Involvement of suppressor for Gal 1 in the ubiquitin/proteasome-mediated degradation of estrogen receptors. *J. Biol. Chem.*, 2004 279, 12020-12026.

[219] Wärnmark, A.; Almlöf, T.; Leers, J.; Gustafsson, J.-Å.; Treuter, E. Differential recruitment of the mammalian subunit TRAP220 by estrogen receptors ERα and ERβ. *J. Biol. Chem.*, 2001 276, 23397-23404.

[220] Brady, M.E.; Ozanne, D.M.; Gaughan, L., Waite, I.; Cook, S.; Neal, D.E.; Robson, C.N. Tip60 is a nuclear hormone receptor co-activator. *J. Biol. Chem.*, 1999 274, 17599-17604.

[221] Le Douarin, B.; You, J.; Nielsen, A.L.; Chambon, P.; Losson, R. TIF1a: a possible link between KRAB zinc finger proteins and nuclear receptors. *J. Steroid. Biochem. Molec. Biol.*, 1998 65, 43-50.

[222] Ding, L.; Yan, J.; Zhu, J.; Zhong, H.; Lu, Q.; Wang, Z.; Huang, C.; Ye, Q. Ligand-independent activation of estrogen receptor α by XBP-1. *Nucleic Acids Res.*, 2003 31, 5266-5274.

[223] Vadlamudi, R.K.; Kumar, R. Functional and biological properties of the nuclear receptor coregulator PELP1/MNAR. *Nucl. Recept. Signal.*, 2007 5, e004.

[224] Vadlamudi, R.K.; Balasenthil, S.; Broaddus, R.R.; Gustafsson, J.-Å.; Kumar, R. Deregulation of estrogen receptor coactivator proline-, glutamic acid-, and leucine-rich protein-1/modulator of nongenomic activity of estrogen receptor in human endometrial tumors. *J. Clin. Endocrinol.*, 2004 89, 6130-6138.

[225] Greger, J.G.; Guo, Y.; Henderson, R.; Ross, J.F.; Cheskis, B.J. Characterization of MNAR expression. *Steroids*, 2006 71, 317-322.

[226] Zhou, D.; Quach, K.M.; Yang, C.; Lee, S.Y.; Pohajdak, B.; Chen, S. PNRC: A proline-rich nuclear receptor coregulatory protein that modulates transcriptional activation of multiple nuclear receptors including orphan receptors SF1 (steroidogenic factor 1) and ERRα1 (estrogen reclated receptor α-1). *Molec. endocrinol.*, 2000 14, 986-998.

[227] Zhou, D.; Chen, S. PNRC2 is a 16 kDa coactivator that interacts with nuclear receptors through an SH3-binding motif. *Nucleic Acids Res.*, 2001 29, 3939-2948.

[228] Lavinsky, R.M.; Jepsen, K.; Heinzel, T.; Torchia, J.; Mullen, T.M.; Schiff, R.; Del-Rio, A.L.; Ricote, M.; Ngo, S.; Gemsch, J.; Hilsenbeck, S.G.; Osborne, C.K.; Glass, C.K.; Rosenfeld, M.G.; Rose, D.W. Diverse signaling pathways modulate nuclear receptor recruitment of N-Cor and SMRT complexes. *Proc. Natl. Acad. Sci. USA*, 1998 95, 2920-2925.

[229] Dobrzycka, K.M.; Townson, S.M.; Jiang, S.; Oesterreich, S. Estrogen receptor corepressors – a role in human breast cancer? *Endocrine-Related Cancer*, 2003 10, 517-536.

[230] Smith, C.L.; Nawaz, Z.; O'Malley, B.W. Coactivator and corepressor regulation of the agonist/antagonist activity of the mixed antiestrogen, 4-hydroxytamoxifen. *Molec. Endocrinol.*, 1997 11, 657-666.

[231] Montano, M.M.; Ekena, M.; Delage-Mourroux, R.; Chang, W.; Martini, P.; Katzenellenbogen, B.S. An estrogen receptor-selective co-regulator that potentiates the effectiveness of antiestrogens and represses the activity of estrogens. *Proc. Natl. Acad. Sci. USA*, 1999 96, 6947-6952.

[232] Fan, S.; Wang, J.; Yuan, R.; Ma, Y.; Meng, Q.; Erdos, M.R.; Pestell, R.G.; Yuan, F.; Auborn, K.J.; Goldberg, I.D.; Rosen, E.M. BRCA1 inhibition of estrogen receptor signaling in transfected cells. *Science*, 1999 284, 1354-1356.

[233] Eakin, C.M.; MacCoss, M.J.; Finney, G.L.; Klevit, R.E. Estrogen receptor α is a putative substrate for the BRCA1 ubiquitin ligase. *Proc. Natl. Acad. Sci. USA*, 2007 104, 5794-5799.

[234] Johansson, L.; Thomsen, J.S.; Damdimopoulos, A.E.; Spyrou, G. Gustafsson, J-Å., Treuter, E. The orphan nuclear receptor SHP inhibits agonist-dependent transcriptional activity of estrogen receptors ERalpha and ERbeta. *J. Biol. Chem.*, 1999 274, 345-353.

[235] Shi, Y.; Downes, M.; Xie, W.; Kao, H.Y.; Ordentlich, P.; Tsai, C.C.; Hon, M.; Evans, R.M. Sharp, an inducible cofactor that integrates nuclear receptor repression and activation. *Genes Dev.*, 2001 15, 1140-1151.

[236] Oesterreich, S.; Zhang, Q.; Hopp, T.; Fuqua, S.A.; Michaelis, M.; Zhao, H.H.; Davie, J.R.; Osborne, C.K.; Lee, A.V. Tamoxifen-bound estrogen receptor (ER) strongly interacts with the nuclear matrix protein HET/SAF-B, a novel inhibitor of ER-mediated transactivation. *Molec. Endocrinol.*, 2000 14, 369-381.

[237] Fernandes, I.; Bastien, Y.; Wai, T.; Nygard, K.; Lin, R.; Cormier, O.; Lee, H.S.; Eng, F.; Bertos, N.R.; Pelletier, N.; Mader, S.; Han, V.K.M.; Yang, X.-J.; White, J.H. Ligand-dependent nuclear receptor corepressor LcoR functions by histone deacetylase-dependent and –independent mechanisms. *Molec. Cell*, 2003 11, 139-150.

[238] Zhang, H.; Thomsen, J.S.; Johansson, L.; Gustafsson, J.A.; Treuter, E. DAX-1 functions as an LXXLL-containing corepressor for activated estrogen receptors. *J. Biol. Chem.*, 2000 275, 39855-39859.

[239] Wu, L.; Wu, Y.; Gathings, B.; Wan, M.; Li, X.; Grizzle, W.; Liu, Z.; Lu, C.; Mao, Z.; Cao, X. Smad4 as a transcription corepressor for estrogen receptor alpha. *J. Biol. Chem.*, 2003 278, 15192-15200.

[240] Hu, Y.C.; Shyr, C.R.; Che, W.; Mu, X.M.; Kim, E.; Chang, C. Suppression of oestrogen receptor-mediated transcription and cell growth by interaction with TR2 orphan receptor. *J. Biol. Chem.*, 2002 277, 33571-33579.

[241] Zhao, H.H.; Herrera, R.E.; Coronado-Heinsohn, E.; Yang, M.C.; Ludes-Meyers, J.H.; Seybold-Tilson, K.J.; Nawaz, Z.; Yee, D.; Barr, F.G.; Diab, S.G.; Brown, P.H.; Fuqua, S.A.W.; Osborne, C.K. Forkhead homologue in rhabdomyosarcoma functions as a bifunctional nuclear receptor-interacting protein with both coactivator and corepressor functions. *J. Biol. Chem.*, 2001 276, 27907-27912.

[242] Norris, J.D.; Fan, D.; Sherk, McDonnell, D.P. A negative coregulator for the human ER. *Molec. Endocrinol.*, 2002 16, 459-468.

[243] Mazumdar, A.; Wang, R.A.; Mishra, S.K.; Adam, L.; Bagheri-Yarmand, R.; Mandal, M.; Vadlamudi, R.K.; Kumar, R. Transcriptional repression of oestrogen receptor by metastasis-associated protein 1 corepressor. *Nat. Cell Biol.*, 2001 3, 30-37.

[244] Kumar, R.; Wang, R.A.; Mazumdar, A.; Talukder, A.H.; Mandal, M.; Yang, Z.; Bagheri-Yarmand, R.; Sahin, A.; Hortobagyi, G.; Adam, L.; Barnes, C.J.; Vadlamudi, R.K. A naturally occuring MTA1 variant sequesters oestrogen receptor-alpha in the cytoplasm. *Nature*, 2002 418, 654-657.

[245] Huang, N.; vomBaur, E.; Garnier, J.M.; Lerouge, T.; Vonesch, J.L.; Lutz, Y.; Chambon, P.; Losson, R. Two distinct nuclear receptor interaction domains in NSD1, a novel SET protein that exhibits characteristics of both corepressors and coactivators. *EMBO J.*, 1998 17, 3398-3412.

[246] Rajendran, R.R.; Nye, A.C.; Frasor, J.; Balsara, R.D.; Martini, P.G.; Katzenellenbogen, B.S. Regulation of nuclear receptor transcriptional activity by a novel DEAE box RNA helicase (DP97). *J. Biol. Chem.*, 2003 278, 4628-4638.

[247] Le Dily, F.; Métivier, R.; Guéguen, M.-M.; Le Péron, C.; Flouriot, G.; Tas, P.; Pakdel, F. COUP-TFI modulates estrogen signaling and influences proliferation, survival and migration of breast cancer cells. *Breast Cancer Res. Treat.*, 2008 110, 69-83.

[248] Métivier, R.; Gay, F.A.; Hübner, M.R.; Flouriot, G.; Salbert, G.; Gannon, F.; Kah, O.; Pakdel, F. Formation of an hERα-COUP-TFI complex enhances hERα AF-1 through Ser118 phosphorylation by MAPK. *EMBO J.*, 2002 21, 3443-3453.

[249] Schubert, E.L.; Lee, M.K.; Newman, B.; King, M.C. Single nucleotide polymorphisms (SNPs) in the estrogen receptor gene and breast cancer susceptibility. *J. Steroid Biochem. Molec. Biol.*, 1999 71, 21-27.

[250] Humphrey, W.; Dalke, A.; Schulten, K. VMD - Visual Molecular Dynamics. *J. Molec. Graph.* 1996 14, 33-38.

[251] Meiyun, F.; Bigsby, R.M.; Nephew, K.P. The NEDD8 pathway is required for proteasome-mediated degradation of human estrogen receptor (ER)-α and essential for the antiproliferative activity of ICI 182,780 in ERα-positive breast cancer cells. *Molec. Endocrinol.* 2003 17, 356-365.

In: Estrogens: Production, Functions and Applications
Editor: James R. Bartos, pp. 273-306
ISBN: 978-1-60741-086-7

Chapter X

Estrogen Receptor Subtype Ligand Selectivity: Molecular Structural Characteristics

Snezana Agatonovic-Kustrin and Joseph V. Turner[5]
School of Pharmacy and Applied Science, La Trobe University, Bendigo, Australia
School of Medicine, University of Queensland, Brisbane, Australia

Abstract

The action of estrogens is mediated through the estrogen receptor alpha (ERα) and the more recently discovered estrogen receptor beta (ERβ). These estrogen receptor (ER) subtypes have distinct functions and differential tissue distribution patterns. Tissue- or cell-specific estrogenic activity of receptor ligands have become targets of drug research due to the potential to affect and control physiological and disease states such as breast and endometrial carcinoma, osteoporosis, and menopause. Receptor-ligand activity can be achieved in different ways such as by selective binding or selective modulation. These, in turn, are governed by the intermolecular interactions between estrogen receptors and their ligands.

The estrogen receptor ligand binding pocket has a degree of flexibility enabling binding of endogenous and synthetically-derived steroids, as well as non-steroidal molecules. Ligand fit is dependent upon aspects of size, polarity, and specific subsitution on ring and sidechain structures. Selectivity of a ligand for the estrogen receptor subtypes can be explained on the basis of differences in ligand-binding affinity, ligand potency, or ligand efficacy. In addition, molecular characteristics can lead to selective antagonism by ligands as well as antiestrogen character. Determinants of selectivity and antagonism have been elucidated using x-ray crystallography revealing various intermolecular and steric features of importance.

[5] Corresponding author: Joseph V Turner, School of Medicine – Rural Clinical Division The University of Queensland Locked Bag 9009 Toowoomba QLD 4350, Australia, Telephone: 61-7-4616 6000, Mobile: 61-419 143 154, Fax: 61-7-4633 9701, Email: josephvturner@ausdoctors.net.

The present review will examine aspects of estrogenic binding including non-selective binding, and ERα/ERβ selectivity. Various chemical classes are critically examined including endogenous compounds, phytoestrogens, and other classes of interest to drug discovery and pharmaceutical product development.

Introduction

Estrogens play key roles in the development and maintenance of normal sexual and reproductive function and exert a vast range of biological effects in the cardiovascular, musculoskeletal, immune, and central nervous systems [1-3]. The action of estrogens is mediated differentially through estrogen receptor alpha (ERα) and the more recently discovered beta (ERβ) [4, 5]. The late discovery of a second estrogen receptor (ER) is not surprising since physiological estrogens (Figure 1) E2 (estradiol-17β), E1 (estrone), and E3 (estriol or 16α-OH-E2) bind equally well to both ER subtypes, whereas some antiestrogens currently on the market, such as tamoxifen and raloxifene, block both receptor subtypes with little selectivity [6].

Estrogen receptors belong to nuclear receptors, a large family of ligand-dependent transcription factors that transform extra- and intracellular signals into cellular responses by triggering the transcription of specific target genes. Nuclear receptors contain three independent but interacting functional domains: NH_2 terminal or A/B domain, DNA-binding or C domain, and ligand-binding or D/E/F domain [7]. Agonists and antagonists differentially position the C-terminal helix of the ligand-binding domain (helix-12) and the F domain (carboxyl terminal domain) [8].

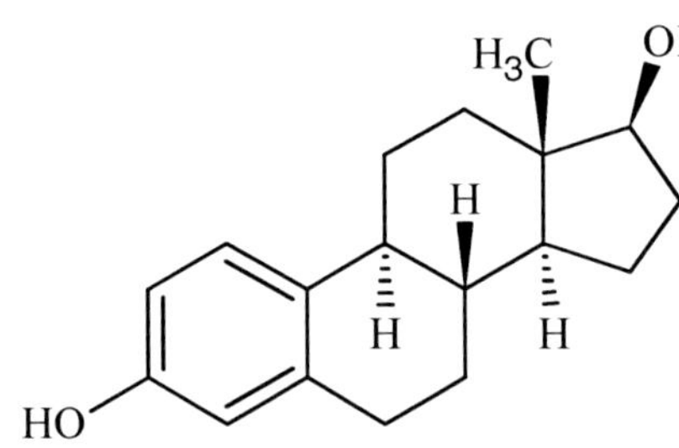

estradiol-17β (E2)

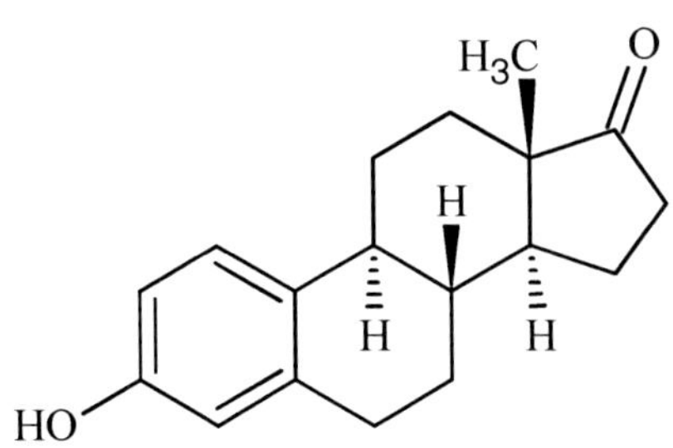

estrone (E1)

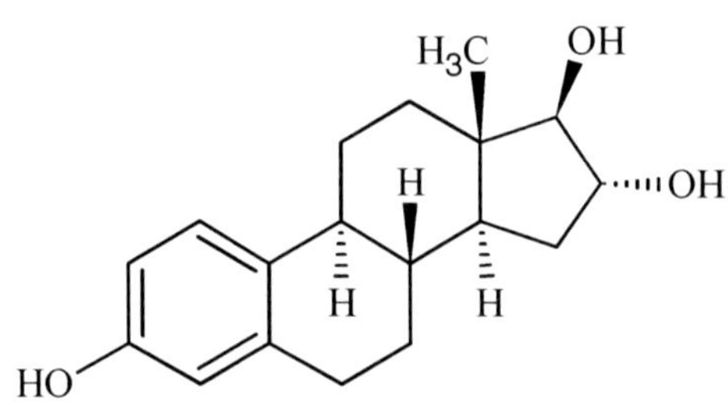

estriol (E3)

Figure 1. Natural steroidal estrogens.

ERα and ERβ differ markedly in the N-terminal A/B domains, with only 20% amino acid identity, and also in the ligand-binding domain. The differences in the A/B domain suggest that the transcriptional activation by ERα and ERβ may play different roles in carcinogenesis. The ratio of ERα/ERβ differs between normal and carcinomatous tissues such that a higher ratio has been observed in breast and endometrial carcinoma [9-11]. ERβ mRNA was detected in 36% of endometrial carcinoma cases, whereas ERα mRNA hybridisation signals were detected in 80% of those cases. Since ERβ is co-expressed with ERα, the estrogenic effects are considered to occur mainly through ERα in endometrial carcinomas [10].

Morover, the two subtypes have differential tissue distribution patterns [2] and different transcriptional activities in certain tissues, cell-types and promoter contexts [12]. Reproductive cells, especially those of the uterus and breast, are abundant in ERα, whereas ERβ is found in brain, bone, bladder and vascular epithelia which are all tissues that are responsive to classical hormone replacement therapy (HRT). The cell proliferative actions of 17β-estradiol (E2) mediated through ERα can be opposed by ERβ [13]. ERβ inhibits ERα-mediated gene transcription in the presence of ERα, whereas in its absence it can partially replace ERα [14]. The two receptor subtypes also play different roles in mammary epithelial cells. ERα induces proliferation while ERβ has a role in apoptosis [13]. Given the complexity of estrogen activity, ER subtype-selective ligands may potentially possess significant clinical utility. For example, ERβ selective modulators would have minimal effect on tissues that contain ERα, and thus exhibit different side-effect profiles than non-selective ligands.

Although specific biological responses have been attributed to the activation of ERα or ERβ, it is also clear that in cells where both receptors are expressed, ERβ functions to reduce ERα transcriptional activity [15]. Thus, the pharmacological response of target cells to estrogens and antiestrogens represents the composite activities of both receptors. From studies aimed at developing new classes of ER agonists and antagonists the selective estrogen receptor modulators (SERMs) have emerged. These are compounds whose relative agonist/antagonist activities are manifest in a cell- and promoter-selective manner. The molecular basis of SERM activity has been attributed to the ability of these molecules to induce different changes in receptor c, an event that engenders the recruitment of functionally distinct cofactors [16].

The falling level of estrogen in post-menopausal women has been considered the main reason for increased osteoporosis and heart disease in ageing women [17]. HRT, such as Premarin (a combination of estrogens and progestins) is used for the relief of estrogenic deficiency symptoms in post-menopausal women. It may reduce the incidence of cardiovascular disease and lower the number of fractures caused by osteoporosis. HRT is associated with a variety of clinical benefits such as bone protection, prevention of hot flushes and and decreased risks of type 2 diabetes mellitus and colorectal cancer. Nevertheless, such therapy also has adverse effects due to the stimulation of breast and uterine tissues leading to associated increases in rates of breast and endometrial carcinoma. Some of these adverse effects are believed to be mediated by ERα or ERβ specific mechanisms [18-20].

It follows that ERβ antagonists or agonists would display different therapeutic profiles than ERα antagonists or agonists, and would be beneficial in tissues expressing high levels of ERβ [21, 22]. Since ERα is the dominant subtype in the breast and uterus, this suggests that

ERβ selective ligands may be used as HRT without increasing the risk of breast or uterine cancer. A combination of a selective ERα antagonist and a selective ERβ agonist would be more potent in breast cancer treatment.

Identification and cloning of the second estrogen receptor (ERβ) in addition to the known receptor (ERα) allowed preparation of new selective ligands with the potential to bind to either ERα and/or ERβ, and with potentially new biologic and pharmacologic applications. Research in this area has already led to ligands exhibiting a greater selectivity for ERα [23, 24] and/or to ERβ [25] than some known synthetic derivatives and natural phytoestrogens.

Structure and Binding

Nonselective Estrogenic Activity

ERs can bind a remarkable number of structurally different compounds. The natural ligand for the ERs is 17β-estradiol (E2), an endogenous steroidal hormone (Figure 1). A number of other endogenous and synthetically derived steroids also activate the receptor, providing evidence for the flexible nature of the receptor ligand binding pocket. In addition to steroidal derivatives, ERs also bind large variety of non-steroidal phenolic compounds. The three well-known non-steroidal stilbene estrogens (Figure 2), diethylstilbesterol (DES), dienestrol, and hexestrol, have very high binding affinities, similar to that of E2.

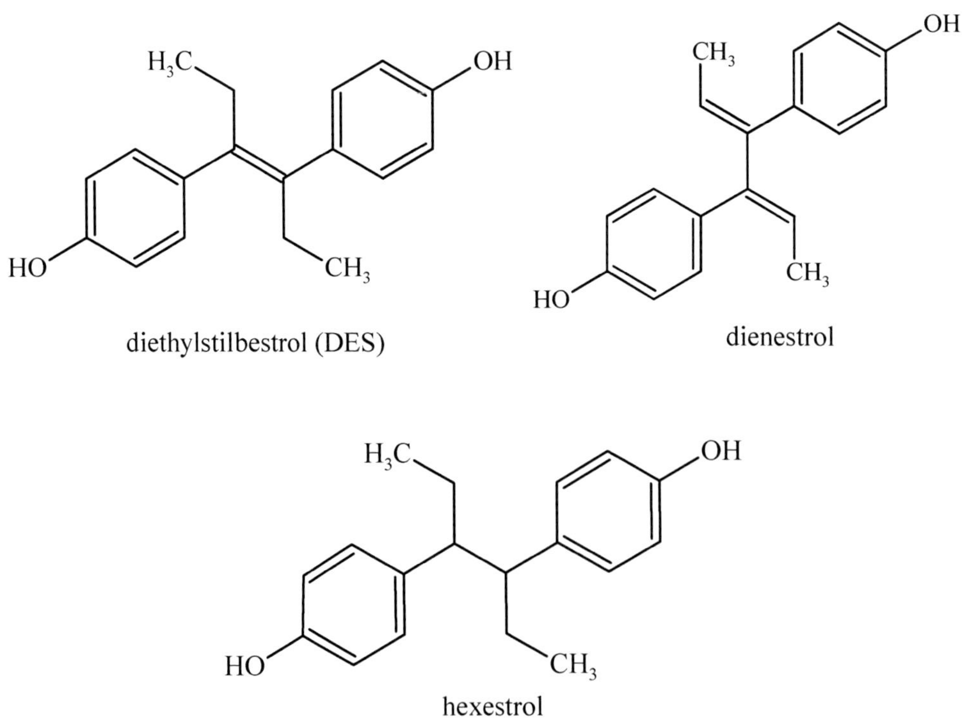

Figure 2. Non-steroidal stilbene estrogens.

The structural analysis of known ER ligands led to the hypothesis that three essential pharmacophore elements arranged on a core scaffold are necessary for effective binding: a phenolic ring important for affinity, a second aromatic group, and another substituent(s) which may be aromatic or aliphatic (Figure 3).

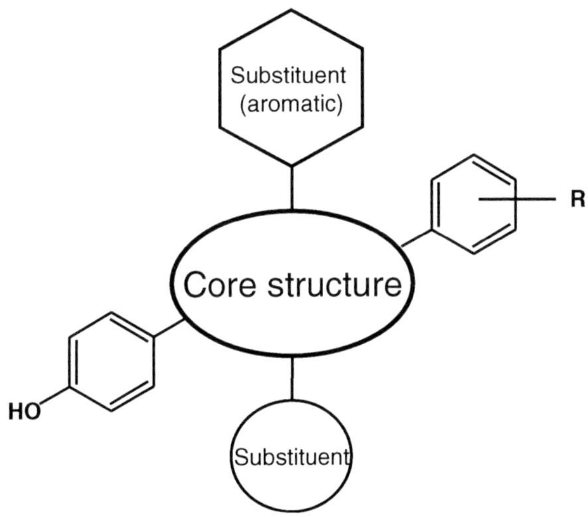

Figure 3. Pharmacophore ligand structure.

The core structure provides necessary structural rigidity and carries the pharmacophore elements in a certain arrangement for binding to a receptor. Important features that enable these compounds to bind to an ER are their steric and hydrophobic properties, as well as the hydrogen bonding between the phenolic hydroxyl group and the ER binding site [26]. While some ER ligands vary in structure, receptor binding seems to be strongly dependent upon the presence of an aromatic hydroxyl group and the conformation of the hydrophobic portion of the molecule [27]. Among all compounds tested to date, there is not a single estrogen-like compound without a ring structure. Rings are usually flat and aromatic, which contributes to molecular rigidity, thereby mimicking the estradiol (E2) ring A. An aromatic ring and an hydroxyl group are important for binding effectiveness, while the remainder of the ER will accept hydrophobic groups [27].

Although the structure of estrogen agonists varies widely, they can be classified as either steroids or non-steroidal synthetic structures. The length and width of both the steroidal and non-steroidal molecules fit well into the receptor binding pocket. The activity of DES analogues was explained in 1946 when it was proposed that the critical structural requirement for the receptor recognition is the distance between two oxygens that should be 12.1Å [28]. Modern medicinal chemistry has shown that the actual distance is 12.1Å in DES and 10.9Å in estradiol. However, in aqueous solution, estradiol has two water molecule hydrogens bonded to the 17-hydroxyl. If one water molecule is included in the distance measurement, there is a perfect fit to 12.1Å [29]. Effective binding requires the presence of the two polar hydroxyl groups at each end of the molecule. Molecules with a distance limitation between the oxygen atoms of the hydroxyl groups on a large inert skeleton have optimal estrogenic activity [30]. Estradiol binds to the receptor using hydrogen bonding as a key interaction. The phenolic A-ring alcohol group makes hydrogen bond contacts with two specific residues of the ER ligand binding domain, Glu-353(-305) and Arg-394(-346) of ERα(ERβ) [31, 32]. By overlaying the crystal structures of four ligand–ER complexes (estradiol–ER, 4-hydroxytamoxifen–ER, raloxifene–ER, and DES–ER complexes) based on their common protein residues at the binding site, it was found that the phenolic rings of all four ligands are closely positioned at the same location to allow hydrogen bond interactions with Glu-353, Arg-394 of the receptor, and a water molecule [33].

The D-ring hydroxyl group binds with His-524. One study analyzing the hydrogen bonding mode of phenolic hydroxyl group of estradiol [27] suggested a donor function of the phenol of estradiol and a high expectation for the 17β-hydroxyl group to be a better hydrogen bond acceptor than donor. These predictions were confirmed by subsequent x-ray crystallographic analysis of the complex of the estrogen receptor ligand-binding domain and estradiol [31]. It was found that the phenol of estradiol binds to the Glu-353 of the receptor as a hydrogen donor, while the 17β-hydroxyl group in the D-ring binds to His-524 as a hydrogen acceptor, either directly or via a water molecule. In addition to hydrogen bonding to Glu-353, the phenolic-hydroxyl group makes direct hydrogen bonds to the guanidium group of Arg-394 and a water molecule. One further study clearly indicated that alkylphenols interact with estrogen receptors only when phenol is conjugated with hydrophobic alkyl groups and that the hydrophobic interfaces of alkylphenols are insufficient to sustain a conformation of estradiol for full receptor binding [34].

The relative binding affinity (RBA) of substituted estradiols is more susceptible to steric and/or electrostatic effects when the substitution is on C2 rather than on C4. Earlier studies have suggested that substitution of small functional groups at the estradiol positions C2 and C4 are tolerated, whereas larger groups may reduce binding affinity due to the formation of an intra-molecular hydrogen bond with the C3 hydroxyl group [27]. Depending on size and polarity, the substituents on C1, by contrast, may cause skeletal alterations of rings B, C, and D, mainly by steric hindrance and through-space electronic induction on C11 and its attached hydrogens. Substitution on C4 does not create major changes in conformation of the alicyclic system since ortho inductive effects are normally minimal [35]. Hydroxylation at specific sites of the estratrien-17β-ol aromatic A-ring is critical. Hydroxylation at the 2 or 3 positions promoted high affinity of a ligand for the ER, while hydroxylation at the 1 or 4 positions attenuated binding affinity. It has been hypothesized that the hydroxyl groups at positions 2 and 3 may share, via hydrogen bonding, a common H-acceptor/-donor site in the receptor cavity [36]. Electron-withdrawing groups such as chlorine or fluorine on the phenyl ring produce a roughly 4-fold improvement in RBA at both receptor subtypes. However, substitution of bromine at the C2 position of estradiol drastically reduces the RBA at ERβ and also ERα to a relatively lesser degree (<0.5% and 4% of estradiol respectively). The position of the substituent appears to have little effect on potency or selectivity as does the addition of a second electron-withdrawing group on the ring. Cyano and trifluoromethyl substituents appear to be slightly less effective in increasing ER affinity than simple halogens. Electron-donating substituents such as methyl are generally equipotent to the unsubstituted phenyl derivatives. It was also suggested that saturation of the phenyl ring leads to a loss in affinity at both receptor subtypes [36].

E1 (estrone), E2 (17β-estradiol), and E3 (estriol or 16α-OH-E2) are the three well-known human estrogens. Although estradiol is the most potent endogenous estrogen with almost equal binding affinity for both human ERs, it is not the major circulating estrogen. Estrone (E1) and estriol (E3), two major metabolites of estradiol (Figure 1), are quantitatively the main circulating estrogens in women under different physiological conditions [6]. Although their binding affinities for ERα and ERβ are much lower than that of estradiol, they may serve unique physiological functions. It is believed that the metabolic conversion of estradiol to estrone or estriol may represent an important mechanism for achieving differential activation of the ERα or ERβ signaling system under different physiological conditions. Notably, while estradiol has nearly the highest and equal binding affinity for ERα and ERβ, estrone and 2-hydroxyestrone (2-OHE$_1$), two quantitatively-predominant endogenous estrogens in nonpregnant woman, have preferential binding affinity for ERα over ERβ. On the other hand, estriol and other D-ring metabolites that are quantitatively-predominant endogenous estrogens formed during pregnancy, have preferential binding affinity for ERβ over ERα [6].

Weak agonists like estriol can activate some, but not all, of the ER responses. This selective regulation of receptor activity by estriol is not correlated with its ability to activate transcription [37]. It is associated with the inability of the estriol-bound receptor to sustain tight nuclear interactions [38]. D-ring substitution of estradiol, particularly at the C16 and C17 positions, results in differential binding affinity for ERα and ERβ. Most of the D-ring metabolites have considerable binding affinity for both ERα and ERβ, and several of them (16α-OH-E2, 16β-OH-E2-17α, and 16-keto-E1) have a distinct, preferential binding affinity for ERβ over ERα (up to 18-fold). Estriol, one of the major metabolites formed during human pregnancy, has a markedly lower binding affinity for ERα compared with estradiol but retains a relatively high binding affinity for ERβ (RBA 11% and 35% of estradiol respectively). Furthermore, while 16β-OH-E2-17α (16,17-epiestriol) has a very low binding affinity for ERα, it has a preferential affinity for ERβ. The difference between these binding affinities is 18-fold [39]. It appears that both ERs are sensitive to the steric hindrance in the vicinity of the 17α position on the steroid ring. QSAR studies of ligand-receptor interactions and comparative molecular field analysis of both ERs revealed that they are sensitive to adding steric bulk at the 17α position on the steroid ring. Hence, it was suggested that substitutions in this region would enhance the binding affinity more for ERα than ERβ [40]. The most interesting difference is found for 17α-estradiol, which has five times higher affinity for ERα than ERβ. The physiological action of 17α-estradiol is quite different from that of the natural hormone, 17β-estradiol (E2). The domain near the 17α position of estradiol is larger for ERα than ERβ suggesting that increasing steric bulk in this region will enhance the binding affinity more for the ERα than for ERβ. Moxestrol (RBA 43 and 5) and norethynodrel (RBA 0.7 and 0.22), both with 17α-ethynil substituent show higher binding affinity to ERα than to ERβ. 17α-ethynylestradiol, a semi-synthetic steroidal estrogen commonly used as an estrogenic component in various oral contraceptives, had very high binding affinity for both ERα and ERβ compared to estradiol. The binding affinity of 17α-ethynylestradiol for ERα is twice as high as that of estradiol, but its affinity for ERβ is only about half of that of estradiol. Accordingly, the relative ratio of preference for binding to ERα and ERβ by 17α-ethynylestradiol is approximately 4 times of that for estradiol. On the other hand, most of the polar D-ring metabolites (16β-OH-E2-17α, 16α-OH-E2-17α, 16-keto-E1, 16α-OH-E2, and 16α-OH-E1) have markedly increased binding affinity for human ERβ over ERα compared with their respective precursors.

Although the steroid estrogen molecule is a rigid structure, its interactions with the receptor and general modulation of activity are highly susceptible to minor skeletal modifications. The volume available in the receptor binding pocket exceeds the size of natural ligand (such as estradiol) leaving empty spaces in the binding pocket below the C7α and above the C11β position of the estradiol B- and C-rings that are not filled by the ligand [6]. Compounds with lipophilic substituents at C11β substitution show high affinities. The preference for C11 substitution is based on its close proximity to the aromatic C1 which can be influenced via steric interaction and through spacial electronic induction. Due to the conformation of the B-ring, substitutions on the α-face on C11 have a more dramatic structural effect than those on the β-face [41]. However, addition of a hydrophilic group (such as a hydroxyl or keto group) at the C11 position (regardless of 11α or 11β) almost completely eliminated the binding affinities for both receptor subtypes. These data indicate that the drastic decrease in binding affinities of 11α-OH-estradiol, 11β-OH-estradiol, or 11-keto-estradiol for human ERα and ERβ is not due to steric hindrance caused by the C11 position substitutions, but is mainly due to alterations of the lipophilicity near the C11 position [6]. A similar situation is seen with non-steroidal estrogens. In the ER-DES structure, these pockets are filled by the two ethyl groups that extend upward and downward from the ligand.

The presence of a planar aromatic six-member ring imparts unique chemical properties to estrogens and is considered more significant than any other structural feature [42], hence a phenolic ring is often associated with estrogenic activity [27]. Steroids lacking an aromatic ring have low binding affinity. Aromatization of A-ring in natural estrogens is the final step in estrogen formation from its precursor androgen. Aromatization alters the overall shape of the molecule. The relative spatial orientation of the A-steroidal ring with respect to the B-ring may be considered important structural characteristics for receptor recognition. A rigid ring structure, as present in estradiol, favors ER binding.

Recently, subtype-selective differences in ligand binding and transcriptional potency of nonphenolic synthetic 19-nor progesterone derivatives between ERα and ERβ were reported. It was found that 19-nor contraceptive progestins, gestodene derivatives (Figure 4), undergo in vivo and in vitro enzyme-mediated A-ring double bond hydrogenation to A-ring reduced metabolites. Bioconversion of 19-nor progestins to their corresponding tetrahydro derivatives resulted in the loss of progestational activity and acquisition of estrogenic activities and binding to the ER [43]. These compounds did not activate gene transcription via ERβ, and none of them showed antagonistic activities through either ER subtype. In summary, two active 3β,5α -tetrahydro derivatives were identified as active selective ERα versus ERβ agonists. This is an important consideration because the relative agonist activity of many selective ER ligands varies by cell and promoter type. The ability to have preferential ligand selectivity for ERα over ERβ receptors can assist in the process of identifying additional synthetic or naturally occurring steroids with different relative affinities for both ER subtypes. In this regard, it is known that only those C19 steroids with an hydroxyl group at C3 and C17 have significant affinity for both ER subtypes [44]. Thus, the relative spatial orientation of the A-ring with respect to the B-ring, as in the case of 5α-reduction and hydroxylation at C3 of steroids, should also be considered as important structural characteristics for ERα ligand recognition.

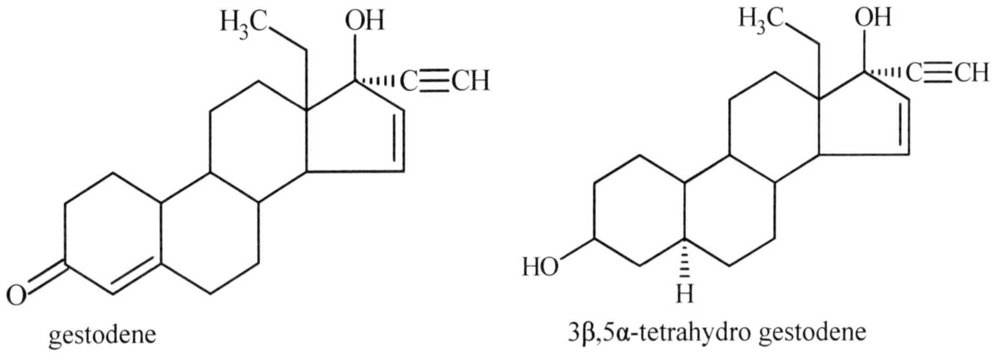

Figure 4. Molecular structures of gestodene and 3β,5α-tetrahydro gestodene.

In an attempt to increase the chemical diversity of estrogen receptor ligands, compounds containing an oxime and a hydroxy- (salicylaldoximes) or amino-moieties (anthranylaldoximes) as alternative to phenolic A-ring were synthesized (Figure 5) [45]. These new classes of compounds showed interesting ER binding properties on both receptor subtypes, demonstrating that the six-member ring formed by an intramolecular hydrogen bond and containing an exocyclic oxime OH may be an effective isosteric replacement of the phenolic ring [46].

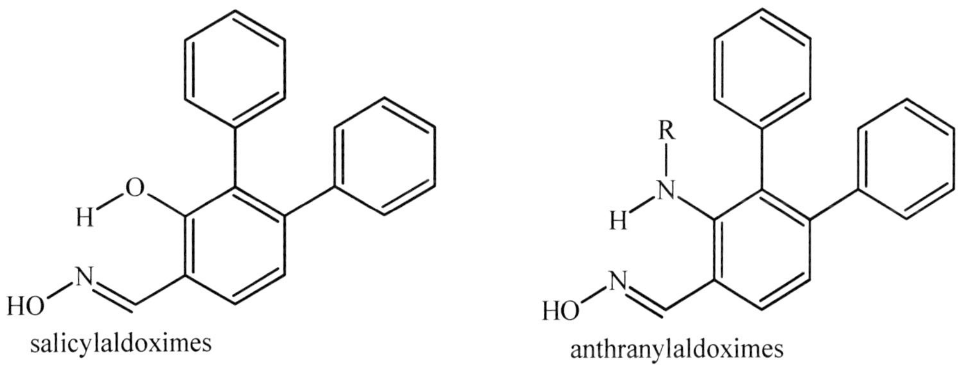

Figure 5. Molecular structures of salicylaldoximes and anthranylaldoximes.

Receptor Selectivity

The physiological hormone 17β-estradiol is not very selective for the two ER subtypes, while the selectivity of some natural ligands (phytoestrogens) is not high enough to be of much practical use. However, individual ligands may differ in their affinity for ERα and ERβ. For example, 17β-estradiol binds equally well to both receptors, while estrone and raloxifene bind preferentially to ERα, and estriol and genistein bind preferentially to ERβ.

Drugs that target the ER can exhibit a variety of effects in different target tissues. Tamoxifen is an estrogen antagonist in breast tissue [47] but an estrogen agonist in bone [48] and uterine tissue [49]. ERα plays an important role in breast cancer and a large fraction of ERα positive breast cancers respond to tamoxifen. Tamoxifen, a selective estrogen receptor modulator (SERM), is the most widely prescribed hormonal therapy treatment for breast cancer. However, despite the benefits of tamoxifen therapy, almost all tamoxifen-responsive breast cancer patients develop resistance to therapy. It was shown that when ERβ is coexpressed with ERα in breast cancer, the tumour sensitivity to 4-hydroxytamoxifen is increased and the overall prognosis of the disease is better than in patients with low or no expression of ERβ [50]. Tamoxifen therapy also has adverse side effects, mainly due to its partial agonist action in endometrium. Similar to tamoxifen, raloxifene is also an estrogen antagonist in breast tissue. In contrast, however, this second-generation SERM has substantially less uterotropic activity than tamoxifen and has been associated with increased bone mineral density [51]. Raloxifene also has several undesirable effects, including hot flushes and venous thrombosis [52]. Tamoxifen has almost identical binding affinities for human ERα and ERβ, although its relative binding affinities are only 3-4% of those of estradiol. In comparison, while raloxifene has a similar binding affinity for ERβ as tamoxifen, it has 16-fold higher binding affinity for ERα. Therefore, raloxifene actually has a strong preferential binding affinity for human ERα over ERβ.

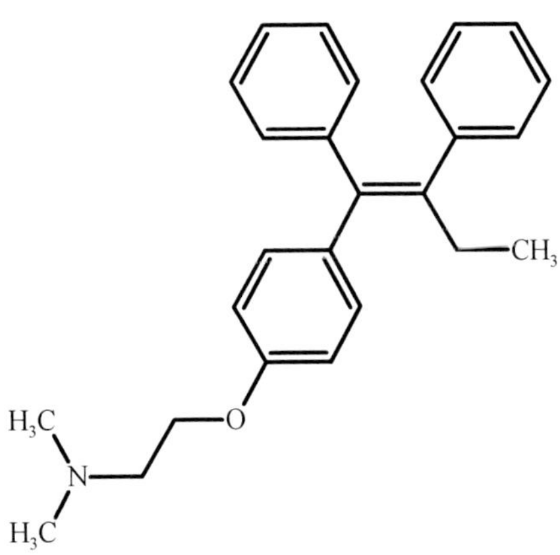

tamoxifen

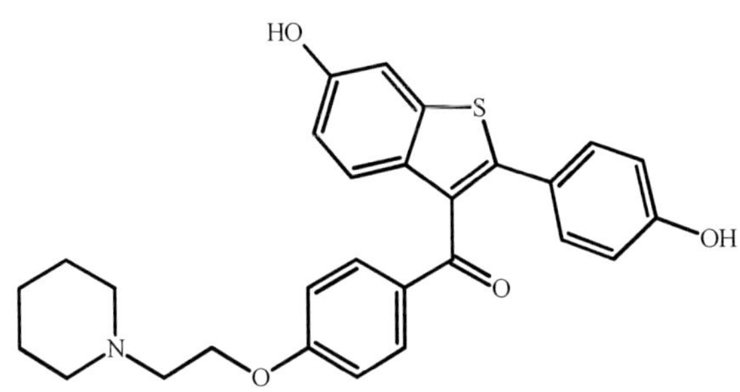

raloxifene

Figure 6. Selected SERM structures.

Selectivity of a ligand for the ER subtypes can be explained on the basis of differences in ligand-binding affinity, ligand potency, or ligand efficacy. Thus, there are three types of ligands: ligands with potency, efficacy and antagonist selectivity. A ligand with potency selectivity is an agonist on both receptor subtypes, but stimulates transcription of one type at a lower concentration. Efficacy selectivity refers to the differences in the level of activity of a ligand. Antagonist selectivity refers to a ligand which is an antagonist on one receptor subtype and has either antagonist or no activity at the other subtype. In addition to specific potency, efficacy and antagonist selectivity, ligands may posses a combination of these three types of selectivities.

Antiestrogen Character and Structural Basis for Antagonisms

Extensive structure activity relationship (SAR) studies were used to propose a molecular model of estrogen and antiestrogen action (Figure 7). This "crocodile model" involved sealing of a ligand within the ligand binding domain to transform the receptor-ligand complex into its active state [53]. Planar estrogens, able to be sealed within the ligand binding domain, transform the receptor-ligand complex into its active state so that gene transcription can be initiated. Binding of estrogens to the receptor induces minor changes in the tertiary structure of the receptor protein so that the estrogens become "locked" into the ligand binding site. Antiestrogens, on the other hand, by virtue of their unique bulky side chain, are jammed into the receptor so that the secondary changes that occur with estrogens cannot occur with antiestrogens due to the steric hindrance. A large bulky side chain locks into the ligand binding domain and prevents full receptor activation by keeping the jaws open. This bulky side chain interacts with an antiestrogenic region of the receptor protein. Alteration in the antiestrogenic side chains will modulate the estrogenic and antiestrogenic actions of the ligand-receptor complex.

The crocodile model was essentially correct, with the planar estrogen sealed within the ligand binding pocket, but the 3D SERM blocked the closure process by relocating helix-12 away from the ligand binding pocket. The bulky side chain for the SERM relocated helix-12, thereby preventing coactivator molecules from binding to the appropriate site on the external surface of a SERM ER complex (AF-2) [54].

X-ray crystal structures for the ligand binding pockets of ERα bound to agonists and antagonists and ERβ bound to a partial agonist and an antagonist showed that the overall structures of both ERα and ERβ are similar [31, 32, 55]. The most striking difference in the liganded and unliganded forms is the positioning of the C-terminal helix-12, the AF-2 region.

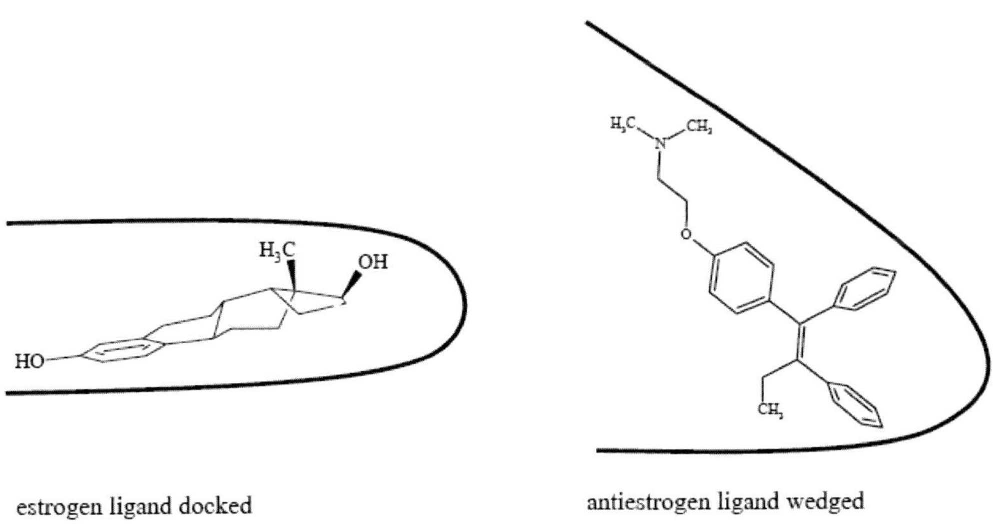

Figure 7. Schematic crocodile model of ER-ligand binding.

In the ERα complexes with agonists, helix-12 is positioned over the ligand binding pocket. The agonist-ERα structure revealed that a portion of a coactivator protein is bound to a hydrophobic channel formed by helices 3, 4, 5, and 12 in an α-helical conformation. This appears to be the mode by which ligand activated ERs transfer their activity.

The molecular basis of agonism and antagonism for ER has been further revised through x-ray crystallography. It has been found that liganded ERα binding domain structures support this theory for agonism and also indicate the mechanism for antagonism [56]. The bulky side chain present in estrogen antagonists exit the binding pocket. Steric hindrance between the basic side chain of these antiestrogens and helix-12 displaces helix-12 from the agonist position to a new position that occludes the coactivator recognition channel. This disorder of the coactivator binding surface is responsible for the antagonism character in both ERa and ERβ ligand binding domain complexes [57]. Binding of the ligand stabilizes specific conformations reflecting the size and shape of the ligand. The rigidified external surface features of the ligand-receptor complex then serves as specific docking sites for coregulators, thereby altering the rate of target gene transcription. When agonists bind, the C-terminal helix-12 folds over the ligand to form a hydrophobic channel in which coactivators may dock. By contrast, antagonist binding reorients helix-12 so that it will interfere with coactivator binding. Without a ligand, helix-12 sticks out from the ligand-bonding pocket; in the presence of ligand it folds back to form a scaled ligand binding pocket. Due to the overall homology in the ligand binding domains of all the nuclear receptors, it is believed that the realignment of helix-12, which forms a new interaction surface with coactivators, is the structural basis for the ligand-dependent transactivation [58].

In contrast to the two structures of ER-agonist complexes, complexes with antiestrogens such as raloxifene and hydroxytamoxifen have an altered helical topology at the C-terminal region of the ligand binding domain [31, 32]. Due to the presence of a large basic side chain, these ligands do not fit into a fully closed ligand binding pocket and the C-terminal helix-12 of the ligand binding domain becomes relocated. Another structural study of the ligand binding domain complex of the pure antiestrogen ICI 164.3S4 bound to ERβ revealed that the bulky polar side chain protrudes from the binding pocket and itself occupies the coactivator binding site [59]. Consequently there is steric prevention of helix-12 from adopting either an agonist or antagonist orientation. Such studies emphasize the role of bulky side chains in achieving antagonism on ER [60].

The recent discovery of *R,R*-tetrahydrochrysene (*R,R*-THC) as an ERβ specific antagonist (Figure 11) breaks the dogma that a bulky side chain is required for ER antagonists, at least for the antagonists on ERβ [61]. This has led to the theory of "passive antagonism" [32]. When a receptor binds to a ligand without a bulky side chain the interaction between the ligand and the receptor still could destabilize helix-12 for its agonist position even though there are no steric contacts physically preventing it [62]. Helix-12 in ER appears to be quite dynamic and destabilization of helix-12 can be initiated by the loss of some contacts between ligand and receptor. It is interesting that the antagonism on ERβ can be more easily achieved than on ERα. It is speculated that the agonist position for helix-12 in ERβ is intrinsically less stable than it is in ERα [31]. The volume of the binding pocket in ERβ is significantly smaller than in ERα (390Å^3 versus 490Å^3 for ERα), although it is still larger than the volume of estradiol. Thus, this difference is not critical for the binding of estradiol, but is important for the binding of larger ligands. Furthermore, ERβ binding pocket is more polar, due to the replacement of Met-336 in ERα with the smaller and more polar Leu-384 in ERβ. [55].

ERα Selectivity

Katzenellenbogen and co-workers have developed several series of non-steroidal compounds based on substituted furans, pyrazoles and tetrahydrochrysenes [63-65] which have been shown to exhibit substantial ER subtype selectivity compared with the classical steroidal compounds.

An interesting comparison can be made among the series of substituted pyrazoles. The 3,5 - disubstituted pyrazoles show very low affinity. Addition of a third substituent causes only 2-3 fold increase in affinity. Addition of a fourth substituent results in 500 -900 increase of affinity. Clearly this is not a simple additive effect suggesting that a detailed and proper match between the peripheral substituent and several sites on the receptor is essential to achieve high binding affinity. It seems that the 5-membered heterocyclic core systems require a tetra-substituted ring for good ER affinity. Generally these are tri-aryl substituted rings. The fourth substituent is usually alkyl (ie ethyl). The structure-activity relationship for the alkyl substituent shows that the affinity increases with the extension of the alkyl chain from methyl to ethyl (furans) or propyl (pyrazole and imidazole series) and decreases with further extension. This is also seen in steroidal systems. Such a trend indicates the filling of a ligand binding pocket of limited volume within the receptor [27]. This pocket is lined with hydrophobic residues and an increase in the alkyl chain results in an unfavourable interaction.

A variety of 5-membered heterocyclic analogs including imidazoles, oxazoles, thiophenes, pyrroles, and furans have been studied. Large differences in binding affinity, up to 50-fold, were found for ligands that had identical peripheral substitution patterns but different core structures (eg pyrazoles versus imidazoles, thiazole or isoxazole). Pyrazole-based ligands with basic side chain substituents have been shown to be selective for ERα in terms of binding affinity as well as its potency. The reason of their superior affinity has not been established. The high-affinity pyrazoles bear close conformational relationship to the non-steroidal ligand raloxifene. Perhaps polarity and dipole interaction, relative to substituents position may contribute to affinity [66]. Several triaryl-substituted five-membered heterocycles show exceptionally large potency and efficacy preferences for ERα [61, 64, 65, 67]. The best of these are triaryl-alkyl-substituted pyrazoles and furans which function as complete ERα agonists but are almost completely inactive at ERβ (Figure 8). The phenol attached to the position 5 of the furan ring or position 3 of the pyrazole ring most likely mimics the A-ring of estradiol. The second phenol, attached to the position 2 of the furan ring, or N(1) in pyrazole ring, does not seem to be very important for high binding affinity. However, this phenol plays a role in selectivity for ERα relative to ERβ. The p-hydroxy group attached on the N(1)-phenyl group enhances affinity and selectivity for ERα. The most selective heterocycle, propyl pyrazole triol (PPT), is approximately 10,000-fold more potent on ERα than on ERβ and shows ERα-selectivity in vivo [64, 68]. PPT is also much larger molecule than estradiol. It can be well accommodated inside the ERα binding pocket, but its fit in ERβ in the same binding manner is poor. Addition of the basic side chain on the third phenol, or C(5) phenol, also increases selectivity to ERα. Basic side chain (BSC) pyrazoles are selective antagonists on ERα. The molecular basis for this ERα selectivity is not fully understood. In fact, other larger ring heterocycles such as tetrasubstituted pyrimidines and pyrazines retain greater potency and efficacy on ERα than on ERβ [69].

Tetra-substituted furans (Figure 8) proved to be ERα selective agents in both RBA (3-fold to 70-fold selectivity) and transcriptional activation assays (10-fold selectivity) [62]. The furans with the highest subtype selectivity were those with 3-alkyl-2,4,5-triaryl substituents, particularly furans with all three aryl groups presents as para-phenols. The highest subtype binding affinity selectivity (71-fold) was observed for 2,3,5-tis(4-hydroxyphenyl)-4-methyl-furan. Both experimental evidence and molecular modeling have been used to help determine the binding mode for the furan series of ligands.

Certain triaryl amides (Figure 9) show potency preferences as agonists for ERα that can be as great as 500 fold. They function as agonists on both ERα and ERβ, but in cell-based assays of gene transcription they activate ERα at much lower concentrations [70]. Bisphenolic amides mimic bibenzyl and homobibenzyl motifs commonly found as substructures in ligands for the ER. ER ligands that have simple amide core structures can be readily prepared. Representative members were prepared from three classes: N- phenyl benzamides, N- phenyl acetamides, and N-benzyl benzamides. Of these three classes, the N-phenylbenzamides had the highest affinity for ER, the N-phenylacetamides had lower, and the N-benzylbenzamides were prone to fragmentation via a quinone methide intermediate. Therefore, high affinity binding requires an appropriate distribution of bulk, polarity, and functionality. The strong conformational preference of the core anilide function in all of these ligands defines a rather rigid geometry for further structural and functional expansion of these series.

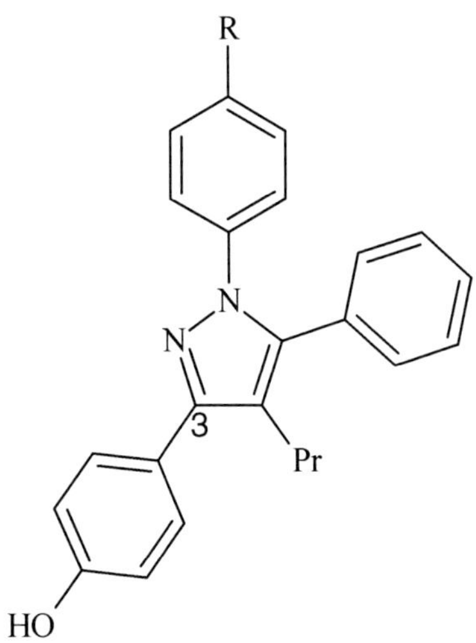

R = H: propylpirazole diol (PPD)
R = OH: propylpyrazole triol (PPT)

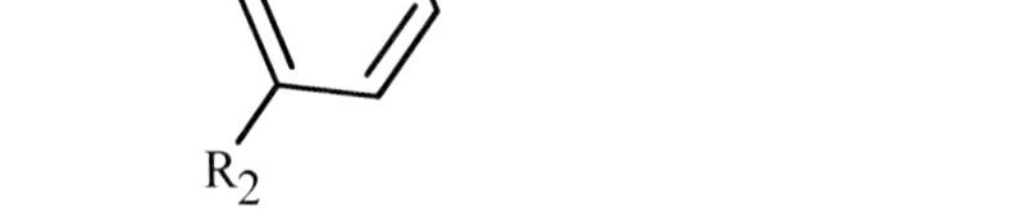

tetra-substituted furan

Figure 8. Selective ERα ligands.

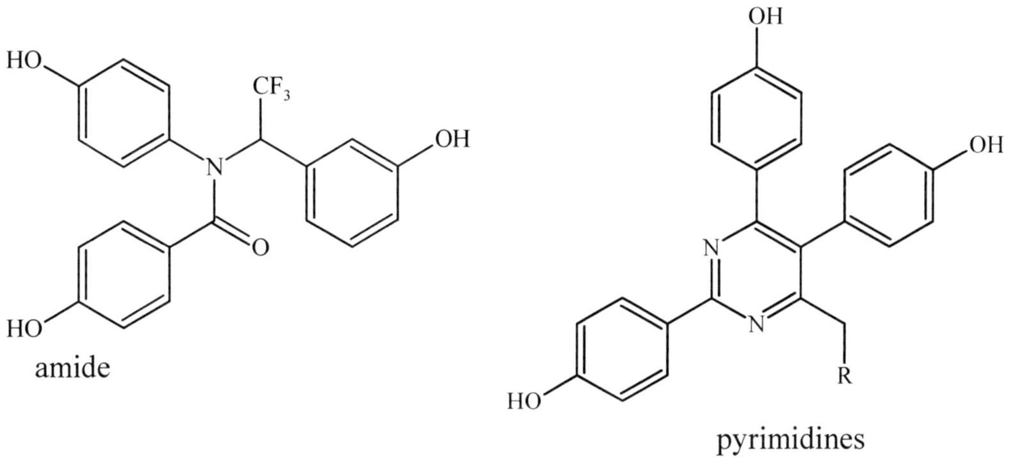

Figure 9. Molecular strucutures of amides and pyrimidines.

Specific chromane analogues were identified as ERα selective ligands with the potential for the treatment of osteoporosis and cancer. X-ray studies revealed that the origin of ERα selectivity was from a C4 trans methyl substitution to the cis-2,3-diphenyl-chromane platform [71].

Vitamin E is a generic term representing two groups of chemically related, lipid-soluble compounds, the tocopherols and tocotrienols [72]. Tocopherols are commonly present in a variety of foods, whereas tocotrienols are relatively rare. It was found that dietary supplementation with the tocotrienol-rich fraction significantly inhibited mammary tumor development and growth. Although tocopherols and tocotrienols are potent antioxidants, the antitumor activity of these compounds is not dependent on their antioxidant activity. The available evidence suggests that these compounds inhibit tumor development and growth by modulating multiple intracellular signaling pathways involved in mitogenesis [73] and apoptosis [74]. The majority of studies have shown that tocotrienols display greater antitumor activity than tocopherols, although the exact mechanism of this is presently unknown [75, 76]. Tocopherols and tocotrienols have the same basic chemical structure characterized by a long phytyl chain attached at the 1-position of a chromane ring, with the major difference being that tocopherols have a saturated, while tocotrienols have an unsaturated, phytyl chain. In addition, specific tocopherol and tocotrienol isoforms differ from each other based on the number of methyl groups bound to their chromane ring. It is possible that the level of phytyl chain saturation and/or chromane ring methylation may be critical in determining the antiproliferative and apoptotic activity of individual tocopherol and tocotrienol isoforms [77]

Substituted tetrahydrochrysene (THC) ligands (Figure 11) are potent agonists on ERα but also potent antagonists on ERβ [78]. This character is a function of substituent size and stereochemistry. THCs can be regarded as ring-fused derivatives of diethylstilbestrol, containing an electron-donating hydroxyl group at C8 and a rigid four-ring structure reminiscent of steroidal estrogens. *RR* and *SS* enantiomers of THC exhibit different activities at ERα and ERβ. Antagonist character depends on the size and special orientation of substituents. ER selective antagonists reside completely in the *RR* enantiomer. *SS* enantiomers have similar agonist activity to ERα and ERβ.

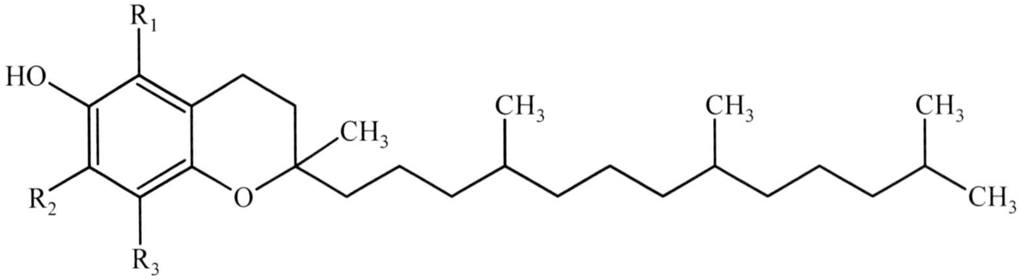

tocopherol

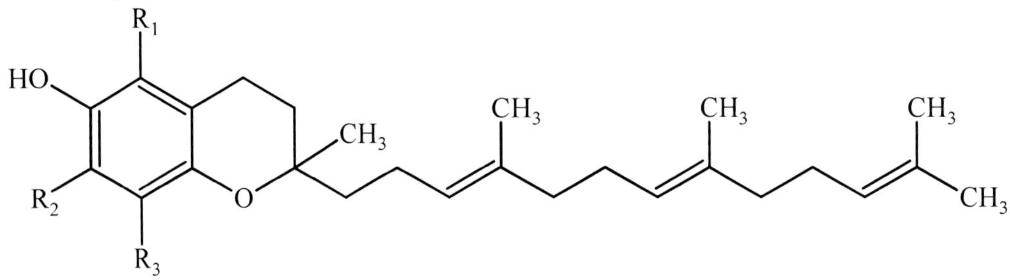

tocotrienols

Figure 10. Tocotrienols and tocopherols.

The difference in efficacy of *R,R*-THC on the two ER subtypes appears to arise from its optimal fit in the ERα ligand-binding pocket and its suboptimal fit in the slightly smaller ERβ pocket [32].

Evaluation of both the RBA and agonist/antagonist selectivity of trans- and cis-THCs suggests that the induction of an antagonist conformation in ERβ can be achieved with these ligands with less steric perturbation than in ERα. Nearly all examined THCs were found to be agonists on ERα, while THCs with small substituents were agonists on both ERα and ERβ. As substituent size was increased, ERβ-selective antagonism was developed first in the *R,R*-cis enantiomer series and finally in the trans diastereomer and *S,S*-cis enantiomer series. The most potent and selective ligand was identified as *R,R*-cis-diethyl THC. All of the trans-THC isomers have significantly greater affinities for both receptor subtypes than the corresponding cis isomers. However, trans-THC isomers and unsubstituted THC show minimal receptor subtype selectivity.

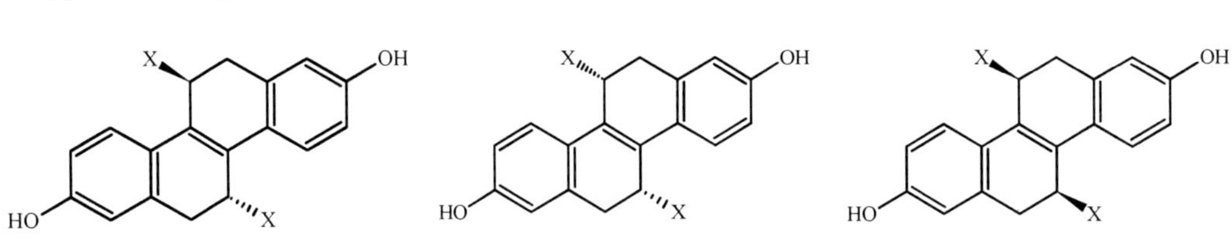

trans-THC cis-(RR)-THC cis-(SS)-THC

Figure 11. Molecular structure of tetrahydrochrysenes.

The most potent and selective ligand was identified as *R,R*-cis-diethyl THC. *R,R*-enantiomers develop ERβ selective antagonism with smaller substituents than do the *S,S*-enantiomers and trans isomers. Furthermore, antagonists that are selectively effective on ERβ can have structures that are very different from the typical antiestrogens that have bulky side chains and are antagonists for both ERα and ERβ.

THC and diethylstilbestrols (DES) both have the stilbene pharmacophore. The estrogen receptor is capable of binding a diverse set of ligands that are broadly categorized as agonists or antagonists. Agonists and antagonists differently position the C-terminal helix of the ligand-binding domain (helix-12). This C-terminal helix of the ligand-binding domain plays a critical role in the activation mechanism. When bound to activating ligands, helix-12 adopts a conformation that promotes the binding of co-activator proteins [79]. Crystal structures of ERα and ERβ ligand binding domain bound to THC revealed that the ERα domain adopts the same conformation when bound to THC as it does when bound to the full agonist E2 and DES. [54] In contrast, binding of THC to ERβ ligand binding domain destabilizes the active ligand binding domain conformation by promoting non-productive interactions between helix-12 and remainder of the domain.

Dihydrobenzoxathiins (Figure 12) were recently synthesized as a novel class of selective ERα modulators (SERAMs) [71, 80-84]. Selectivity of the dihydrobenzoxathiins is highly dependent on the size, location and stereochemistry of side chain substituents. Although the magnitude of receptor subtype selectivity (ERβ/ERα ratio) varied considerably, all of the novel analogs remained ERα selective. Dihydrobenzoxathiins with alkyl substituted pyrrolidine side chains are ERα selective ligands with antagonist activity. Addition of a methyl group to the side chain, at the appropriate position and with the correct orientation, generates substantial steric effects, causing the pyrrolidine ring to twist. Stereochemistry substantially increased estrogen antagonist activity in uterine tissue.

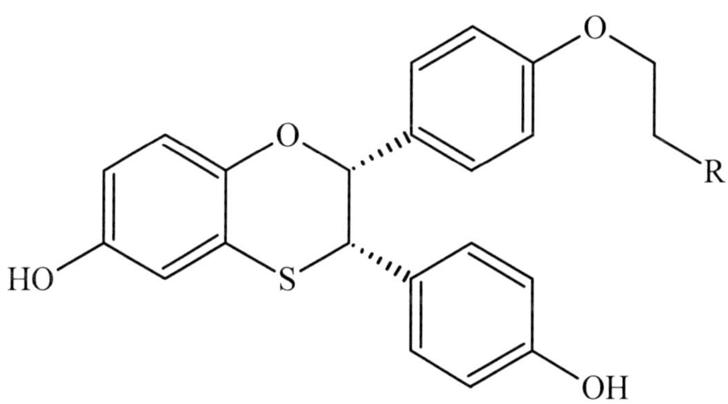

dihydrobenzoxanthiin

Figure 12. Molecular structure of dihydrobenzoxanthiin.

Tetrahydroisoquinoline derivatives (Figure 13) have been investigated for selective ER binding [85]. Since the binding pocket of the ER is rather lipophilic, increasing the lipophilicity of the tetrahydroisoquinoline by adding an alkyl substituent at the 1-position of the tetrahydroisoquinoline nucleus lead to the development of a pure antiestrogen with high affinity for ERα [86]. Tetrahydroisoquinolines bind to ER with high affinity. Studies have shown that modification of the substitution pattern of the N-phenyl ring has a modest impact on potency in most instances but significantly influences the selectivity. The pyrrolidine and piperidine were found to exhibit up to 50-fold specificities for ERα over ERβ. In addition, the nitrogen atom of the aminoethoxyphenyl substituent and 6-hydroxy substituent of the tetrahydroisoquinoline nucleus play important roles in ERα/ERβ selectivity in addition to R1 and R2 substituents.

To gain further insight into the ligand-receptor interaction, the x-ray crystallographic structure of the 1-H tetrahydroisoquinoline derivative–ER complex was solved. An overlay of this x-ray crystal structure with that reported for the complex of ER and raloxifene showed that both compounds bind to the same cleft of the receptor and display comparable binding modes. The differences observed were in the conformation of their phenyl groups corresponding to the D-ring of estradiol.

ERα exhibits stereo-selective ligand binding and transactivation for several structural derivatives and metabolites of the synthetic estrogen diethylstilbestrol (DES). DES (Figure 2) is a known carcinogen which is oxidatively metabolized to a variety of metabolites with varying degrees of hormonal activity [87]. Indenestrol A (IA) is a metabolite with high binding affinity for ERα but with weak biological activity [88]. It exists as a racemic mixture of the enantiomers *S*-indenestrol A and *R*-indenestrol A [89], which have a methyl substitution on the chiral carbon (Figure 13).

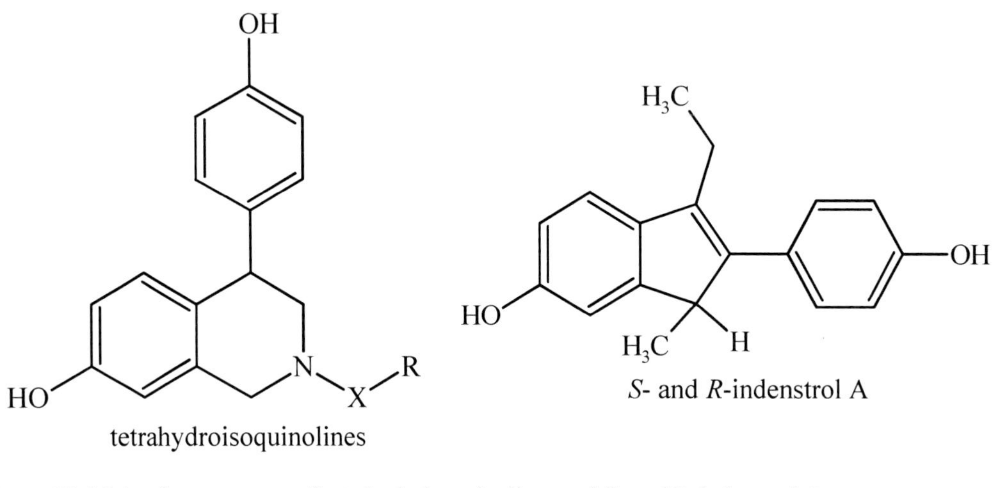

Figure 13. Molecular structures of tetrahydroisoquinolines and S- and R-indenstrol A.

Both enantiomers have agonistic properties. *S*-IA is a strong agonist, whereas *R*-IA displayed only weak agonistic activity for ERα and is a potency-selective agonist for ERβ in a cell-type specific manner. One single residue in the ligand binding domain of ERα and ERβ modulates their transcriptional activity in a cell type-independent fashion. These demonstrates that a single residue in the ligand binding domain determines the stereoselectivity of ERα and ERβ for indenestrol ligands, and that *R*-IA shows cell-type selectivity through ERβ [90].

ERβ Selectivity

Phytoestrogens as well as some androstanediols show selectivity towards ERβ even though they activate both ERα and ERβ [57]. The literature demonstrates that it is more difficult to develop ligands that stimulate ERβ to a greater extent than ERα than the converse. There are a number of estrogens with good selectivity for ERα but fewer compounds with good selectivity for ERβ. All environmental estrogenic chemicals compete with estradiol for binding to both ER subtypes with a similar preference and degree. In most instances the RBAs are at least 1000-fold lower than that of natural estrogens. Some phytoestrogens such as coumestrol, genistein (Figure 14), apigenin, naringenin, and kaempferol compete more strongly with estradiol for binding to ERβ than to ERα. While certain isoflavone phytoestrogens including genistein and coumestrol have higher affinity for ERβ than ERα [66], they do not show much difference in potency in cell-based transcription assays [91], although metabolism of isoflavones may have been a confounding factor [92]. Genistein is a relatively potent agonist for ERβ with an affinity approximately equal to that of estradiol. The relative selective binding of genistein to the ERβ indicates that the isoflavones may produce different clinical effects from that of estrogens by selectively triggering ERβ-mediated transcriptional pathways or differentially triggering transcriptional activation or repression pathways by ER [91]. Similar selectivity is reported for some aryl benzothiophene derivatives [93] and 4-hydroxy-N-phenylubstituted phthalimides [94].

Phytoestrogens

Some fifty years ago, researchers became aware that phytoestrogens (ie estrogens from plant sources) in alfalfa and clovers could affect the fertility of livestock. More recently, multiple epidemiological studies have found a relationship between high dietary intake of isoflavones and lignans and lower rates of certain cancers, cardiovascular problems, and menopausal symptoms [95]. The scientific literature contains conflicting reports regarding the relative "estrogenicities" of phytoestrogens compared with endogenous estrogens. Many in vitro studies have indicated that phytoestrogens have some 1/100 to 1/1000 the binding affinity of estradiol for cellular ERs leading to the conclusion that phytoestrogens are 100 to 1000 times weaker than estradiol [96]. However some of the reports on binding affinity did not distinguish between affinities for ERα and the more recently discovered ERβ. Although inconclusive, scientific evidence is accumulating to suggest that phytoestrogens may have a role in preventing chronic disease. There is increasing evidence that they may also be effective in preventing and treating prostate cancer, due to their antiandrogenic properties [97].

Phytoestrogens are made via biosynthetic pathways that are different from those for human estrogens and, consequently, they are not closely related chemically. Dietary estrogens are either produced by plants themselves (phytoestrogens) or by fungi that infect plants (mycoestrogens). The majority of phytoestrogens belong to a large group of polyphenolic compounds known as flavonoids. Flavonoids are low molecular weight hydrophobic compounds with molecular weights and structures similar to those of steroids.

Phytoestrogens can be divided into three main classes: isoflavones such as genistein and daidzein; coumestans such as coumestrol; and lignans such as enterodiol and enterolactone (Figure 14). Both human estrogens and phytoestrogens have certain structural similarities that enable them to bind with mammalian estrogen receptors. These similarities include: (a) the A and C rings of the isoflavones are similar to the A and B rings of estradiol; (b) the actual distance between the two hydroxyl groups (blue) on both molecules is nearly identical; (c) these hydroxyl groups are critically located to enable binding to the estrogen receptor protein; and (d) both molecules have similar polarities and molecular weights. The chemical structure of phytoestrogens resemble the estradiol structure in that they are composed of a planar ring system that includes a *p*-hydroxy-substituted aromatic ring approximately 12Å away from a second planar hydroxyl group. Two ring structures separated by two carbon atoms as well as spacing between hydrophobic and hydrogen bond interactions are also important in determining the binding affinity to ERs [98].

Recently, the prenylated flavanone, 8-prenylnaringenin (8-PN) derived from hops (Humulus lupulus L.), has been identified as a potent estrogen showing the highest in vitro estrogenic activity to date among all phytoestrogens known [99]. The biological activity of phytoestrogens varies due to structural features and deviations in the structure. Current research suggests that phytoestrogens may be natural SERMs [100]. Genistein, a well-known isoflavone phytoestrogen abundantly present in soy products, has very high binding affinity for human ERβ almost comparable to that of estradiol, but with a binding affinity for human ERα that is only 6% of this value. Coumestrol has a very high binding affinity for ERα and ERβ, with a slightly greater RBA for ERβ than for ERα. Myricetin and dibenzoylmethane both have weak overall binding affinities for ERα and ERβ. Similarly, daidzein has very weak binding affinities for both ERα and ERβ, but its RBA for ERβ is significantly higher than its RBA for ERα..

Isoflavones and flavones are the most well known of the phytoestrogens, and are capable of binding to both ERs. However, ERβ exhibits a 7- to 30-fold greater binding affinity for the isoflavone genistein (Figure 14), whereas estradiol binds to both ERα and ERβ with equal affinity. [101] The relatively selective binding of genistein to the ER indicates that the isoflavones may produce different clinical effects from that of the estrogens by selectively triggering ERβ-mediated transcriptional pathways or differentially triggering transcriptional activation or repression pathways by ER. One small study utilized a set of 21 flavonoids exhibiting estrogenic activity to develop a QSAR. Although selective binding was not evaluated, spatial, electronic and topological properties of the molecules were investigated in order to identify basic pharmacophore features of flavonoids for ER binding. The models that was generated highlighted the importance of atoms C2', C4' (ring C) and C7 (ring A), along with orientation and conformational rigidity of flavonoids for estrogenic activity [102]. Of importance are the partial charges at atoms C2' and C4' in the phenyl ring C, and molecular orientation and conformational stringency factors. It has been proposed that substitution by an electron donating group in the phenyl ring at C2', electron withdrawing groups at C4' and C7 of the molecule in conjunction with minimal conformational rigidity could be important for estrogenic activity.

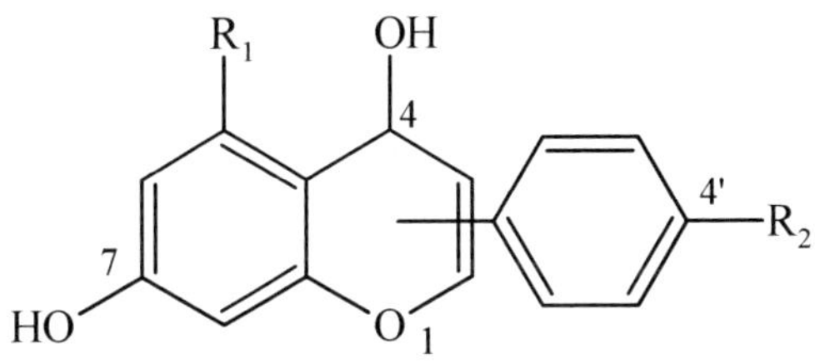

flavones and isoflavones

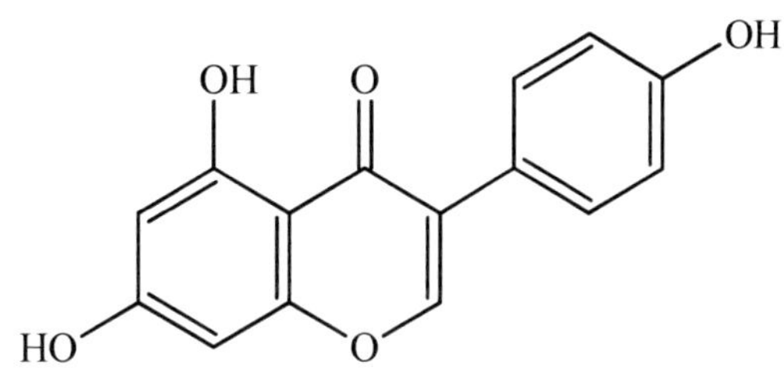

genistein

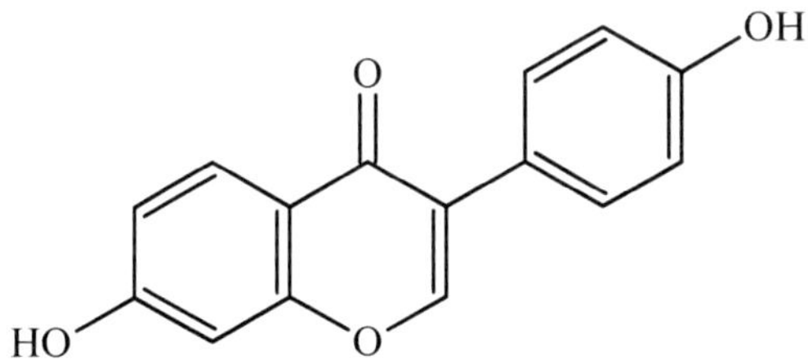

daidzein

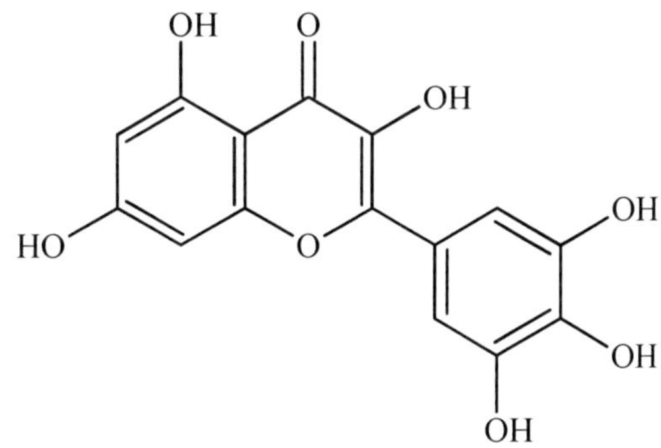

myricetin

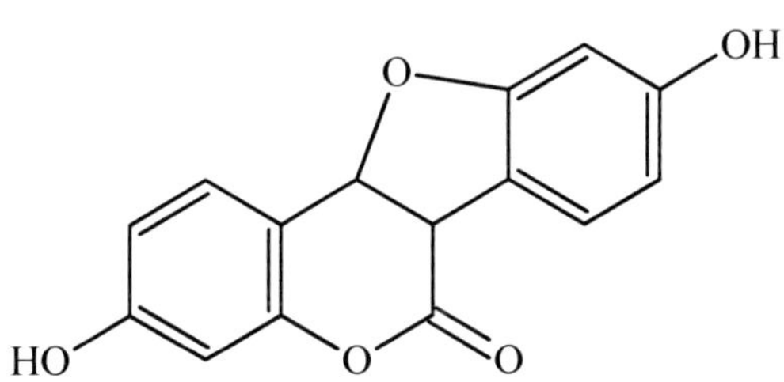

coumestrol

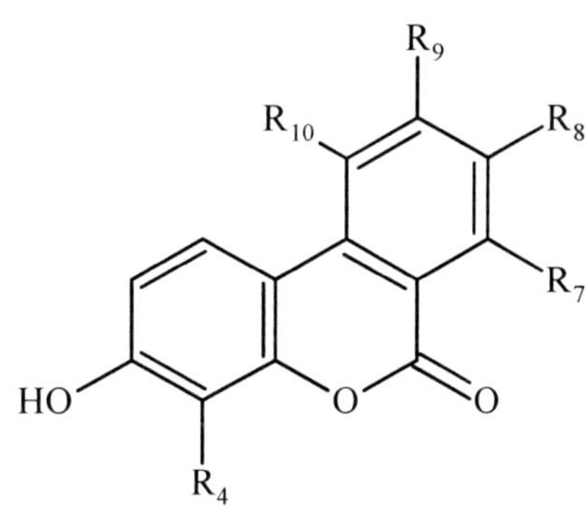

phenanthrenes

Figure 14. Molecular structures of certain phytoestrogens.

In a SAR study of natural and synthetic phenanthrenes (Figure 14), it was shown that an increase in the number of small hydrophobic substituents on the phenyl rings gave better ERβ binding affinity along with a significant increase in selectivity [103]. Small hydrophobic groups, such as methyl and ethyl groups are required for optimum binding affinity and selectivity, while hydroxy groups are essential for activity. An hydroxyl substituent in position 8 along with the hydroxyl at position 3 improves activity, while a polar amino group lowers the binding affinity and selectivity. Position 7 needs to be substituted with a methyl, ethyl or bromine to improve the ERβ-binding affinity as well as selectivity. The significance of lipophilic side-chains was also demonstrated in another QSAR study of phytoestrogen selective binding [104]. Previous research on the coumarins showed that estrogenic activity was related to their structural similarity to estradiol [105].

A study of the relationships between the structure of various substituted coumarins and their RBAs to the ERs showed the importance of the substituents at positions 3 and 7 [106]. More potent affinity for ERβ than for ERα, up to five-times the RBAs in the case of 3-(4-hydroxyphenyl)-7-hydroxycoumarin, was also demonstrated. The synthesis and SAR study of various substituted coumarins indicated that in comparison to estradiol, the 3-phenyl-4-ethyl-7-hydroxycoumarins and 3-(4-hydroxyphenyl)-4,7-dihydroxycoumarin present weak RBAs to both ERα and ERβ, thus lacking in selectivity. Substitution by a second phenyl group at position 4 as for 3,4-diphenyl-7-hydroxycoumarin increased the RBAs to both ERs, but with more selectivity for ERα than ERβ.

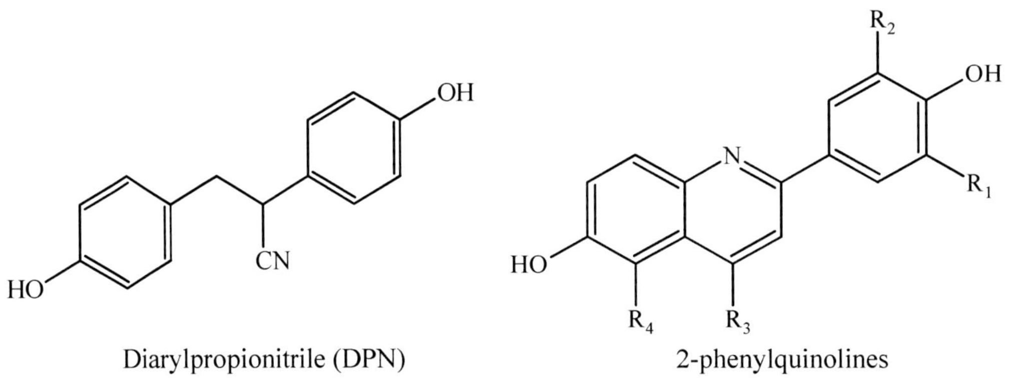

Figure 15. Structures of DPN and 2-phenylquinolines.

While certain phytoestrogens such as genistein and coumestrol have higher affinity for ERβ than ERα in cell-based transcription assays, they do not show much difference in potency. Even so, some simple diarylethane systems do show considerable affinity and potency preferences as agonists for ERβ [25, 107]. The best of these, diarylpropionitrile (DPN), Figure 15, activates ERβ at 100-fold lower concentrations than ERα. A single ERα point mutation (L384M vs Met-336) is sufficient to switch the DPN preferential binding to the ERβ type, but residues in helix-3 are also important in achieving the full ERβ selectivity of DPN. An energetically and structurally satisfying fit was found with the S-enantiomer of DPN, in which the β-ring of DPN functions as the mimic of the phenolic A-ring of estradiol and the nitrile projects toward the β face of the ligand-binding pocket. In this orientation, the nitrile is positioned where it might engage in energetically productive interactions with Met-336 and Thr-299 in ERβ, but the corresponding interactions in ERα (with Leu-384 and Thr-347) are not possible. Therefore, the ERβ selectivity of DPN seems to result from its preferential dynamic interaction of the nitrile moiety with a key methionine residue (Met-336) that is present only in the ERβ ligand binding pocket [108]. In addition, some differences in helix-3 constrain a portion of the ER ligand binding pocket, which can improve interactions between receptor and this rather small ligand [108]. The differential interaction of the nitrile with Met-336 in ERβ versus Leu-384 in ERα appears to be simply a consequence of residue differences. However, the potential interaction of the nitrile with Thr-299 in ERβ versus its lack of possible interaction with Thr-347 in ERα seems to result from sequence differences at the start of helix-3 that are rather remote from the ligand and that reshape the ligand binding pocket, making it smaller in ERβ than in ERα. S-DPN, being a small ligand, fits more tightly in the ERβ ligand pocket in a manner that positions its nitrile rather close to Thr-299, whereas the larger pocket in ERα does not engender such a nitrile-threonine approximation.

New synthetic bis-benzylnitriles and related compounds have up to 170-fold potency selectivity at ERβ [107]. While nitriles are not a common functionality in non-steroidal estrogens, cyanoestrogens have been known since the middle of last century [109]. In 1956, a series of bisphenolic alkanonitriles were patented for the treatment of cardiovascular disease [110]. The compounds were claimed to have no estrogenic effects even in high doses. Prior to 1996, it was assumed that only one ER existed and a common analytical assay measuring RBA was done on uterine tissue that mostly contained ERα [111]. Recently a number of diarylpropionitriles, diarylsuccinonitriles as well as acetylene and polar analogues of these nitriles were also found to be ERβ selective agonists. The acetylene analogues had higher binding affinities but lower selectivities than their nitrile analogues. This study suggested that the nitrile functionality is critical to ER selectivity in this series of ligands. Furthermore, the addition of a second nitrile group to the nitrile in DPN, or the addition of a methyl substitutent at an ortho position on the aromatic ring increased the affinity and selectivity of these compounds for ERβ. Structure-activity relationship results of these studies suggested that the nitrile functionality represents the optimal combination of linear *sp* geometry and local polarity, and it is the best functional group for ligands of this type in respect to ER binding affinity, more so for ERα than for ERβ. It appears that ERα has a lesser ability to tolerate the polar nature of the nitrile functionality, while the ERβ is less affected by the polar nature of the nitrile function than by the geometric requirement of the *sp* hybridization. As a result, ligands with linear groups show high selectivity for ERβ, and the increased polarity of the nitrile group reduces the affinity of the ligand for ERα, resulting in higher ERβ binding selectivities. Thus, their selectivity depends on the presence of nitrile, while their affinity to both receptors depends on the presence of both phenolic hydroxyl groups. If either hydroxyl group is removed, the affinity for both receptors falls significantly but more for ERβ than for ERα. If either OH group is moved to meta position there is a only a moderate drop in affinity. However, addition of a methyl group in the ortho position relative to hydroxy of either ring increases affinity probably due to the restricted rotation and increased rigidity of the molecular scaffold. Binding affinities for succinonitriles depends on their relative stereochemistry. Selectivity, on the onther hand is not influenced by stereochemistry.

The 2-phenylquinolines (Figure 15) have been identified as a new series of potential ERβ-selective agonists [112]. Substitution at the C4 position, particularly with electronegative groups, is required for ERβ selectivity. The SAR study has shown that selectivity enhancement could be achieved by incorporating a fluoro group at the 3' position of the phenyl ring. A number of substituted 2-phenylquinolines displayed superior ERβ affinity and selectivity compared to that of genistein. The best compound of this study (compound 13b) contained both fluoro and bromo substitutions and was found to be a selective partial agonist at ERβ in a cell-based transcriptional assay. Its uterine weight bioassay showed no significant uterine stimulation, suggesting that this compound would not activate ERα in vivo.

Over the last decade several groups have developed ERβ selective ligands using structure based design methods along with inspiration from the well-known ERβ-selective isoflavone phytoestrogens daidzein and genistein. All of these ligands have in common two phenols which bind to the Glu-Arg-water triad at one end of the ERβ receptor binding pocket and His-475 at the other end. These two critical features of the ERβ pharmacophore require a separation of the phenol oxygen atoms by a distance of about 10-12Å (roughly 10 atoms). The benzopyran scaffold (Figure 16) served as an excellent starting point to build ERβ selective ligands because the benzopyran substructure provides a rigid platform with a distance between the phenol oxygens of 11.9Å. This distance positions the phenol oxygen atoms between the genistein distance of 12.2Å and the estradiol distance of 10.9Å. Fusing a cyclopentane ring to the 3,4-positions of benzopyran dramatically improved binding affinity and afforded a compound with 9-fold selectivity for ERβ over ER. Increasing the ring size of the ring fused to cyclohexane or cycloheptane did not improve ERβ binding potency. Removal of the hydoxyl group from the pendant 4'-aryl ring resulted in a 60-fold and a 100-fold loss in binding affinity for ERα and ERβ, respectively, demonstrating the importance of this phenol in the ER pharmacophore [113]. Benzopyrans are selective estrogen receptor (ER) beta agonists (SERBAs), which bind ERα and ERβ in opposite orientations.

Recently, other more polar heterocyclic core systems, benzothiazoles, benzimidazoles, and benzoxazoles have been described as ERβ-selective agents [114-116]. Notable in these ligands is a relatively narrow structural profile and a core system enriched in heteroatoms: characteristics that appear favor ERβ selective binding although that also do not appear to be essential. Recently, deoxyhexestrol (Figure 17), a compound that was first examined long before the discovery of ERβ, was tested again for its binding to both ERs.

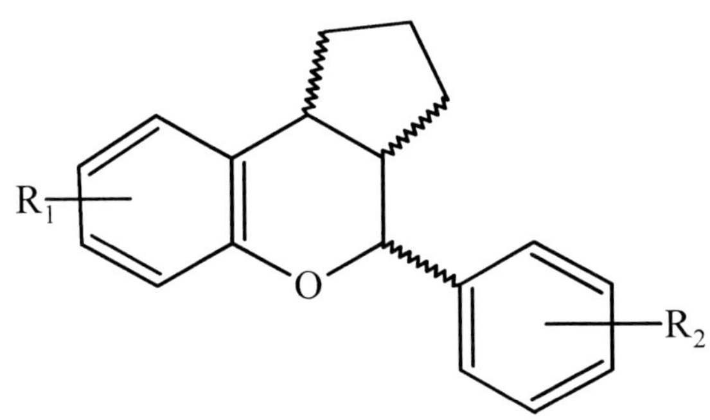

Figure 16. Molecular scaffold of benzopyrans.

It had good affinity, especially for ERβ, being in this regard more preferential than its congeners hexestrol and diethylstilbestrol. In order to develop compounds selective for ERβ, pyridine and pyrimidine analogs (Figure 17) of the non-steroidal estrogen deoxyhexestrol were synthesized. Their low affinity for the ER was attributed to resonance enforcement of a conformation unfavorable for binding. Resonance-enforced conformational constraint prevents optimal accommodation in the ER ligand binding pocket [117]. DES and hexestrol fit very well in the ER binding pocket. One phenol fits in the narrow A-ring binding pocket as does the A-ring of estradiol, and the two ethyl groups can nicely fill the major 7α, 11β subpockets. By contrast, because of the more pronounced amine-heterocycle resonance, the pyridine and pyrimidine analogs of deoxyhexestrol appear to be forced to adopt a conformation in which the backbone is almost coplanar with the hydroxy-containing heteroarene, with the result that the two ethyl groups are not well disposed to fill the 7α, 11β subpockets. Thus, introduction of nitrogen heteroatoms within the flexible structure of a high affinity all-carbon ligand, deoxyhexestrol, can dramatically reduce binding affinity, even without altering the overall hydrophobicity of the ligand.

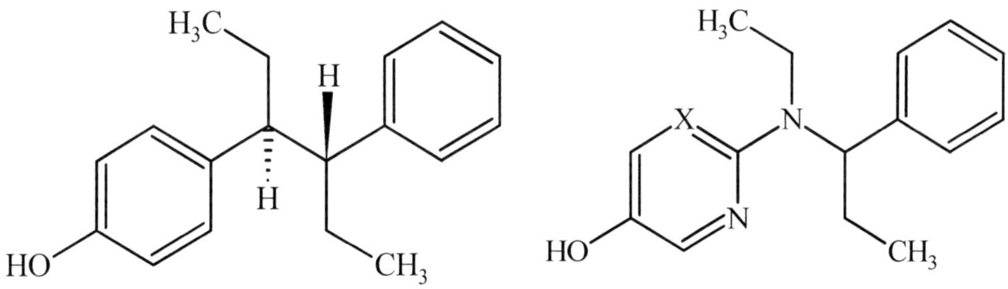

deoxyhexestrol

X = C: purine analogue
X = N: pyrimidine analogue

Figure 17. Pyridine and pyrimidine analogs of the phenol in deoxyhexestrol.

Conclusion

As the molecular mechanisms of the action of SERMs become more completely understood, rational drug design will replace the current empirical method for the discovery of new drugs that will selectively express desirable actions and suppress undesirable actions of the various steroid hormones. A tissue-selective drug would have all the beneficial effects of estrogen, none of its side effects, and might therefore offer protection against numerous human physiological and pathological conditions. Current research has identified ligands with selective potency, efficacy and antagonist properties at ER subtypes. There is value in deciphering the target site and specific actions of ligands at ERα and ERβ. Advances have been made in identifying both ligand and ligand binding domain structural requirements for selectivity. As our understanding grows there is the potential for selective ER modulators to be developed as useful clinical medicines.

References

[1] Farhat, M. Y.; Lavigne, M. C.; Ramwell, P. W. The vascular protective effects of estrogen. *FASEB J.* 1996, *10*, 615-24.

[2] Nilsson, S.; Gustafsson, J. A. Biological role of estrogen and estrogen receptors. *Crit. Rev. Biochem. Mol. Biol.* 2002, *37*, 1-28.

[3] Turner, R. T.; Riggs, B. L.; Spelsberg, T. C. Skeletal effects of estrogen. *Endocr. Rev.* 1994, *15*, 275-300.

[4] Cowley, S. M.; Hoare, S.; Mosselman, S.; Parker, M. G. Estrogen receptors alpha and beta form heterodimers on DNA. *Journal of Biological Chemistry* 1997, *272*, 19858-62.

[5] Katzenellenbogen, B. S.; Korach, K. S. A new actor in the estrogen receptor drama - Enter ER-beta. *Endocrinology* 1997, *138*, 861-2.

[6] Zhu, B. T.; Han, G. Z.; Shim, J. Y.; Wen, Y.; Jiang, X. R. Quantitative structure-activity relationship of various endogenous estrogen metabolites for human estrogen receptor alpha and beta subtypes: Insights into the structural determinants favoring a differential subtype binding. *Endocrinology* 2006, *147*, 4132-50.

[7] Kumar, V.; Green, S.; Stack, G.; Berry, M.; Jin, J. R.; Chambon, P. Functional Domains of the Human Estrogen-Receptor. *Cell* 1987, *51*, 941-51.

[8] Kraus, W. L.; McInerney, E. M.; Katzenellenbogen, B. S. Ligand-dependent, transcriptionally productive association of the amino- and carboxyl-terminal regions of a steroid hormone nuclear receptor. *Proc. Natl. Acad. Sci. U. S. A.* 1995, *92*, 12314-8.

[9] Sasano, H.; Suzuki, T.; Matsuzaki, Y.; Fukaya, T.; Endoh, M.; Nagura, H.; Kimura, M. Messenger ribonucleic acid in situ hybridization analysis of estrogen receptors alpha and beta in human breast carcinoma. *J. Clin. Endocrinol. Metab.* 1999, *84*, 781-5.

[10] Utsunomiya, H.; Suzuki, T.; Harada, N.; Ito, K.; Matsuzaki, S.; Konno, R.; Sato, S.; Yajima, A.; Sasano, H. Analysis of estrogen receptor alpha and beta in endometrial carcinomas: correlation with ER beta and clinicopathologic findings in 45 cases. *Int. J. Gynecol. Pathol.* 2000, *19*, 335-41.

[11] Bardin, A.; Boulle, N.; Lazennec, G.; Vignon, F.; Pujol, P. Loss of ERbeta expression as a common step in estrogen-dependent tumor progression. *Endocr. Relat. Cancer* 2004, *11*, 537-51.

[12] Matthews, J.; Gustafsson, J.-A. Estrogen Signaling: A Subtle Balance Between ER{alpha} and ER{beta}. *Mol. Interv.* 2003, *3*, 281-92.

[13] Helguero, L. A.; Faulds, M. H.; Gustafsson, J.-A.; Haldosen, L.-A. Estrogen receptors alfa (ER[alpha]) and beta (ER[beta]) differentially regulate proliferation and apoptosis of the normal murine mammary epithelial cell line HC11. *Oncogene* 2005, *24*, 6605-16.

[14] Lindberg, M. K.; Moverare, S.; Skrtic, S.; Gao, H.; Dahlman-Wright, K.; Gustafsson, J.-A.; Ohlsson, C. Estrogen Receptor (ER)-{beta} Reduces ER{alpha}-Regulated Gene Transcription, Supporting a "Ying Yang" Relationship between ER{alpha} and ER{beta} in Mice. *Mol Endocrinol* 2003, *17*, 203-8.

[15] Hall, J. M.; McDonnell, D. P. The estrogen receptor beta-isoform (ERbeta) of the human estrogen receptor modulates ERalpha transcriptional activity and is a key regulator of the cellular response to estrogens and antiestrogens. *Endocrinology* 1999, *140*, 5566-78.

[16] Dusell, C. D.; Umetani, M.; Shaul, P. W.; Mangelsdorf, D. J.; McDonnell, D. P. 27-hydroxycholesterol is an endogenous selective estrogen receptor modulator. *Mol. Endocrinol.* 2008, *22*, 65-77. Epub 2007 Sep 13.

[17] Davidson, N. E. Hormone-replacement therapy--breast versus heart versus bone. *N. Engl. J. Med.* 1995, *332*, 1638-9.

[18] Stampfer, M. J.; Colditz, G. A.; Willett, W. C.; Manson, J. E.; Rosner, B.; Speizer, F. E.; Hennekens, C. H. Postmenopausal estrogen therapy and cardiovascular disease. Ten-year follow-up from the nurses' health study. *N. Engl. J. Med.* 1991, *325*, 756-62.

[19] Barrett-Connor, E.; Bush, T. L. Estrogen and coronary heart disease in women. *J. Am. Med. Soc.* 1991, *265*, 1861-7.

[20] Rice, M. M.; Graves, A. B.; McCurry, S. M.; Larson, E. B. Estrogen replacement therapy and cognitive function in postmenopausal women without dementia. *Am. J. Med.* 1997, *103*, 26S-35S.

[21] Chang, W. Y.; Prins, G. S. Estrogen receptor-beta: Implications for the prostate gland. *Prostate* 1999, *40*, 115-24.

[22] Nilsson, S.; Kuiper, G.; Gustafsson, J. A. ERb a novel estrogen receptor offers the potential for new drug development. *Trends Endocrinol. Metab.* 1998, *9*, 387-95.

[23] Kim, S.; Wu, J. Y.; Birzin, E. T.; Frisch, K.; Chan, W.; Pai, L. Y.; Yang, Y. T.; Mosley, R. T.; Fitzgerald, P. M. D.; Sharma, N.; Dahllund, J.; Thorsell, A. G.; DiNinno, F.; Rohrer, S. P.; Schaeffer, J. M.; Hammond, M. L. Estrogen Receptor Ligands. II. Discovery of Benzoxathiins as Potent, Selective Estrogen Receptor and#x03B1; Modulators. *J. Med. Chem.* 2004, *47*, 2171-5.

[24] Mortensen, D. S.; Rodriguez, A. L.; Carlson, K. E.; Sun, J.; Katzenellenbogen, B. S.; Katzenellenbogen, J. A. Synthesis and Biological Evaluation of a Novel Series of Furans: Ligands Selective for Estrogen Receptor and#x03B1. *J. Med. Chem.* 2001, *44*, 3838-48.

[25] Meyers, M. J.; Sun, J.; Carlson, K. E.; Marriner, G. A.; Katzenellenbogen, B. S.; Katzenellenbogen, J. A. Estrogen Receptor-and#x03B2; Potency-Selective Ligands: Structure-Activity Relationship Studies of Diarylpropionitriles and Their Acetylene and Polar Analogues. *J. Med. Chem.* 2001, *44*, 4230-51.

[26] Hu, J.-Y.; Aizawa, T. Quantitative structure-activity relationships for estrogen receptor binding affinity of phenolic chemicals. *Water Research* 2003, *37*, 1213-22.

[27] Anstead, G. M.; Carlson, K. E.; Katzenellenbogen, J. A. The estradiol pharmacophore: Ligand structure-estrogen receptor binding affinity relationships and a model for the receptor binding site. *Steroids* 1997, *62*, 268-303.

[28] Schueler, F. W. Sex hormonal Action and Chemical constitution. *Science* 1946, *103*, 213-40.

[29] Précigoux, G.; Marsau, P.; Leroy, F.; Busetta, B. 17-Hydroxymethyl-1,3,5(10)-estratrien-3-ol monohydrate. *Acta Cryst.* 1980, *B36*, 749-51.

[30] Schueler, F. W. Sex Hormonal Action and Chemical Constitution. *Science* 1946, *103*, 221-3.

[31] Brzozowski, A. M.; Pike, A. C.; Dauter, Z.; Hubbard, R. E.; Bonn, T.; Engstrom, O.; Ohman, L.; Greene, G. L.; Gustafsson, J. A.; Carlquist, M. Molecular basis of agonism and antagonism in the oestrogen receptor. *Nature* 1997, *389*, 753-8.

[32] Shiau, A. K.; Barstad, D.; Radek, J. L.; Meyers, M. J.; Nettles, K. W.; Katzenellenbogen, B. S.; Katzenellenbogen, J. A.; Agard, D. A.; Greene, G. L. Structural characterization of a subtype-selective ligand reveals a novel mode of estrogen receptor antagonism. *Nat. Struct. Biol.* 2002, *9*, 359-64.

[33] Shi, L. M.; Fang, H.; Tong, W.; Wu, J.; Perkins, R.; Blair, R. M.; Branham, W. S.; Dial, S. L.; Moland, C. L.; Sheehan, D. M. QSAR models using a large diverse set of estrogens. *J. Chem. Inf. Comput. Sci.* 2001, *41*, 186-95.

[34] Tabira, Y.; Nakai, M.; Asai, D.; Yakabe, Y.; Tahara, Y.; Shinmyozu, T.; Noguchi, M.; Takatsuki, M.; Shimohigashi, Y. Structural requirements of para-alkylphenols to bind to estrogen receptor. *Eur. J. Biochem.* 1999, *262*, 240-5.

[35] Rozhin, J.; Huo, A.; Zemlicka, J.; Brooks, S. C. Studies on bovine adrenal estrogen sulfotransferase. Inhibition and possible involvement of adenine-estrogen stacking. *J. Biol. Chem.* 1977, *252*, 7214-20.

[36] Bradbury, S.; Mekenyan, O.; Ankley, G. Quantitative structure-activity relationships for polychlorinated hydroxybiphenyl estrogen receptor binding affinity - an assessment of conformer flexibility. *Environ. Toxicol. Chem.* 1996, *15*, 1945–54.

[37] Melamed, M.; Castano, E.; Notides, A. C.; Sasson, S. Molecular and kinetic basis for the mixed agonist/antagonist activity of estriol. *Mol. Endocrinol.* 1997, *11*, 1868-78.

[38] Clark, J. H.; Paszko, Z.; Peck, E. J., Jr. Nuclear binding and retention of the receptor estrogen complex: relation to the agonistic and antagonistic properties of estriol. *Endocrinology* 1977, *100*, 91-6.

[39] Kuiper, G. G.; Carlsson, B.; Grandien, K.; Enmark, E.; Haggblad, J.; Nilsson, S.; Gustafsson, J. A. Comparison of the ligand binding specificity and transcript tissue distribution of estrogen receptors alpha and beta. *Endocrinology* 1997, *138*, 863-70.

[40] Tong, W.; Perkins, R.; Xing, L.; Welsh, W. J.; Sheehan, D. M. QSAR Models for Binding of Estrogenic Compounds to Estrogen Receptor {alpha} and {beta} Subtypes. *Endocrinology* 1997, *138*, 4022-5.

[41] Palomino, E.; Heeg, M. J.; Horwitz, J. P.; Polin, L.; Brooks, S. C. Skeletal Conformations and Receptor-Binding of Some 9,11-Modified Estradiols. *Journal of Steroid Biochemistry and Molecular Biology* 1994, *50*, 75-84.

[42] Fang, H.; Tong, W. D.; Shi, L. M.; Blair, R.; Perkins, R.; Branham, W.; Hass, B. S.; Xie, Q.; Dial, S. L.; Moland, C. L.; Sheehan, D. M. Structure-activity relationships for a large diverse set of natural, synthetic, and environmental estrogens. *Chemical Research in Toxicology* 2001, *14*, 280-94.

[43] Perez-Palacios, G.; Santillan, R.; Garcia-Becerra, R.; Borja-Cacho, E.; Larrea, F.; Damian-Matsumura, P.; Gonzalez, L.; Lemus, A. E. Enhanced formation of non-phenolic androgen metabolites with intrinsic oestrogen-like gene transactivation potency in human breast cancer cells: a distinctive metabolic pattern. *J Endocrinol* 2006, *190*, 805-18.

[44] Larrea, F.; Garcia-Becerra, R.; Lemus, A. E.; Garcia, G. A.; Perez-Palacios, G.; Jackson, K. J.; Coleman, K. M.; Dace, R.; Smith, C. L.; Cooney, A. J. A-Ring Reduced Metabolites of 19-nor Synthetic Progestins as Subtype Selective Agonists for ER{alpha}. *Endocrinology* 2001, *142*, 3791-9.

[45] Minutolo, F.; Antonello, M.; Bertini, S.; Ortore, G.; Placanica, G.; Rapposelli, S.; Sheng, S.; Carlson, K. E.; Katzenellenbogen, B. S.; Katzenellenbogen, J. A.; Macchia, M. Novel Estrogen Receptor Ligands Based on an Anthranylaldoxime Structure: Role of the Phenol-Type Pseudocycle in the Binding Process. *J. Med. Chem.* 2003, *46*, 4032-42.

[46] Minutolo, F.; Bertini, S.; Martinelli, A.; Ortore, G.; Placanica, G.; Prota, G.; Rapposelli, S.; Tuccinardi, T.; Sheng, S.; Carlson, K. E.; Katzenellenbogen, B. S.; Katzenellenbogen, J. A.; Macchia, M. Salicylaldoximes and anthranylaldoximes as alternative to phenol-based estrogen receptor ligands. *Arkivoc* 2006, *viii*, 83-94.

[47] Jordan, V. C. The Strategic Use of Antiestrogens to Control the Development and Growth of Breast-Cancer. *Cancer* 1992, *70*, 977-82.

[48] Love, R. R.; Mazess, R. B.; Barden, H. S.; Epstein, S.; Newcomb, P. A.; Jordan, V. C.; Carbone, P. P.; Demets, D. L. Effects of Tamoxifen on Bone-Mineral Density in Postmenopausal Women with Breast-Cancer. *New England Journal of Medicine* 1992, *326*, 852-6.

[49] Kedar, R. P.; Bourne, T. H.; Powles, T. J.; Collins, W. P.; Ashley, S. E.; Cosgrove, D. O.; Campbell, S. Effects of tamoxifen on uterus and ovaries of postmenopausal women in a randomised breast cancer prevention trial. *Lancet* 1994, *343*, 1318-21.

[50] Murphy, L. C.; Peng, B.; Lewis, A.; Davie, J. R.; Leygue, E.; Kemp, A.; Ung, K.; Vendetti, M.; Shiu, R. Inducible upregulation of oestrogen receptor-{beta}1 affects oestrogen and tamoxifen responsiveness in MCF7 human breast cancer cells. *J Mol Endocrinol* 2005, *34*, 553-66.

[51] Black, L. J.; Sato, M.; Rowley, E. R.; Magee, D. E.; Bekele, A.; Williams, D. C.; Cullinan, G. J.; Bendele, R.; Kauffman, R. F.; Bensch, W. R.; et al. Raloxifene (LY139481 HCI) prevents bone loss and reduces serum cholesterol without causing uterine hypertrophy in ovariectomized rats. *J Clin Invest* 1994, *93*, 63-9.

[52] Dunn, B.; Anthony, M.; Arun, B. The search for the ideal SERM. *Expert Opinion on Pharmacotherapy* 2002, *3*, 681-91.

[53] Tate, A. C.; Greene, G. L.; DeSombre, E. R.; Jensen, E. V.; Jordan, V. C. Differences between estrogen- and antiestrogen-estrogen receptor complexes from human breast tumors identified with an antibody raised against the estrogen receptor. *Cancer Res.* 1984, *44*, 1012-8.

[54] Shiau, A. K.; Barstad, D.; Loria, P. M.; Cheng, L.; Kushner, P. J.; Agard, D. A.; Greene, G. L. The Structural Basis of Estrogen Receptor/Coactivator Recognition and the Antagonism of This Interaction by Tamoxifen. *Cell* 1998, *95*, 927-37.

[55] Pike, A. C. W.; Brzozowski, A. M.; Hubbard, R. E.; Bonn, T.; Thorsell, A. G.; Engstrom, O.; Ljunggren, J.; Gustafsson, J. K.; Carlquist, M. Structure of the ligand-binding domain of oestrogen receptor beta in the presence of a partial agonist and a full antagonist. *EMBO J.* 1999, *18*, 4608-18.

[56] Kraichely, D. M.; Sun, J.; Katzenellenbogen, J. A.; Katzenellenbogen, B. S. Conformational changes and coactivator recruitment by novel ligands for estrogen receptor-alpha and estrogen receptor-beta: Correlations with biological character and distinct differences among SRC coactivator family members. *Endocrinology* 2000, *141*, 3534-45.

[57] Kuiper, G. G. J. M.; Lemmen, J. G.; Carlsson, B.; Corton, J. C.; Safe, S. H.; van der Saag, P. T.; van der Burg, P.; Gustafsson, J. A. Interaction of estrogenic chemicals and phytoestrogens with estrogen receptor beta. *Endocrinology* 1998, *139*, 4252-63.

[58] Pike, A. C. W.; Brzozowski, A. M.; Hubbard, R. E.; Bonn, T.; Thorsell, A. G.; Engstrom, O.; Ljunggren, J.; Gustafsson, J. K.; Carlquist, M. Structure of the ligand-

binding domain of oestrogen receptor beta in the presence of a partial agonist and a full antagonist. *Embo Journal* 1999, *18*, 4608-18.

[59] Pike, A. C.; Brzozowski, A. M.; Walton, J.; Hubbard, R. E.; Thorsell, A. G.; Li, Y. L.; Gustafsson, J. A.; Carlquist, M. Structural insights into the mode of action of a pure antiestrogen. *Structure* 2001, *9*, 145-53.

[60] Heldring, N.; Pike, A.; Andersson, S.; Matthews, J.; Cheng, G.; Hartman, J.; Tujague, M.; Strom, A.; Treuter, E.; Warner, M.; Gustafsson, J. A. Estrogen receptors: how do they signal and what are their targets. *Physiol. Rev.* 2007, *87*, 905-31.

[61] Sun, J.; Meyers, M. J.; Fink, B. E.; Rajendran, R.; Katzenellenbogen, J. A.; Katzenellenbogen, B. S. Novel ligands that function as selective estrogens or antiestrogens for estrogen receptor-alpha or estrogen receptor-beta. *Endocrinology* 1999, *140*, 800-4.

[62] Shiau, A. K.; Barstad, D.; Radek, J. T.; Meyers, M. J.; Nettles, K. W.; Katzenellenbogen, B. S.; Katzenellenbogen, J. A.; Agard, D. A.; Greene, G. L. Structural characterization of a subtype-selective ligand reveals a novel mode of estrogen receptor antagonism. *Nat Struct Biol* 2002, *9*, 359-64.

[63] Mortensen, D. S.; Rodriguez, A. L.; Sun, J.; Katzenellenbogen, B. S.; Katzenellenbogen, J. A. Furans with basic side chains: Synthesis and biological evaluation of a novel series of antagonists with selectivity for the estrogen receptor alpha. *Bioorg. Med. Chem. Lett.* 2001, *11*, 2521-4.

[64] Stauffer, S. R.; Coletta, C. J.; Tedesco, R.; Nishiguchi, G.; Carlson, K.; Sun, J.; Katzenellenbogen, B. S.; Katzenellenbogen, J. A. Pyrazole ligands: Structure-affinity/activity relationships and estrogen receptor-alpha-selective agonists. *Journal of Medicinal Chemistry* 2000, *43*, 4934-47.

[65] Stauffer, S. R.; Huang, Y.; Coletta, C. J.; Tedesco, R.; Katzenellenbogen, J. A. Estrogen pyrazoles: defining the pyrazole core structure and the orientation of substituents in the ligand binding pocket of the estrogen receptor. *Bioorg Med Chem* 2001, *9*, 141-50.

[66] Kuiper, G. G.; Lemmen, J. G.; Carlsson, B.; Corton, J. C.; Safe, S. H.; van der Saag, P. T.; van der Burg, B.; Gustafsson, J. A. Interaction of estrogenic chemicals and phytoestrogens with estrogen receptor beta. *Endocrinology* 1998, *139*, 4252-63.

[67] Mortensen, D. S.; Rodriguez, A. L.; Carlson, K. E.; Sun, J.; Katzenellenbogen, B. S.; Katzenellenbogen, J. A. Synthesis and biological evaluation of a novel series of furans: ligands selective for estrogen receptor alpha. *J Med Chem* 2001, *44*, 3838-48.

[68] Harris, H. A.; Katzenellenbogen, J. A.; Katzenellenbogen, B. S. Characterization of the biological roles of the estrogen receptors, ERalpha and ERbeta, in estrogen target tissues in vivo through the use of an ERalpha-selective ligand. *Endocrinology* 2002, *143*, 4172-7.

[69] Ghosh, U.; Ganessunker, D.; Sattigeri, V. J.; Carlson, K. E.; Mortensen, D. J.; Katzenellenbogen, B. S.; Katzenellenbogen, J. A. Estrogenic diazenes: heterocyclic non-steroidal estrogens of unusual structure with selectivity for estrogen receptor subtypes. *Bioorg Med Chem* 2003, *11*, 629-57.

[70] Stauffer, S. R.; Sun, J.; Katzenellenbogen, B. S.; Katzenellenbogen, J. A. Acyclic amides as estrogen receptor ligands: synthesis, binding, activity and receptor interaction. *Bioorg Med Chem* 2000, *8*, 1293-316.

[71] Tan, Q.; Blizzard, T. A.; Morgan, J. D., 2nd; Birzin, E. T.; Chan, W.; Yang, Y. T.; Pai, L. Y.; Hayes, E. C.; DaSilva, C. A.; Warrier, S.; Yudkovitz, J.; Wilkinson, H. A.; Sharma, N.; Fitzgerald, P. M.; Li, S.; Colwell, L.; Fisher, J. E.; Adamski, S.; Reszka, A. A.; Kimmel, D.; DiNinno, F.; Rohrer, S. P.; Freedman, L. P.; Schaeffer, J. M.; Hammond, M. L. Estrogen receptor ligands. Part 10: Chromanes: old scaffolds for new SERAMs. *Bioorg. Med. Chem. Lett.* 2005, *15*, 1675-81.

[72] Packer, L. Protective role of vitamin E in biological systems. *Am J Clin Nutr* 1991, *53*, 1050S-5.

[73] Stäuble, B.; Boscoboinik, D.; Tasinato, A.; Azzi, A. Modulation of Activator Protein-1 (AP-1) Transcription Factor and Protein Kinase C by Hydrogen Peroxide and d-and#x03B1;-Tocopherol in Vascular Smooth Muscle Cells. *European Journal of Biochemistry* 1994, *226*, 393-402.

[74] Turley, J. M.; Fu, T.; Ruscetti, F. W.; Mikovits, J. A.; Bertolette, D. C., III; Birchenall-Roberts, M. C. Vitamin E Succinate Induces Fas-mediated Apoptosis in Estrogen Receptor-Negative Human Breast Cancer Cells. *Cancer Res* 1997, *57*, 881-90.

[75] Nesaretnam, K.; Guthrie, N.; Chambers, A.; Carroll, K. Effect of tocotrienols on the growth of a human breast cancer cell line in culture. *Lipids* 1995, *30*, 1139-43.

[76] Gould, M. N.; Haag, J. D.; Kennan, W. S.; Tanner, M. A.; Elson, C. E. A comparison of tocopherol and tocotrienol for the chemoprevention of chemically induced rat mammary tumors. *Am J Clin Nutr* 1991, *53*, 1068S-70.

[77] McIntyre, B.; Briski, K.; Tirmenstein, M.; Fariss, M.; Gapor, A.; Sylvester, P. Antiproliferative and apoptotic effects of tocopherols and tocotrienols on normal mouse mammary epithelial cells. *Lipids* 2000, *35*, 171-80.

[78] Meyers, M. J.; Sun, J.; Carlson, K. E.; Katzenellenbogen, B. S.; Katzenellenbogen, J. A. Estrogen receptor subtype-selective ligands: asymmetric synthesis and biological evaluation of cis- and trans-5,11-dialkyl- 5,6,11, 12-tetrahydrochrysenes. *J Med Chem* 1999, *42*, 2456-68.

[79] Lonard, D. M.; Smith, C. L. Molecular perspectives on selective estrogen receptor modulators (SERMs): progress in understanding their tissue-specific agonist and antagonist actions. *Steroids* 2002, *67*, 15-24.

[80] Blizzard, T. A.; DiNinno, F.; Chen, H. Y.; Kim, S.; Wu, J. Y.; Chan, W.; Birzin, E. T.; Yang, Y. T.; Pai, L. Y.; Hayes, E. C.; DaSilva, C. A.; Rohrer, S. P.; Schaeffer, J. M.; Hammond, M. L. Estrogen receptor ligands. Part 13: Dihydrobenzoxathiin SERAMs with an optimized antagonist side chain. *Bioorg. Med. Chem. Lett.* 2005, *15*, 3912-6.

[81] Blizzard, T. A.; DiNinno, F.; Morgan, J. D., 2nd; Chen, H. Y.; Wu, J. Y.; Gude, C.; Kim, S.; Chan, W.; Birzin, E. T.; Tien Yang, Y.; Pai, L. Y.; Zhang, Z.; Hayes, E. C.; DaSilva, C. A.; Tang, W.; Rohrer, S. P.; Schaeffer, J. M.; Hammond, M. L. Estrogen receptor ligands. Part 7: Dihydrobenzoxathiin SERAMs with bicyclic amine side chains. *Bioorg. Med. Chem. Lett.* 2004, *14*, 3861-4.

[82] Blizzard, T. A.; Dininno, F.; Morgan, J. D., 2nd; Chen, H. Y.; Wu, J. Y.; Kim, S.; Chan, W.; Birzin, E. T.; Yang, Y. T.; Pai, L. Y.; Fitzgerald, P. M.; Sharma, N.; Li, Y.;

Zhang, Z.; Hayes, E. C.; Dasilva, C. A.; Tang, W.; Rohrer, S. P.; Schaeffer, J. M.; Hammond, M. L. Estrogen receptor ligands. Part 9: Dihydrobenzoxathiin SERAMs with alkyl substituted pyrrolidine side chains and linkers. *Bioorg. Med. Chem. Lett.* 2005, *15*, 107-13.

[83] Blizzard, T. A.; DiNinno, F.; Morgan, J. D., 2nd; Wu, J. Y.; Chen, H. Y.; Kim, S.; Chan, W.; Birzin, E. T.; Yang, Y. T.; Pai, L. Y.; Zhang, Z.; Hayes, E. C.; DaSilva, C. A.; Tang, W.; Rohrer, S. P.; Schaeffer, J. M.; Hammond, M. L. Estrogen receptor ligands. Part 8: Dihydrobenzoxathiin SERAMs with heteroatom-substituted side chains. *Bioorg. Med. Chem. Lett.* 2004, *14*, 3865-8.

[84] Chen, H. Y.; Kim, S.; Wu, J. Y.; Birzin, E. T.; Chan, W.; Yang, Y. T.; Dahllund, J.; DiNinno, F.; Rohrer, S. P.; Schaeffer, J. M.; Hammond, M. L. Estrogen receptor ligands. Part 3: The SAR of dihydrobenzoxathiin SERMs. *Bioorg. Med. Chem. Lett.* 2004, *14*, 2551-4.

[85] Mukherjee, S.; Saha, A.; Roy, K. QSAR of estrogen receptor modulators: exploring selectivity requirements for ER(alpha) versus ER(beta) binding of tetrahydroisoquinoline derivatives using E-state and physicochemical parameters. *Bioorg. Med. Chem. Lett.* 2005, *15*, 957-61.

[86] Renaud, J.; Bischoff, S. F.; Buhl, T.; Floersheim, P.; Fournier, B.; Halleux, C.; Kallen, J.; Keller, H.; Schlaeppi, J. M.; Stark, W. Estrogen receptor modulators: identification and structure-activity relationships of potent ERalpha-selective tetrahydroisoquinoline ligands. *J. Med. Chem.* 2003, *46*, 2945-57.

[87] Kohno, H.; Bocchinfuso, W. P.; Gandini, O.; Curtis, S. W.; Korach, K. S. Mutational analysis of the estrogen receptor ligand-binding domain: Influence of ligand structure and stereochemistry on transactivation. *J. Mol. Endocrinol.* 1996, *16*, 277-85.

[88] Barkhem, T.; Carlsson, B.; Nilsson, Y.; Enmark, E.; Gustafsson, J. A.; Nilsson, S. Differential response of estrogen receptor alpha and estrogen receptor beta to partial estrogen agonists/antagonists. *Mol. Pharmacol.* 1998, *54*, 105-12.

[89] Couse, J. F.; Lindzey, J.; Grandien, K.; Gustafsson, J. A.; Korach, K. S. Tissue distribution and quantitative analysis of estrogen receptor-alpha (ER alpha) and estrogen receptor-beta (ER beta) messenger ribonucleic acid in the wild-type and ER alpha-knockout mouse. *Endocrinology* 1997, *138*, 4613-21.

[90] Mueller, S. O.; Hall, J. M.; Swope, D. L.; Pedersen, L. C.; Korach, K. S. Molecular determinants of the stereoselectivity of agonist activity of estrogen receptors (ER) alpha and beta. *J Biol Chem* 2003, *278*, 12255-62.

[91] Kuiper, G. G.; Carlsson, B.; Grandien, K.; Enmark, E.; Haggblad, J.; Nilsson, S.; Gustafsson, J. A. Comparison of the ligand binding specificity and transcript tissue distribution of estrogen receptors alpha and beta. *Endocrinology* 1997, *138*, 863-70.

[92] Barnes, S.; Kim, H.; Darley-Usmar, V.; Patel, R.; Xu, J.; Boersma, B.; Luo, M. Beyond ERalpha and ERbeta: estrogen receptor binding is only part of the isoflavone story. *J. Nutr.* 2000, *130*, 656S-7S.

[93] Schopfer, U.; Schoeffter, P.; Bischoff, S. F.; Nozulak, J.; Feuerbach, D.; Floersheim, P. Toward selective ERbeta agonists for central nervous system disorders: synthesis and characterization of aryl benzthiophenes. *J. Med. Chem.* 2002, *45*, 1399-401.

[94] Ullrich, J. W.; Unwalla, R. J.; Singhaus, R. R., Jr.; Harris, H. A.; Mewshaw, R. E. Estrogen receptor beta ligands: design and synthesis of new 2-phenyl-isoindole-1,3-diones. *Bioorg. Med. Chem. Lett.* 2007, *17*, 118-22.

[95] Deapen, D.; Liu, L.; Perkin, C.; Bernstein, L.; Ross, R. K. Rapidly rising breast cancer incidence rates among Asian-American women. *International Journal of Cancer* 2002, *99*, 747-50.

[96] Branham, W. S.; Dial, S. L.; Moland, C. L.; Hass, B. S.; Blair, R. M.; Fang, H.; Shi, L.; Tong, W.; Perkins, R. G.; Sheehan, D. M. Phytoestrogens and Mycoestrogens Bind to the Rat Uterine Estrogen Receptor. *J. Nutr.* 2002, *132*, 658-64.

[97] Adlercreutz, H.; Mazur, W.; Bartels, P.; Elomaa, V. V.; Watanabe, S.; Wahala, K.; Landstrom, M.; Lundin, E.; Bergh, A.; Damber, J. E.; Aman, P.; Widmark, A.; Johansson, A.; Zhang, J. X.; Hallmans, G. Phytoestrogens and Prostate Disease. *J. Nutr.* 2000, *130*, 658-.

[98] Brzozowski, A. M.; Pike, A. C. W.; Dauter, Z.; Hubbard, R. E.; Bonn, T.; Engstrom, O.; Ohman, L.; Greene, G. L.; Gustafsson, J.-A.; Carlquist, M. Molecular basis of agonism and antagonism in the oestrogen receptor. *Nature* 1997, *389*, 753-8.

[99] Skaltsounis, A. L.; Pratsinis, H.; Mikros, E.; Alexis, M. N. A new class of phytoestrogens; evaluation of the estrogenic activity of deoxybenzoins. *Chem. Biol.* 2004, *11*, 397-406.

[100] Setchell, K. D. R. Soy Isoflavones--Benefits and Risks from Nature's Selective Estrogen Receptor Modulators (SERMs). *J Am Coll Nutr* 2001, *20*, 354S-62.

[101] Kuiper, G. G. J. M.; Carlsson, B.; Grandien, K.; Enmark, E.; Haggblad, J.; Nilsson, S.; Gustafsson, J. A. Comparison of the ligand binding specificity and transcript tissue distribution of estrogen receptors alpha and beta. *Endocrinology* 1997, *138*, 863-70.

[102] Mukherjee, S.; Mukherjee, A.; Saha, A. QSAR modeling on binding affinity of diverse estrogenic flavonoids: electronic, topological and spatial functions in quantitative approximation. *Journal of Molecular Structure-Theochem* 2005, *715*, 85-90.

[103] Sun, W.; Cama, L. D.; Birzin, E. T.; Warrier, S.; Locco, L.; Mosley, R.; Hammond, M. L.; Rohrer, S. P. 6H-Benzo[c]chromen-6-one derivatives as selective ERbeta agonists. *Bioorg Med Chem Lett* 2006, *16*, 1468-72. Epub 2006 Jan 18.

[104] Agatonovic-Kustrin, S.; Turner, J. V. Artificial neural network modeling of phytoestrogen binding to estrogen receptors. *Lett. Drug Des. Discov.* 2006, *7*, 436-42.

[105] Bickoff, E. M.; Booth, A. N.; Lyman, R. L.; Livingston, A. L.; Thompson, C. R.; Deeds, F. Coumestrol, a New Estrogen Isolated from Forage Crops. *Science* 1957, *126*, 969-a-70.

[106] Bakhchinian, R.; Terrier, F.; Kirkiacharian, S.; Resche-Rigon, M.; Bouchoux, F.; Cerede, E. Synthesis and relative binding affinity to human steroid receptors of substituted 3-aryloxycoumarins. *Il Farmaco* 2003, *58*, 1201-7.

[107] B. S.; Katzenellenbogen, J. A. Estrogen receptor-beta potency-selective ligands: structure-activity relationship studies of diarylpropionitriles and their acetylene and polar analogues. *J. Mol. Model.* 2001, *44*, 4230-51.

[108] Sun, J.; Baudry, J.; Katzenellenbogen, J. A.; Katzenellenbogen, B. S. Molecular basis for the subtype discrimination of the estrogen receptor-beta-selective ligand, diarylpropionitrile. *Mol. Endocrinol.* 2003, *17*, 247-58.

[109] Schaub, R. E.; Kissman, H. M.; Weiss, M. J. The Synthesis of Certain 16alpha-Substituted Derivatives of the 3-Methyl Ethers of 16beta-Cyanoestrone and 16beta-Cyanoestradiol. *J. Org. Chem.* 1964, *29*, 2775-7.

[110] Diphenylalkanonitriles. U.S. patent 2,740.806, 1956.

[111] Makela, S.; Savolainen, H.; Aavik, E.; Myllarniemi, M.; Strauss, L.; Taskinen, E.; Gustafsson, J. A.; Hayry, P. Differentiation between vasculoprotective and uterotrophic effects of ligands with different binding affinities to estrogen receptors alpha and beta. *Proc Natl Acad Sci U S A* 1999, *96*, 7077-82.

[112] Vu, A. T.; Cohn, S. T.; Manas, E. S.; Harris, H. A.; Mewshaw, R. E. ERbeta ligands. Part 4: Synthesis and structure-activity relationships of a series of 2-phenylquinoline derivatives. *Bioorg. Med. Chem. Lett.* 2005, *15*, 4520-5.

[113] Grese, T. A.; Cho, S.; Finley, D. R.; Godfrey, A. G.; Jones, C. D.; Lugar, C. W.; Martin, M. J.; Matsumoto, K.; Pennington, L. D.; Winter, M. A.; Adrian, M. D.; Cole, H. W.; Magee, D. E.; Phillips, D. L.; Rowley, E. R.; Short, L. L.; Glasebrook, A. L.; Bryant, H. U. Structure-Activity Relationships of Selective Estrogen Receptor Modulators: Modifications to the 2-Arylbenzothiophene Core of Raloxifene. *J. Med. Chem.* 1997, *40*, 146-67.

[114] AstraZeneca, A. B. WO Patent 02/051821-A1. 2002.

[115] AstraZeneca, A. B. WO Patent 02/46168-A1. 2002.

[116] Wyeth WO Patent 03/050095-A1. 2003.

[117] De Angelis, M.; Katzenellenbogen, J. A. Ring nitrogen-substituted non-steroidal estrogens: pyridine and pyrimidine analogs of the phenol in deoxyhexestrol experience resonance constraints on preferred ligand conformation. *Bioorg Med Chem Lett* 2004, *14*, 5835-9.

In: Estrogens: Production, Functions and Applications
Editor: James R. Bartos, pp. 307-317
ISBN: 978-1-60741-086-7

Chapter XI

Estrogen Receptor: Structure and Clinical Importance

Viroj Wiwanitkit
Wiwanitkit House, Bangkhae, Bangkok, Thailand 10160

Abstract

The estrogen receptor is an important receptor in human beings. It relates to the physiological function of estrogen as well as to some specific pathological disorders. In this article, the author will briefly review and discuss the estrogen receptor. The structure of the estrogen receptor will be focused upon in depth. Important analyses of the structural component of an estrogen receptor will be demonstrated and presented. In addition, details on the clinical importance of an estrogen receptor laboratory test and examples of experience in cases of breast cancer will be reported in this article.

Introduction to Estrogen Receptor

Estrogen is an important female hormone that plays a big role in gynecology and obstetrics. The estrogen receptor is an important receptor in human beings. It relates to the physiological function of estrogen as well as to some specific pathological disorders.

Estrogen receptors, both alpha and beta types, are members of the steroid/thyroid nuclear receptors superfamily of ligand-dependent transcription factors [1]. The impact of the alpha isoform of estrogen receptor (ER) on breast cancer etiology and progression is now well mentioned [1–2]. In this article, the author will discuss and give a brief review of estrogen receptors.

Estrogen Receptor Gene

The ER gene has been continuously studied in many clinical conditions. Pathological alterations of the ER structure and function are the main cause of estrogen insensitivity in women and a possible underlying aspect of breast cancer. Indeed, estrogen has some significant roles in the proliferation of cancer cells in reproductive organs such as the breast and uterus [3]. Based on the observation of bilateral risks and frequent multifocality with atypical ductal hyperplasia, atypical lobular hyperplasia and lobular carcinoma in situ, it is proposed that ER may represent risk factors as well as precursors [4]. ER beta-positive and ER alpha-negative expression characterizes the highest levels of proliferative abnormal oncological cell activity [4]. Of interest, a large number of naturally occurring splice variants of both ER have been identified in normal epithelium and pathological or cancerous tissues [5]. However, only a few point mutations have been confirmed in human patient samples from a variety of disease status, especially for breast carcinoma, endometrial carcinoma, and psychiatric diseases [5].

There are many reports on the estrogen receptor genes that should be mentioned. Some important reports are hereby listed in Table 1.

Table 1. Important reports on the estrogen receptor genes

Authors	Details
Orikasa et al. [6]	Orikasa et al. reported that ER alpha, but not beta, was expressed in the interneurons of the hippocampus in prepubertal rats by an in situ hybridization study [6].
Bergner et al. [7]	Bergner et al. reported that point mutations of ER-alpha and ER-beta were not necessary for metastatic prostate cancer, alterations in different areas of the ER genes are more often found [7]. Bergner et al. also noted that these polymorphisms are a part of genetic influences that might accumulate to contribute to men's overall risk for developing prostate cancer [7].
Creekmore et al. [8]	Creekmore et al. used a chromatin immunoprecipitation (ChIP)-based cloning strategy to isolate and identify genes associated with ER alpha in MCF-7 human breast cancer cells [8]. Creekmore et al. demonstrated that chromatin immunoprecipitation cloning strategies might be utilized to successfully isolate regulatory regions that are far removed from the transcription start site and could assist in identifying cis elements involved in conferring estrogen responsiveness [8].
Thellenberg-Karlsson et al. [9]	Thellenberg-Karlsson et al. found an association between a SNP located in the promoter region of the ER beta gene and the risk of developing prostate cancer [9].

Authors	Details
	Thellenberg-Karlsson et al. concluded that the biological significance of this finding was not clear, but it might support a specific hypothesis that sequence variation in the promoter region of ER beta was of importance for risk of prostate cancer in men[9].
Tanaka et al. [10]	Tanaka et al. studied polymorphisms of ER alpha in prostate cancer [10]. Tanaka et al. found that polymorphism in codon 10 of ER alpha might be a risk factor for prostate cancer in men [10]. Tanaka et al. concluded that these results were important in understanding the role of ER alpha polymorphism in the pathogenesis of prostate cancer [10].
Cancel-Tassin et al. [11]	Cancel-Tassin et al. reported that variants of the GGGA polymorphism from the ER alpha gene might be associated with an increased risk of developing prostate cancer [11].
Schausi et al. [12]	Schausi et al. characterized the intronic promoter of the rat ER alpha gene, responsible for the lactotrope-specific truncated ER product (TERP)-1 isoform expression [12]. Schausi et al. demonstrated that TERP promoter regulation related to estrogen-responsive element and Pit-1 cis-elements and corresponding trans-acting factors, which could play a role in the physiological changes that happened in TERP-1 transcription in lactotrope cells [12].
Sasaki et al. [13]	Sasaki et al. demonstrated for a protective effect of 10C allele against endometrial cancer [13]. Sasaki et al. said that inherited alterations in ERalpha might be associated with changes in estrogen metabolism, therefore, it could possibly explain inter-individual differences in disease incidences of endometrial cancer [13].
Andersen et al. [14]	Anderson et al. studied ER polymorphisms and breast cancer susceptibility [14]. Anderson found that there was no significant association between any of the ER polymorphisms and the ER status of the primary tumors [14]. Anderson et al. indicated that the ER gene or a gene closely linked to it was involved in the development of at least a subset of breast carcinomas [14].
Ponglikitmongkol et al. [15]	Ponglikitmongkol et al. reported that the human ER gene was greater than 140 kb in length, split into eight exons and that the positions of these introns were highly conserved when compared with the chicken progesterone receptor and were similar to those of one of the chicken thyroid hormone receptor genes [15].

Genomics Approach for Estrogen Receptor

Genomics analysis on the ER in depth helps us to better understand the pathogenesis of an estrogen receptor disorder.

A. Mutation in Estrogen Receptor

The prevalence of mutations in the estrogen receptor gene is not presently known. Analysis for ER mutated prone points can be the first useful step for further research on the ER mutation, while the next step is the study of the functional characterization. Presently, prediction of a protein structure and its function can be a great challenge in the proteomics and genomics era. To identify the point vulnerable to mutate is a new scientific approach to expand the knowledge on disorders at the genomic and proteomic level of diseases [16–17]. Basically, any disordered regions in proteins often contain short linear peptide motifs that can be important for protein function. Identification of the peptide motifs in the amino acid sequence can give a good prediction for the weak linkages in a protein [16–17]. Fortunately, this analysis is possible based on the advancement of the genomics technique. Here, the author performs a bioinformatics analysis to study the prone positions that tend to apply peptide motifs in the amino acid sequence of ER.

Considering materials and methods in this report, the database Expert Protein Analysis System (ExPASY) [18] was used for searching for the amino acid sequence of AR. Briefly, the ExPASy is a proteomics server of the Swiss Institute of Bioinformatics (SIB) dedicated to the analysis of protein sequences and structures as well as 2-D PAGE [19]. After that the gotten sequences were used for further study on weak linkage using a new genomics tool namely GlobPlot [19]. Briefly, GlobPlot is a web service that allows the user to plot the tendency within the query protein for order/globularity and disorder [19]. The interface is straight forward to use; the user can paste a sequence or enter the SWISS-PROT/SWALL accession or entry code [19].

MTMPLPNKTT gvtflhqiqs seletltrpp lkislerplg emyvennrtg **IFNYP**egtty dfaaaaapvy ssaslsyaas set**FGSSSLT GLHTLNNVPP S**pvvflaklp qlspfihhhg qqvpyylese qgtfavreaa ppt**FYRSSSD NRRQSGRERM SSANDKGPPS MES**tketryc avcsdyasgy hygvwscegc kaffkrsiqg h**NDYMCPAT**n qctidknrrk scqacrlrkc yevgmmkggi rkdrrggrll khkrqkeeqe qkndvdpsei rtasiwvnps vksmklspvl sltaeqlisa lmeaeapivy sehdstkpls easmmtlltn ladrelvhmi nwakrvpgfv dltlhdqvhl lecawleilm vgliwrsveh pgklsfapnl lldrnqgrcv eglveifdml vttatrfrmm rlrgeeficl ksiillnsgv ytflsstles ledtdlihii ldkiidtlvh fmaksglslq qqrrlaqll lilshirhms nkgmehlysm kcknvvplyd lllemldahr ihtpkdk**TTT QEEDSRSPPT TTVNGASPCL Q**pyytntee**V SLQS**tv

* Each alphabet letter within the figure represents an amino acid. The capital alphabet letters represent the amino acid with resistance to mutation.

Figure 1. Identified positions (in capital) that apply peptide motifs in amino acid sequence of ER.

The GlobPlot server fetches the sequence and description of the polypeptide from an ExPASy server using Biopython.org software [19]. With the already described process, identification of inter-domain segments containing linear motifs was done [19]. The identified motifs are the weak linkages in a protein which are prone to mutation [16–17]. Wiwanitkit reported that the positions 1-10, 51-55, 84-101, 144-173, 212-219, 548-571, 580-584 could be identified as the motif positions which are resistant to mutation.

Physiologically, the temporal and tissue-specific actions of estrogen are mediated by ERs alpha and beta [20]. The ERs are classified as steroid hormone receptors that modulate the transcription of target genes when attached to a ligand [20]. There is a large and increasing body of experimental and clinical data supporting the existence or variant ER proteins in both normal and neoplastic estrogen target tissues especially for the human breast [21]. The functions of variant ER proteins, either physiological or pathological, remain unclear, although roles for some ER variants in breast oncogenesis would be consistent with the accumulated data [21]. On one hand, ER mutations are connected with some rare syndromes of estrogen disorder, and on the other hand it is the post-receptor modifications that very well explain the molecular pathogenesis of ER defect, breast cancer and prostate cancer. Identification of the mutation points within ER can be useful for further research to understand the pathogenesis of many estrogen disorders. However, the finding on the mutation points with classical in vitro experiments takes a long time and is based on the low possibility of getting a positive case. To solve this problem, the advanced bioinformatics technology can be applied [22–23]. To search for the mutation, the GlobPlot was used. This new technique is acceptable and used for identification of a mutation in globins of a previous research [24]. A reliable result can be derived [25]. The mutant analysis data will be useful for further functional characterization prediction, which can be presently performed by a gene ontology technology technique [26–27]. The functional significance of identified mutation-resisting locations should also be further tested on its possible functional characterization.

B. Functional Change Due to Estrogen Receptor Variant

The single substitution in the amino acid chain is the more common form of many protein variants. However, the functional aberrations according to the structural aberration of ER are not well documented. Here, the author performed a functional analysis on some minor prothrombin deficiency variants using a novel bioinformatic tool. This work can be a good model and basic information for further experimental studies on the ER variants. A novel bioinformatic simulation tool, PolyPhen [28], was used for mutation study.

A famous ER variant, ER-alpha36 [29], was selected for further investigation.

Briefly, the author studied the effect of each mutation on ER structure and function. Briefly, PolyPhen is an automatic tool for prediction of possible impact of an amino acid substitution on the structure and function of a human protein. This prediction is based on straightforward empirical rules, which are applied to the sequence, phylogenetic and structural information characterizing the substitution. Concerning the input, PolyPhen works with human proteins and identifies them by the amino acid sequence itself. Amino acid replacement is characterized by position number and substitution. For a given amino acid substitution in a human protein, PolyPhen performs several steps: a) sequence-based characterisation of the substitution site, b) calculation for the degree of functional change, PSIC scores, c) calculation for structural parameters and contacts, and d) prediction. The main outputs are PSIC score, implying degree of damaging. Grading of degree of damaging is referred to in the Ramensky et al. reference [28]. According to this in silico mutation study, the functional change in the studied ER variant is determined as PSIC difference score equal to 0.4 which range in the degree of benign which means most likely lacking any phenotypic effect [28].

Proteomics Approach for Estrogen Receptor

Proteomics analysis on the ER in depth could also help better understand the pathogenesis of an estrogen receptor disorder.

A. Secondary and Tertiary Structure of Estrogen Receptor

Although the primary structure of ER is well-known the secondary and tertiary structures of ER are not well documented. Here, the author performs a bioinformatics analysis for nanoscience to study the secondary and tertiary structures of this abnormal based on the amino acid sequence in the database. Answering this question, a computer-based study for protein structure modeling is performed. The database Expert Protein analysis System (ExPASY) [18] was used to search for the amino acid sequence of normal human ER. The ExPASY server of the Swiss Institute of Bioinformatics (SIB) is dedicated to the analysis of protein sequences and structures as well as 2-D PAGE. It allows you to browse through a number of databases produced in Geneva, such as Swiss-Prot, PROSITE, SWISS-2DPAGE, SWISS-3D IMAGE, ENYME, as well as other cross-referenced databases (such as EMBL/GenBank/DDBJ, OMIM, Medline, FlyBase, ProDom, SGD, SubtiList, etc).

Concerning secondary structure modeling, the author performed protein secondary structure predictions of ER from its primary sequence using the NNPREDICT server [30]. The NNPREDICT server is a program that predicts the secondary structure type for each residue in an amino acid sequence. The basis of the prediction is a two-layer, feed-forward neural network [30]. It takes input as a sequence consisting of one-letter amino acid codes or three-letter amino acid codes separated by spaces [30]. The output is a secondary structure prediction for each position in the sequence. The predicted type will be either: 'H', a helix element; 'E', a beta strand element, or '-', a turn element [30]. The calculated secondary structures were presented in Figure 2.

```
---EE------HHHHHH----------------------EEE--------E------HH
HHHHHHHHHHHHHE------------HHHH-------------------E-----------
----------E--------EE----------------------EE--------HHHHH--
H--EEEE--------EEEE------HHHHHH---------------------------H
------HH--------H--H---HHH------------EE-----HHH--------HHH-
-----HHHHH-HHHHHHH---------------------HHHHHHH--HHHHHHHHHHHH
-------E-E-HHH-HHHHHHHHHHHHHHHHHH-HH---------HH-------------
HHHHHHHHHH-----HEE-----HHHHHH-EEEE----EEEEH--H-HH-HHHHHHHHHH
-HHHHHHHHHHHH-HHHHHHHHHHHHHHHHHHHHHH------HHHHH---------HHHHH
HHHHHHH------------E-HH-H-HHEE----------EEEE-----------
```

Figure 2. Predicted secondary structure of human ER.

Concerning tertiary structure modeling, the author performed protein tertiary structure predictions of ER from its primary sequence using CPH models 2.0 Server [31]. CHH models 2.0 server is a homology modeling. It takes input as a sequence consisting of one-letter amino acid codes [31]. The template for building the model is sought by iteratively building up a profile by aligning the query sequence to a non-redundant database of protein sequences and then searching a database of proteins with known structure (pdb) to find a suitable template for making a model [31]. The output is a tertiary structure prediction for each position in the sequence [31]. The calculated tertiary structures were presented in Figure 3.

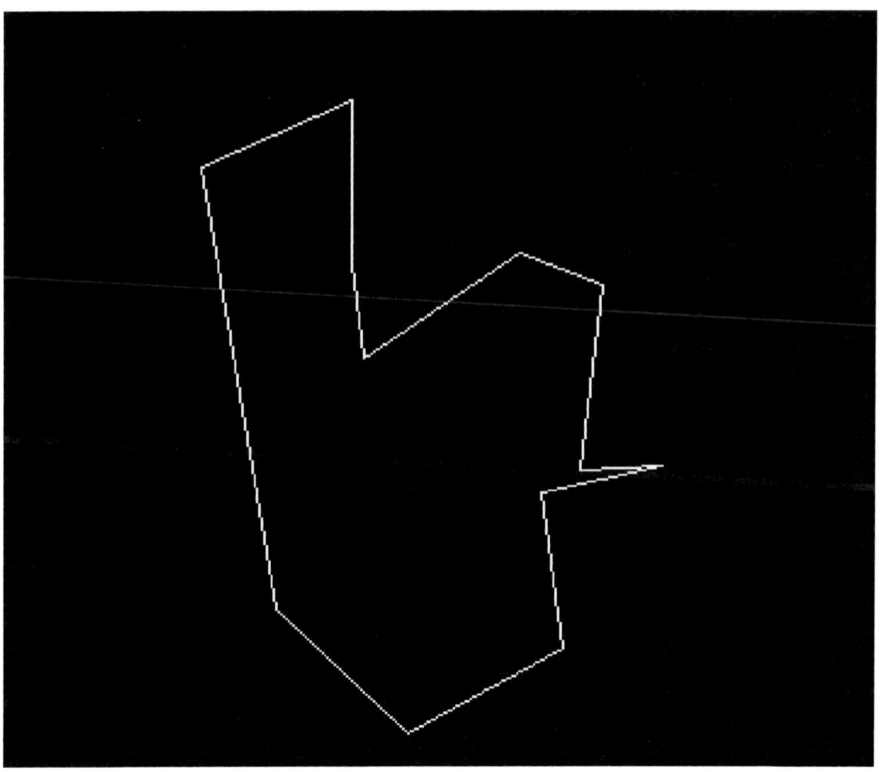

Figure 3. Predicted tertiary structure of human ER.

Clinical Importance of Estrogen Receptor Laboratory Test

ER laboratory test is an important group of immunohistochemistry study. There are many reports on this immunohistochemistry test especially for breast cancer specimens. The presence of ERs, as detected by immunohistochemistry, is a weak prognostic marker of clinical outcome in breast cancer, but a strong predictive marker for response, for example, to tamoxifen-based therapy [32]. Some important reports are presented in Table 2.

Table 2. Important reports on immunohistochemistry test for estrogen receptor.

Authors	Details
Pan et al. [33]	Pan et al. studied the influence of superovulation by GnRHa protocol and a pregnant mare's serum gonadotropin (PMSG) alone on the expression of ER, progesterone receptor (PR) and leukemia inhibitory factor (LIF) mRNA on endometrium in mouse model [33]. Pan et al. found that the protocol with GnRHa down regulated the expressions of ER, PR and the LIF mRNA on the mice of secretive phase endometrium, suggesting it might have an adverse effect on the endometrial receptivity in mice, but it might still be better than PMSG alone [33].
Andre et al. [34]	The aim of the study was to assess the efficacy of adjuvant docetaxel and anthracycline therapy according to ER expression [34]. Andre et al. reported that docetaxel did not have a statistically significantly different effect on the risk of recurrence or death in ER-positive and ER-negative patients [34].
Kalayarasan et al. [35]	Kalayarasan et al. proposed that ER beta might be a marker for poor biological behavior, that was dedifferentiation or higher stage of disease [35].
Real et al. [36]	Real et al. analyzed the presence of the ERR beta protein in the mouse brain by means of immunohistochemistry [36]. Real et al. revealed numerous ERR beta immunoreactive fibers in the retinal efferent projections in the brain, which was in agreement with the presence of intense ERR beta immunoreactivity in the cell bodies and axonal processes of the retinal ganglion cells [36]. In addition, ERR beta immunoreactive fibers were distributed in a pattern which perfectly matched the retinal efferent projections: optic tract, supraoptic commissure, hypothalamic suprachiasmatic nucleus, ventral and dorsal geniculate nuclei, pretectal nuclei,
Rocha et al [37]	

Authors	Details
	and superior colliculus in both postnatal and adult brains [36].
	Rocha et al. compared the novel RabMab anti-ER and anti-PR antibodies with the mouse monoclonal antibodies using a tissue microarray of breast carcinomas [37]. Rocha et al. concluded that both ER and PR rabbit antibodies could allow a lower cost per test because of higher working dilutions compared to mouse antibodies using the same procedure [37].
Journe et al. [38]	Journe et al. mentioned that ER-positive breast tumors could be stimulated to proliferate via a crosstalk between FXR and ER, particularly in a state of estrogen deprivation (menopause, aromatase inhibitors) [38].
Cho and Hsu [39]	Cho and Hsu revealed that mucinous carcinoma samples from the breast had some distinct clinicopathologic and hormone receptor expression features compared to non-mucinous carcinoma [39].
Talman et al. [40]	Talman et al. concluded that immunohistochemistry in analysing ER was a rapid, reliable and easy method, and recommended the use of external quality control program [40].

References

[1] Leclercq G, Lacroix M, Laios I, Laurent G. Estrogen receptor alpha: impact of ligands on intracellular shuttling and turnover rate in breast cancer cells. *Curr Cancer Drug Targets*. 2006;6:39-64.

[2] Cordera F, Jordan VC. Steroid receptors and their role in the biology and control of breast cancer growth. *Semin Oncol*. 2006;33:631-41.

[3] Ikeda K, Inoue S. Estrogen receptors and their downstream targets in cancer. *Arch Histol Cytol*. 2004;67:435-42.

[4] Schneider HP, Bocker W. Hormones and progeny of breast tumor cells. *Climacteric*. 2006;9:88-107.

[5] Herynk MH, Fuqua SA. Estrogen receptor mutations in human disease. *Endocr Rev*. 2004;25:869-98.

[6] Orikasa C, McEwen BS, Hayashi H, Sakuma Y, Hayashi S. Estrogen receptor alpha, but not beta, is expressed in the interneurons of the hippocampus in prepubertal rats: an in situ hybridization study. *Brain Res Dev Brain Res*. 2000 Apr 14;120(2):245-54.

[7] Bergner CC, Krause FS, Zugor V, Rith T, Schrott KM, Endele S, Engehausen DG. Polymorphisms of human estrogen receptor (ER) gene alpha and beta in prostate cancer PC-EW and PC-OR cell lines. *Anticancer Res*. 2007 Jul-Aug;27(4A):2071-4.

[8] Creekmore AL, Ziegler YS, Boney JL, Nardulli AM. Estrogen receptor alpha regulates expression of the breast cancer 1 associated ring domain 1 (BARD1) gene through intronic DNA sequence. *Mol Cell Endocrinol.* 2007 Mar 15;267(1-2):106-15.

[9] Thellenberg-Karlsson C, Lindström S, Malmer B, Wiklund F, Augustsson-Bälter K, Adami HO, Stattin P, Nilsson M, Dahlman-Wright K, Gustafsson JA, Grönberg H. Estrogen receptor beta polymorphism is associated with prostate cancer risk. *Clin Cancer Res.* 2006 Mar 15;12(6):1936-41.

[10] Tanaka Y, Sasaki M, Kaneuchi M, Shiina H, Igawa M, Dahiya R. Polymorphisms of estrogen receptor alpha in prostate cancer. *Mol Carcinog.* 2003 Aug;37(4):202-8.

[11] Cancel-Tassin G, Latil A, Rousseau F, Mangin P, Bottius E, Escary JL, Berthon P, Cussenot O. Association study of polymorphisms in the human estrogen receptor alpha gene and prostate cancer risk. *Eur Urol.* 2003 Oct;44(4):487-90.

[12] Schausi D, Tiffoche C, Thieulant ML. Regulation of the intronic promoter of rat estrogen receptor alpha gene, responsible for truncated estrogen receptor product-1 expression. *Endocrinology.* 2003 Jul;144(7):2845-55.

[13] Sasaki M, Tanaka Y, Kaneuchi M, Sakuragi N, Dahiya R. Polymorphisms of estrogen receptor alpha gene in endometrial cancer. *Biochem Biophys Res Commun.* 2002 Sep 27;297(3):558-64.

[14] Andersen TI, Heimdal KR, Skrede M, Tveit K, Berg K, Børresen AL. Oestrogen receptor (ESR) polymorphisms and breast cancer susceptibility. *Hum Genet.* 1994 Dec;94(6):665-70.

[15] Ponglikitmongkol M, Green S, Chambon P. Genomic organization of the human oestrogen receptor gene. *EMBO J.* 1988 Nov;7(11):3385-8.

[16] Lee C, Wang Q. Bioinformatics analysis of alternative splicing. *Brief Bioinform* 2005;6:23-33.

[17] Levin JM, Penland RC, Stamps AT, Cho CR. Using in silico biology to facilitate drug development. *Novartis Found Symp* 2002;247:222-38.

[18] Gasteiger E, Gattiker A, Hoogland C, Ivanyi I, Appel RD, Bairoch A. ExPASy: The proteomics server for in-depth protein knowledge and analysis. *Nucleic Acids Res* 2003;31:3784-8.

[19] Linding R, Russell RB, Neduva V, Gibson TJ. GlobPlot: Exploring protein sequences for globularity and disorder. *Nucleic Acids Res* 2003 ;31:3701-8.

[20] Pearce ST, Jordan VC. The biological role of estrogen receptors alpha and beta in cancer. Crit Rev Oncol Hematol. 2004;50:3-22.

[21] Murphy LC, Dotzlaw H, Leygue E, Douglas D, Coutts A, Watson PH. Estrogen receptor variants and mutations. *J Steroid Biochem Mol Biol.* 1997;62:363-72.

[22] Gogarten JP, Olendzenski L. Orthologs, paralogs and genome comparisons. *Curr Opin Genet Dev.* 1999;9:630-6.

[23] Golaz O, Wilkins MR, Sanchez JC, Appel RD, Hochstrasser DF, Williams KL. Identification of proteins by their amino acid composition: an evaluation of the method. *Electrophoresis.* 1996;17:573-9.

[24] Wiwanitkit V. Where is the weak linkage in the globin chain? *Int J Nanomed* 2006; 1: 109 – 110.

[25] Linding R, Schymkowitz J, Rousseau F, Diella F, Serrano L. A comparative study of the relationship between protein structure and beta-aggregation in globular and intrinsically disordered proteins. *J Mol Biol.* 2004;342:345-53.

[26] Azuaje F, Al-Shahrour F, Dopazo J. Ontology-driven approaches to analyzing data in functional genomics. *Methods Mol Biol.* 2006;316:67-86.

[27] Khan S, Situ G, Decker K, Schmidt CJ. GoFigure: automated Gene Ontology annotation. *Bioinformatics* 2003;19:2484-5.

[28] Ramensky V, Bork P, Sunyaev S. Human non-synonymous SNPs: server and survey. *Nucleic Acids Res* 2002; 30: 3894-900

[29] Lee LM, Cao J, Deng H, Chen P, Gatalica Z, Wang ZY. ER-alpha36, a novel variant of ER-alpha, is expressed in ER-positive and -negative human breast carcinomas.*Anticancer Res.* 2008 Jan-Feb;28(1B):479-83.

[30] Kneller G, Cohen FE, Langridge R. Improvements in protein secondary structure prediction by an enhanced neural network. *J Mol Bio.* 1990; 214 (1): 171-182.

[31] Lund O, Nielsen M, Lundegaard C, Worning P. "CPHmodels 2.0: X3M a Computer Program to Extract 3D Models," Abstract at the CASP5 conferenceA102, 2002.

[32] Gown AM. Current issues in ER and HER2 testing by IHC in breast cancer.*Mod Pathol.* 2008 May;21 Suppl 2:S8-S15.

[33] Pan YM, Shi YF, Chen HZ, Zhou CY. Expression of estrogen receptor, progesterone receptor and leukemia inhibitory factor on endometrium during different ovarian stimulation protocols in mice.Zhejiang Da Xue Xue Bao Yi Xue Ban. 2008 May;37(3):300-3.

[34] Andre F, Broglio K, Roche H, Martin M, Mackey JR, Penault-Llorca F, Hortobagyi GN, Pusztai L. Estrogen receptor expression and efficacy of docetaxel-containing adjuvant chemotherapy in patients with node-positive breast cancer: results from a pooled analysis. *J Clin Oncol.* 2008 Jun 1;26(16):2636-43.

[35] Kalayarasan R, Ananthakrishnan N, Kate V, Basu D. Estrogen and progesterone receptors in esophageal carcinoma. *Dis Esophagus.* 2008;21(4):298-303.

[36] Real MA, Heredia R, Dávila JC, Guirado S. Efferent retinal projections visualized by immunohistochemical detection of the estrogen-related receptor beta in the postnatal and adult mouse brain. *Neurosci Lett.* 2008 Jun 13;438(1):48-53.

[37] Rocha R, Nunes C, Rocha G, Oliveira F, Sanches F, Gobbi H. Rabbit monoclonal antibodies show higher sensitivity than mouse monoclonals for estrogen and progesterone receptor evaluation in breast cancer by immunohistochemistry.*Pathol Res Pract.* 2008 Jun 17. [Epub ahead of print]

[38] Journe F, Durbecq V, Chaboteaux C, Rouas G, Laurent G, Nonclercq D, Sotiriou C, Body JJ, Larsimont D. Association between farnesoid X receptor expression and cell proliferation in estrogen receptor-positive luminal-like breast cancer from postmenopausal patients. *Breast Cancer Res Treat.* 2008 Jun 19. [Epub ahead of print]

[39] Cho LC, Hsu YH. Expression of androgen, estrogen and progesterone receptors in mucinous carcinoma of the breast. *Kaohsiung J Med Sci.* 2008 May;24(5):227-32.

[40] Talman ML, Rasmussen BB, Andersen J, Christensen IJ. Estrogen Receptor analyses in the Danish Breast Cancer Cooperative Group. History, methods, prognosis and clinical implications. *Acta Oncol.* 2008;47(4):789-94.

In: Estrogens: Production, Functions and Applications
Editor: James R. Bartos, pp. 319-325
ISBN: 978-1-60741-086-7

Chapter XII

Estrogen Usage in Gays: Extraordinary Application

Viroj Wiwanitkit
Wiwanitkit House, Bangkhae, Bangkok, Thailand 10160

Abstract

Estrogen is classified as a feminine hormone although it can be found in both sexes. Excessive estrogen in men can be problematic. However, in some situations, intended administration of estrogen in men can be seen. The best scenario is the use of estrogen in gays, with the aim of achieving a feminine appearance. In this article, the author will focus on this extraordinary application and other transsexual procedures for gays.

Introduction

Estrogen is classified as a feminine hormone although it can be found in both sexes. Excessive estrogen in men can be problematic. Testis cancer is an example [1]. In testis cancer, environmental factors may have a role in the etiology with high estrogen concentrations implicated [1]. Prostate is another cancerous example. Lycette et al. said that whereas oral estrogen therapy was known to be associated with thromboembolic complications, studies of parenteral estrogen in men with prostate cancer suggested that the use of parenteral estrogen achieved target androgen suppression [2]. Gynecomastia is another common problem in men with excessive estrogen. About half the cases of gynecomastia are known as physiological gynecomastia, connected with the neonatal period, puberty or aging, but gynecomastia can also be the first symptom of a serious disease such as liver disorders [3]. However, in some situations, intended administration of estrogen in men can be seen. The best scenario is the usage of estrogen in gays, with the aim of achieving a feminine appearance. In this article, the author will focus on this extraordinary application.

Gays and a Feminine Appearance

Gays are a population of males that have an underlying psychological drive to act in feminine ways. A feminine appearance is the psychological target for many gays. Many different formats for treating gay men with sexual dysfunctions are described [4]. There are many ways to get a feminine appearance, which will be further discussed.

A. Surgical Procedure

Surgical procedure is the choice of many to get a feminine appearance. A sex change operation is the most well-known surgical procedure to achieve that goal. Penis amputation or castration is the classical technique. In ancient China, this procedure was used for male workers in the central palace; these workers were called "Khun-Tee" (However, these workers are not gays with a psychological drive to have a sex change surgery). There is another famous scenario of penis amputation in the Middle East. Genital self-mutilation, whether partial or complete, is an uncommon condition, which usually occurs in psychotic patients and occasionally has a religious background [5]. A common complication of penis amputation is the destruction of nearby structures especially the urogenital diaphragm, which can cause incontinence.

Table 1. Reports of self penis amputation

Authors	Details
Stunell et al. [6]	Stunell et al. reported a male brought to the emergency department having removed both testicles and amputated his penis using a bread knife [6]. This patient was taken to see where the perineal wound was debrided and the remaining urethra brought down as a perineal urethrostomy, with a local cutaneous flap rotated to provide coverage for the urethra [6].
Aboseif et al. [7]	Aboseif et al. reported a series of 14 patients with 19 self-inflicted genital injuries during a period of 10 years and of the patients 65% were psychotic and 35% were not psychotic [7].
Keil et al. [8]	In this paper, suicide of a 31 year old man with multiple slashes and stab wounds including complete amputation of penis, scrotum and testicles is reported [8]. Keil et al. noted that self-castrations as well as other self-inflicted genital mutilations were usually associated with psychiatric disorders and transsexuality or hypersexuality [8].
Tomita et al. [9]	A 69-year-old man admitted after having amputated his own penis completely from its root was reported [9]. The patient was treated by a psychiatrist under a diagnosis of alcoholic dementia [9].
Schweitzer [10]	Schweitzer said that psychotic patients with delusions, sexual

Authors	Details
	conflict associated with guilt, past suicide attempts or other self-destructive behaviour and depression, severe childhood deprivation, and major premorbid personality disorder, were the group at risk for genital self-amputation.
Mitsui et al. [11]	Mitsui et al. reported a male resected his own scrotum and both testes by himself with a small knife, since he thought that his testes had developed necrosis [11].
Tomita et al. [12]	Tomita et al. reported a case of self-amputation of the penis with subsequent complication of myiasis [12].

Additional common procedures include breast reconstruction and construction of a neovagina by inversion of the penis skin [13]. For breast construction, silicone injection is common for gay men. There are many reports on silicone injection for gay men in the literature as seen in Table 2.

Table 2. Reports of silicone injection in gay men

Authors	Details
Chastre et al. [14]	Chastre et al. reported a case of acute pneumonitis after subcutaneous injections of silicone in transsexual men [14].
Hage et al. [15]	In this work, the outcome of massive subcutaneous injection of highly viscous fluids in male-to-female transsexuals was reported [15]. Hage et al. said that feminization by the injection of high-viscosity fluids should be soundly condemned [15].
Sanz-Herrero et al. [16]	Sanz-Herrero et al. reported a case of acute pneumonitis after subcutaneous injection of liquid silicone as a breast implant in a male-to-female transsexual [16].
Fox et al. [17]	Fox et al. reported a case of *Mycobacterium abscessus* cellulitis and multifocal abscesses of the breasts in a transsexual from illicit intramammary injections of silicone [17]. Fox et al. said that all physicians should be alerted to the current cluster of *M. abscessus* infections after injections for cosmetic purposes by nonmedical practitioners [17].
Kaczynski et al. [18]	A case of reduction mammaplasty in a male-to-female transsexual was presented using a combination of conventional resection and implant change surgery [18]. This is the first reduction mammaplasty in a male [18].
Bejerno et al. [19]	Bejerno et al. reported 2 cases of self-inflicted injection of paraffin and silicone in the male chest to modify chest contour [19]. Both patients were followed by subsequent inflammation and necrosis [19].

Considering neovagina construction, development of feminizing genitoplasty for gender dysphoria has a long history. Improved function and cosmesis continue to be the main aim of the surgery for gays [20].The neovagina can be developed from a cosmetic swelling into an innovated organ, derived from the glans penis and harvested penile neurovascular bundle [20]. There are many reports on neovagina construction for gays in the literature as seen in Table 3.

Table 3. Reports of neovagina construction in gays

Authors	Details
Meyer et al. [21]	Meyer et al. presented a one-step method for neovagina construction; the labia are shaped with scrotal skin, using two Z-plasties; a small bud of corpus cavernosum covered by penile skin substitutes for a clitoris [21].
Blanchard et al. [22]	Vaginoplasty outcome in male-to-female transsexuals was reported [22]. Blanchard et al. concluded that transsexuals accomplished coitus, despite short vaginas, by assuming positions that limited the depth of their partners' thrusting [22].
Small [23]	Technique for penile and scrotal inversion vaginoplasty for male to female transsexuals was reported [23].
Stein et al. [24]	Stein et al. reported follow-up observations of operated male-to-female transsexuals [24]. Stein et al. reported that the majority of the patients were able to lubricate the neovagina and have painless intercourse with a potential for orgasm [24].
Marten-Perolino et al. [25]	Male-female transsexualization with glandular preservation technique was reported [25]. Neuro-vascular bundle preservation is the hallmark of this technique [25].
Stanojević et al. [26]	Stanojević et al. reported on fixation of the vagina and neovagina with the sacrospinal ligament [26]. The technique is as follows: after making the tunnel between the bladder and rectum, under the control of the left hand fingers the vagina, or neovagina is fixed to sacrospinous ligament [26].
Liguori et al. [27]	Luguori et al. reported on acute peritonitis due to introital stenosis and perforation of a bowel neovagina in a transsexual [27].
Perovic et al. [28]	Perovic et al. reported on vaginoplasty in male transsexuals using penile skin and a urethral flap [28]. Perovic et al. said that this technique could produce a vagina with more normal anatomical and physiological characteristics than those produced by other methods, as all the penile components are used to form almost normal external female genitalia [28]. Perovic et al. also mentioned that vaginoplasty using pedicled penile skin with a urethral flap was a good alternative to other methods of vaginoplasty in male-to-female sex reassignment surgery [28].
Haustein [29]	Haustein reported on pruritus of the artificial vagina of a

Authors	Details
	transsexual patient caused by gonococcal infection [29].
Bodsworth et al. [30]	Bodsworth et al. reported on a case of asymptomatic gonococcal infection of the surgically constructed vagina of a male-to-female transsexual prostitute [30].
Freundt et al. [31]	Freundt et al. reported on prolapse of the sigmoid neovagina [31]. Freundt et al. said that prolapse of an artificially created vagina was a rare occurrence, without a standard treatment and noted that both abdominal and vaginal approaches might be needed to restore the neovagina without compromising its function [31].
Freundt et al. [32]	Freundt et al. reported on long-term psychosexual and psychosocial performance of patients with a sigmoid neovagina [32]. Freundt et al. said that the creation of a sigmoid neovagina resulted in a long-term anatomically satisfactory situation and sexual and social adjustment was good or satisfactory [32].

B. Medical Procedure

Medical procedure is a way of choice for many gays. The ingestion of estrogen and injection of estrogen are widely used. Estrogen ingestion in men can result in a feminine appearance and long-term usage can induce gynecomastia, which is the preferable side effect for gays. Ingestion of higher quantities of hormones than prescribed is therefore an extraordinary usage of estrogen. However, there are some interesting reports on specific cases of non-gay males who used excessive estrogen ingestion. A well-known case was reported by Kremer et al. [33]. This patient did not feel himself to be homosexual or transsexual but considered himself incomplete without female breasts and nipples [33]. An additional reported way to increase breast size is to encourage breast-tissue development using a sink plunger or breast suction [34].

However, since estrogen ingestion relies on long-term treatment to derive a large breast and depends on daily ingestion, gays consider the estrogen injection more preferable. Goh et al. reported effects of sex steroids on the positive estrogen feedback mechanism in castrated men that prolonged estrogen priming might be involved in activation of the positive feedback mechanism in humans [35]. Dörner et al. reported that an intravenous injection of 20 mg Presomen (Premarin) produced a significant decrease of serum LH levels followed by a significant increase above the initial LH values in homosexual transsexual men. By contrast, intravenous oestrogen administration, while producing a significant decrease of serum LH levels, was not followed by an increase above the initial LH values in hetero- or bisexual transsexual men [36].

References

[1] Khan O, Protheroe A. Testis cancer. *Postgrad Med J.* 2007 Oct;83(984):624-32.

[2] Lycette JL, Bland LB, Garzotto M, Beer TM. Parenteral estrogens for prostate cancer: can a new route of administration overcome old toxicities? *Clin. Genitourin. Cancer.* 2006 Dec;5(3):198-205.

[3] Karczewska-Kupczewska M, Kowalska I, Gorska M. Gynecomastia--a frequent clinical problem. *Med Wieku. Rozwoj.* 2006 Jul-Sep;10(3 Pt 2):973-83.

[4] Reece R. Group treatment of sexual dysfunction in gay men. *J Homosex.* 1981-1982 Winter-Spring;7(2-3):113-29.

[5] Shirodkar SS, Hammad FT, Qureshi NA. Male genital self-amputation in the Middle East. A simple repair by anterior urethrostomy. *Saudi Med J.* 2007 May;28(5):791-3.

[6] Stunell H, Power RE, Floyd M Jr, Quinlan DM. Genital self-mutilation. *Int. J. Urol.* 2006 Oct;13(10):1358-60.

[7] Aboseif S, Gomez R, McAninch JW. Genital self-mutilation. *J. Urol.* 1993 Oct;150(4):1143-6.

[8] Keil W, Betz P, Penning R. Self-castration with suicide. *Arch. Kriminol.* 1994 Jul-Aug;194(1-2):8-14.

[9] Tomita M, Maeda S, Kimura T, Ikemoto I, Oishi Y. A case of complete self-mutilation of penis. *Hinyokika Kiyo.* 2002 Apr;48(4):247-9.

[10] Schweitzer I. Genital self-amputation and the Klingsor syndrome. *Aust. N. Z. J. Psychiatry.* 1990 Dec;24(4):566-9

[11] Mitsui K, Kokubo H, Kato K, Nakamura K, Aoki S, Taki T, Yamada Y, Honda N, Fukatsu H. A case of self-mutilation of testis. *Hinyokika Kiyo.* 2002 May;48(5):281-3.

[12] Tomita M, Uchijima Y, Okada K, Yamaguchi N. A report of self-amputation of the penis with subsequent complication of myiasis. *Hinyokika Kiyo.* 1984 Sep;30(9):1293-6.

[13] Eicher W. Transsexualism. *Rev. Fr. Gynecol .Obstet.* 1990 Oct;85(10):507-11

[14] Chastre J, Basset F, Viau F, Dournovo P, Bouchama A, Akesbi A, Gibert C. Acute pneumonitis after subcutaneous injections of silicone in transsexual men. *N. Engl. J. Med.* 1983 Mar 31;308(13):764-7.

[15] Hage JJ, Kanhai RC, Oen AL, van Diest PJ, Karim RB. The devastating outcome of massive subcutaneous injection of highly viscous fluids in male-to-female transsexuals. *Plast Reconstr Surg.* 2001 Mar;107(3):734-41.

[16] Sanz-Herrero F, de Casimiro-Calabuig E, López-Miguel P. Acute pneumonitis after subcutaneous injection of liquid silicone as a breast implant in a male-to-female transsexual. *Arch Bronconeumol.* 2006 Apr;42(4):205-6.

[17] Fox LP, Geyer AS, Husain S, Della-Latta P, Grossman ME. Mycobacterium abscessus cellulitis and multifocal abscesses of the breasts in a transsexual from illicit intramammary injections of silicone. *J. Am. Acad. Dermatol.* 2004 Mar;50(3):450-4.

[18] Kaczynski A, McKissock PK, Dubrow T, Lesavoy MA. Breast reduction in the male-to-female transsexual. *Ann Plast Surg.* 1989 Oct;23(4):323-6.

[19] Bjerno T, Basse PN, Siemssen PA, Møller TD. Injection of high viscosity liquids. Acute or delayed excision? *Ugeskr Laeger.* 1993 Jun 14;155(24):1876-8.

[20] Goddard JC, Vickery RM, Terry TR. Development of feminizing genitoplasty for gender dysphoria. *J. Sex Med.* 2007 Jul;4(4 Pt 1):981-9.
[21] Meyer R, Kesselring UK. One-stage reconstruction of the vagina with penile skin as an island flap in male transsexuals. *Plast Reconstr. Surg.* 1980 Sep;66(3):401-6.
[22] Blanchard R, Legault S, Lindsay WR. Vaginoplasty outcome in male-to-female transsexuals. *J. Sex Marital Ther.* 1987 Winter;13(4):265-75.
[23] Small MP. Penile and scrotal inversion vaginoplasty for male to female transsexuals. *Urology.* 1987 Jun;29(6):593-7.
[24] Stein M, Tiefer L, Melman A. Followup observations of operated male-to-female transsexuals. *J. Urol.* 1990 Jun;143(6):1188-92.
[25] Marten-Perolino R, Cocimano V, Marino G. Male-female transsexualization with glandular preservation. *Arch Ital. Urol. Nefrol. Androl.* 1990 Mar;62(1):101-5.
[26] Stanojević D, Perović S, Djordjević M. Fixation of the vagina and neovagina with the sacrospinal ligament. *Acta Chir. Iugosl.* 2001;48(2):33-5.
[27] Liguori G, Trombetta C, Buttazzi L, Belgrano E. Acute peritonitis due to introital stenosis and perforation of a bowel neovagina in a transsexual. *Obstet Gynecol.* 2001 May;97(5 Pt 2):828-9.
[28] Perovic SV, Stanojevic DS, Djordjevic ML. Vaginoplasty in male transsexuals using penile skin and a urethral flap. *BJU Int.* 2000 Nov;86(7):843-50.
[29] Haustein UF. Pruritus of the artificial vagina of a transsexual patient caused by gonococcal infection. *Hautarzt.* 1995 Dec;46(12):858-9.
[30] Bodsworth NJ, Price R, Davies SC. Gonococcal infection of the neovagina in a male-to-female transsexual. *Sex Transm Dis.* 1994 Jul-Aug;21(4):211-2.
[31] Freundt I, Toolenaar TA, Jeekel H, Drogendijk AC, Huikeshoven FJ. Prolapse of the sigmoid neovagina: report of three cases. *Obstet Gynecol.* 1994 May;83(5 Pt 2):876-9.
[32] Freundt I, Toolenaar TA, Huikeshoven FJ, Jeekel H, Drogendijk AC. Long-term psychosexual and psychosocial performance of patients with a sigmoid neovagina. Am *J. Obstet. Gynecol.* 1993 Nov;169(5):1210-4.
[33] Kremer J, den Daas HP. Case report: a man with breast dysphoria. *Arch. Sex. Behav.* 1990 Apr;19(2):179-81.
[34] Wylie KR. Suction to the breasts of a transsexual male. *J. Sex. Marital. Ther.* 2000 Oct-Dec;26(4):353-6.
[35] Goh HH, Wong PC, Ratnam SS. Effects of sex steroids on the positive estrogen feedback mechanism in intact women and castrate men. *J. Clin .Endocrinol. Metab.* 1985 Dec;61(6):1158-64.
[36] Dörner G, Rohde W, Schott G, Schnabl C. On the LH response to oestrogen and LH-RH in transsexual men. *Exp. Clin. Endocrinol. 1*983 Nov;82(3):257-67.

Index

4

A

B

C

D

E

F

G

H

J

K

L

M

N

O

P

S

T

X

Y

Z